Sociology
of
Mental Disorder

FOURTH EDITION

Sociology of Mental Disorder

William C. Cockerham

University of Alabama at Birmingham

Prentice Hall, Upper Saddle River, New Jersey 07458

Library of Congress Cataloging-in-Publication Data

Cockerham, William C.
   Sociology of mental disorder / William C. Cockerham.—4th ed.
     p. cm.
   Includes bibliographical references and index.
   ISBN 0–13–125469–3
   1. Social psychiatry. 2. Mentally ill—Social conditions.
 I. Title.
RC455.C57   1996
616.89—dc20   95–12725
                                          CIP

Acquisitions editor: Sharon Chambliss
Editorial/production supervision: Cecile Joyner
Buyer: Mary Ann Gloriande
Interior design: Joan Stone

To Bruce
"Le Brave des Braves"

© 1996, 1992, 1989, 1981 by Prentice-Hall, Inc.
Simon & Schuster/A Viacom Company
Upper Saddle River, New Jersey 07458

Printed in the United States of America

10 9 8 7 6 5 4 3

ISBN 0-13-125469-3

PRENTICE-HALL INTERNATIONAL (UK) LIMITED, *London*
PRENTICE-HALL OF AUSTRALIA PTY. LIMITED, *Sydney*
PRENTICE-HALL CANADA INC., *Toronto*
PRENTICE-HALL HISPANOAMERICANA, S.A., *Mexico*
PRENTICE-HALL OF INDIA PRIVATE LIMITED, *New Delhi*
PRENTICE-HALL OF JAPAN, INC., *Tokyo*
SIMON & SCHUSTER ASIA PTE. LTD., *Singapore*
EDITORA PRENTICE-HALL DO BRASIL, LTDA., *Rio de Janeiro*

Contents

___ *3* ___

Mental Disorder: Concepts of Causes and Cures   56

___ *4* ___

Mental Disorder as Deviant Behavior   92

___ *5* ___

Mental Disorder: Social Epidemiology   126

___ *15* ___

Preface

This book underscores the increasing interest in the problem of mental disorder by sociologists. A contents analysis of the American Sociological Association's *Journal of Health and Social Behavior* for the past few years would disclose that nearly as many articles are published on some aspect of mental health as are published on physical health. Increase in the number of sociologists and the amount of sociological research oriented toward mental disorder has meant a corresponding increase in the number of courses taught on the subject in American colleges and universities. Yet it has only been since the mid-1960s that a substantial body of literature has emerged to establish firmly the sociology of mental disorder as a major subfield. It is appropriate that an effort be made to summarize and analyze the direction of the field. This book represents a continuing personal attempt to accomplish that end.

Although the conclusions expressed in this book are solely the responsibility of the author, other individuals provided extremely helpful comments. A note of appreciation is due to the following colleagues who read all or part of the manuscript: Norman Denzin, University of Illinois; Sharon Guten, Case Western Reserve University; Stephan P. Spitzer, University of Minnesota; Raymond M. Weinstein, University of South Carolina at Aiken; Paul M. Roman, Tulane University; Robert Emerick, San Diego State University; R. Blair Wheaton, University of Toronto; Neil J. Smelser, Center for Advanced Study in the Behavioral Sciences, Stanford; David D. Franks, Virginia Commonwealth University; Michael Radelet, University of Florida; Michael Hughes, Virginia Polytechnic Institute and State University; Hugh Floyd, University of New Orleans; Jeffrey Kamakahi, University of Central Arkansas; Matt Kinkley, Lima Technical College; Fred O. Rasmussen, Rutgers University; and Mark Winton, University of Central Florida.

William C. Cockerham
Birmingham, Alabama

1

The Problem of Mental Disorder

Mental disorder affects the lives and well-being of millions of people throughout the world. The exact number of persons who suffer from some form of it is not known, because many afflicted people do not come to the attention of reporting agencies. Moreover, community investigators face a multitude of problems in obtaining fully reliable data on the extent of mental disorders in noninstitutionalized populations. But enough data are available in advanced societies to make relatively accurate assessments, and it is clear that mental disorder is a major social problem. For example, the Center for Mental Health Services (1994a; Narrow et al. 1993) estimates that 28.1 percent of the total population of the United States suffers from a mental or addictive disorder in the course of a year. Symptoms range from relatively mild distress to severe cases of highly disabling mental abnormalities. Most likely some 1.8 percent of this population has a serious mental disorder (Center for Mental Health Services 1992). Other estimates suggest that as much as 48 percent of the total population will experience symptoms of a mental disorder during their lifetime, with depression and alcohol abuse the two common problems (Kessler et al. 1994).

The extent of mental disorder and the high social and economic cost associated with it are substantial in modern societies. An estimated $67 billion was spent on treating mental disorders in the United States alone in 1992. But what is truly the most damaging aspect of mental illness is its shattering effect upon the lives of its victims and their families. Suicide, divorce, alcoholism and drug abuse, unemployment, child abuse, damaged social relationships, and wasted lives, not to mention the incalculable pain and mental anguish suffered by those involved, are among the consequences of mental illness. In these respects, mental disorder can be regarded as a terrible affliction for many people in the United States and elsewhere.

With increasing numbers of studies uncovering a significant relationship between social factors and many psychiatric conditions, the study of mentally disturbed behavior has become an important area of research in sociology. Unlike psychiatrists and clinical psychologists, who usually focus on individual cases of mental disorder, sociologists approach the subject from the standpoint of its collective nature; that is, they typically analyze mental disorder in terms of group and larger societal processes that affect people and their mental state.

In a social context, mental disorder is seen as a significant deviation from standards of behavior generally regarded as normal by a majority of people in a society. The relevance of this perspective for our understanding of mental disorder is that, even though a pathological mental condition is something that exists within the mind of an individual, the basis for determining whether a person is mentally ill often involves criteria that are also sociological. A psychiatric finding of generalized impairment in social functioning requires an understanding of such sociological concepts as norms, roles, and social status that establish and define appropriate behavior in particular social situations and settings. It is the disruption or disregard of the taken-for-granted understandings of how people should conduct themselves socially that causes a person's state of mind to be questioned. Consequently, it is the overt expression of a person's disordered thinking and activity as social behavior that ultimately determines the need for psychiatric treatment in most cases.

This situation has attracted sociologists to the study of mental disorder and has led to its development as a specialized area of sociological research. The sociology of mental disorder is generally viewed as a subfield of medical sociology, which itself is a fairly new field. In fact, it was the funding and encouragement of the National Institute of Mental Health during the late 1940s that stimulated the development and rapid expansion of medical sociology in the United States. Therefore, from its most important beginnings, the sociology of mental disorder has been linked to medical sociology. But despite its status as a subfield within medical sociology, the sociology of mental disorder has acquired an extensive literature containing significant theoretical concepts and applied knowledge of the human condition. It is the purpose of this book to provide an overview of that knowledge for students, sociologists, health practitioners, and others interested in and concerned with the social aspects of mental disorder.

DEFINING MENTAL DISORDER

Before proceeding, we first should define mental disorder. This is no easy task, since there is considerable disagreement over what constitutes mental disorder, even among mental health professionals. For example, in 1993, the United States government officially defined a serious mental illness as a diagnosable mental, behavioral, or emotional disorder that substantially interferes with one or more major activities in life, including basic living skills such as dressing, eating, or working. For children, the disorder must interfere with activities such as family relationships or school or community functions. This definition, however, may be too broad, because it could include people who are perhaps adjusting to stress rather than experiencing symptoms of schizophrenia, manic-depression, and the like.

In developing a more precise definition of mental disorder for the American Psychiatric Association, Robert Spitzer and Paul Wilson (1975) began by asking (1) whether certain mental conditions should be regarded as undesirable; (2) how undesirable these mental conditions should be to warrant being classified as mental disorders; and (3) even if undesirable, whether the conditions in question should be treated within the domain of psychiatry or by some other discipline.

Some psychiatrists define mental disorder very broadly as practically any significant deviation from some ideal standard of positive mental health. This view, as pointed out by Thomas Szasz (1974, 1987), a psychiatrist and critic of his profession, would regard any kind of human experience or behavior (for example, divorce, bachelorhood, childlessness) as mental illness if mental suffering or malfunction could be detected. Other psychiatrists, in contrast, subscribe to a more narrow definition of mental disorder, which views the condition as being *only* those behaviors that clearly are highly undesirable. Behaviors that are merely unpleasant would not be mental illness. This narrower definition would encompass those mental abnormalities like schizophrenia, mood or anxiety disorders, or an antisocial personality, which Spitzer and Wilson (1975:827) describe as "manifestations which no one wants to experience— either those persons with the conditions or those without them." This latter approach appears more realistic.

The problem of defining mental disorder is further complicated by the fact that concepts of mental disorder often change and are even changing now. For example, homosexuality was considered a mental disorder by American psychiatrists until the early 1970s but is not considered such today. Terms such as melancholia (depression), amentia (mental retardation), hysteria (conversion disorder), and moral insanity (for people who were not truly insane but were thought to be perverted, such as nymphomaniacs) are no longer used. Yet they were major classifications of mental disorders at one time or another during periods ranging from ancient Greece to the twentieth century. A recent example is neurosis, which used to be a major behavioral disorder characterized by chronic anxiety, but now has its various subtypes classified under mood, anxiety, somatoform, or dissociative disorders.

Surprisingly, neither standard textbooks in psychiatry nor the first and second editions of the *Diagnostic and Statistical Manual of Mental Disorders* (DSM) generally defined mental disorder. Spitzer, a research psychiatrist who headed the American Psychiatric Association's Task Force on Nomenclature and Statistics charged with developing DSM-III, addressed this problem. According to Spitzer (Spitzer and Wilson 1975:829), mental disorder can be defined as follows: (1) It is a condition that is primarily psychological and that alters behavior, including changes in physiological functioning if such changes can be explained by psychological concepts, such as personality, motivation, or conflict. (2) It is a condition that in its "full-blown" state is regularly and intrinsically associated with subjective stress, generalized impairment in social functioning, or behavior that one would like to stop voluntarily because it is associated with threats to physical health. (3) It is a condition that is distinct from other conditions and that responds to treatment.

Of the three criteria just described, the first separates psychiatric from nonpsychiatric conditions. The second specifies that the disorder may be recognizable only in a later stage of its development ("full-blown") and that its identification depends upon consistent symptomatology ("regularly associated with"). Spitzer also says that the disorder must arise from an inherent condition and that the impairment in functioning must not be limited to a single situation, but should include an inability to function in several social contexts ("generalized impairment in social functioning"). The second criterion also includes "behavior that one would like to stop voluntarily," for instance, compulsive eating or smoking. The third criterion places the definition within a medical perspective by limiting it to distinct treatable conditions. This definition was continued in DSM-III-R (1987) and is currently followed in DSM-IV (1994).

MADNESS THROUGH THE AGES

Throughout history, people have attempted to cope with the problem of behavior that was irrational, purposeless, and unintelligible. Ideas about the nature of mental illness have been intrinsic to ideas about the nature of human beings and their mode of civilization. What people have thought about mental illness has revealed what they have thought about themselves and the world they lived in. To better understand contemporary approaches to the problem of mental disorder, it is useful to review the evolution of those approaches from humankind's preliterate past up to the present. Present measures on the part of human societies to cope with mental disorder as a social problem are grounded in the experiences of the past.

Witch Doctors

Primitive attempts to explain both physical and mental disorders were based largely upon intuition. Sometimes, early humans noted a cause-and-effect relationship between taking a certain action and alleviating a certain symptom or curing a wound. Primitive people could certainly understand the effect caused by striking someone with a spear or a large rock. The effect could be death. Most often, an illness, however, especially if its cause could not be directly observed, was ascribed to supernatural powers. In essence, primitive medical practice was primitive psychiatry, as humans applied subjective notions about their environment to ailments whose origin and prognosis were beyond their comprehension.

In most preliterate cultures, an illness would be defined as a problem brought on because those who were sick (1) had lost a vital substance (such as their soul) from their body, (2) had had a foreign substance (such as an evil spirit) introduced into their body, (3) had violated a taboo and were being punished, or (4) were victims of witchcraft (Abel, Metraux, and Roll 1987; Kiev 1964, 1972; Mora 1985). All of these explanations of disease causation are clearly bound up in ideas about magic and the supernatural. Because there was so much that was mysterious about the world around them and the functioning of their own bodies, primitive humans attempted to explain the unexplainable by applying human motivations to the unknown. Yet, as Ari Kiev (1972) observes, these etiological concepts were not random ideas but were derived from linking particular symptoms to particular beliefs and customs prevalent within a society. Widely held taboos among primitive groups, for example, are murder and incest. Violations of these taboos are thought to have deleterious effects on the mind of the perpetrator. Thus, in this situation, insanity is believed to be a form of punishment by God, or whatever deities are common to that society, for misdeeds that violate collective morals. According to Kiev (1972), taboo violations seem to be universally a primitive explanation for mental illness.

Another example is found in Haiti, where the belief still prevails among some superstitious persons that a sorcerer can force the soul from a victim's head through the use of magic and replace it with the soul of an animal or an insane dead person. This act is thought responsible for the victim's then disordered behavior. There is also a belief that a curse can cause death. Here one is dealing with a cultural belief that a curse is "real." The result can be a state of extreme anxiety on the part of the person cursed, who eventually dies from shock induced by prolonged and intense emotion associated with believing in the reality of the curse. This reaction is reinforced by the response of others who seek to avoid contact with the person who has been cursed. Such an event demonstrates the possible psychological leverage that a group can have over an individual in certain circumstances and the significance of the role assigned to that person. According to local customs, being cursed might result in interaction that could hasten a person's death. Of course, this is dependent on the belief of all concerned, especially the victim, that the curse is fatal.

If evil spirits and *black* magic are believed to cause death and illness, then it is perfectly permissible to employ *white* magic to counter the work of the evil person or supernatural entity causing the suffering. This belief created the need for healers known as witch doctors or shamans, who work at producing a cure by applying magical arts grounded in folk medicine and prevailing religious beliefs. The most commonly held image of a shaman is that of a medicine man who is susceptible to possession by spirits and through whom the spirits are able to communicate (Abel et al. 1987; Mora 1985). Shamans can be either men or women, although men apparently are more likely to be extraordinarily successful (Murphy 1964). This is probably because men can "act" more violently during rituals and thereby appear more powerful. Advanced age, high intellect, and sometimes sexual deviance, such as transvestism and homosexuality, are characteristics of shamans. Also, being an orphan, being physically disabled, or even being mentally ill is not uncommon.

The most important equipment for a shaman is a strong imagination, for the shaman theoretically gains his strength by mentally drawing upon power that he believes exists outside himself in nature or in the cosmos. He tries to accomplish this through deep concentration while engaging in a mind set stimulated by chants, prayers, drugs, drinking, ritual dancing, or perhaps sex. The shaman works himself into a frenzy until he senses he has become the very force he seeks; when this happens, he projects his supposedly powerful thoughts out of his mind toward the intended target. The extent of his influence depends upon the belief that other people have in his ability to conjure up and control supernatural forces for either good or evil.

Although witch doctors have often had considerable power and prestige among their fellows, they by no means have always occupied a desirable role in society. They may have been viewed as deviant and odd, a condition perhaps reinforced by the need to work with undesirable people and matter (for example, snakes, insects, human organs, and excretion). Kiev (1972:99) notes that primitive shamans were often recruited from the ranks of the mentally disturbed. Skill in performance is apparently the most significant criterion in shamanism, rather than heredity or special experience, although the latter can be particularly important. In this occupation, a degree of craziness can be an advantage for the performer.

Typically, the shaman's performance reflects certain principles of magic, such as similarity or "sympathetic magic" and solidarity or "contagious magic." *Sympathetic magic* is based upon the idea that two things at a distance can produce an effect upon each other through a secret relationship. That is, two things that look alike affect each other through their similarity because the shared likeness places them in "sympathy" with each other. Thus, "like" is believed to produce "like." A well-known example of this notion comes from voodoo and is the sticking of pins into a doll made in the image of a certain person to inflict pain on that individual. In healing, a shaman might act out a sick person's symptoms and recovery, supposedly to "orient" the illness toward recovery. An example of sympathetic magic in relatively recent times comes from the Shona tribe living in southern Zimbabwe in Africa. Here a usual practice of witch doctors is to administer the shell of a tortoise in some form to a patient to give that patient a general feeling of strength and security; or a portion of bone removed from a python's back may be used to try to restore strength in a patient's back by having the patient eat the bone fragments.

Contagious magic is based on the idea that things that have once been in contact continue to be related to each other. Hence, a shaman might use a fingernail, a tooth, or a hair as the object of a magical act to affect the source of that part in some way. Among the Shona, all shamans practice contagion. A member of the Shona group might, for example, obtain some article of clothing that an enemy has worn close to his or her body, take it to a shaman who can produce a spell on it, and supposedly cause the enemy to become ill (Gelfand 1964).

Other measures used by witch doctors include the prescription of drugs made from parts of people, animals, or plants and prepared secretly according to a prescribed ritual. Sometimes, an evil spirit might be forced to leave a body by inducing vomiting, through bloodletting, or as bodily waste. For instance, the following ritual is used by Yoruba witch doctors in Nigeria for treating a psychosis diagnosed as being due to a curse *(epe)* or sorcery *(asasi):*

> The patient's head is shaved. Shea butter, palm oil, pap, and banana are kneaded together and then generously plastered on the scalp; next juices of certain leafy plants are squeezed into a pail of water to make a cooling shampoo. This shampoo is used to wash off the oily plaster. Finally, a series of shallow razor cuts is made over the scalp in the form of a cross. Into these cuts is rubbed a medicine composed of certain roots, the filings of a human tooth, and a small quantity of fluid collected from a putrifying human corpse. The oily mixture soothes the patient's agitation, while the shampoo cools his overheated brain. The medicine enters the patient's blood through the cuts, "fights" with the toxic agents caused by the *epe* or *asasi*, and expels them into the feces and urine. This technique of cutting to introduce substances into the blood is widely used. The cuts are made near the seat of the trouble, that is, in the case described above, in the head; in cases of visual hallucinations or the nightmares of children, they are made under the eyes; for auditory hallucinations, they may be made in front of the ears.[1]

---

[1]Raymond Prince, "Indigenous Yoruba Psychiatry," in *Magic, Faith, and Healing: Studies in Primitive Psychiatry Today,* ed. A. Kiev (Glencoe, IL: Free Press, 1964), pp. 100–101.

Another method employed by early humans to rid the mind of evil spirits was skull trepanning. No longer performed, skull trepanning was done in the eastern Mediterranean and North Africa during the Neolithic Age some four thousand to five thousand years ago and reached its highest state of development in Stone Age Peru one thousand to two thousand years ago. This procedure consisted of boring a hole into the skull to liberate an evil spirit supposedly contained in the person's head. The discoveries by anthropologists of more than one hole in some skulls and the lack of erosion of bone tissue suggest that the operation was not always fatal. Some estimates are that the mortality rate from skull trepanation was as low as 10 percent in some cultures, an amazing feat, considering the difficulty of the procedure and the crude conditions under which it must have been performed (Mora 1985).

However, despite the various techniques, the shaman's principal contribution to therapy appears to be that of anxiety reduction, which draws upon the cultural background of his patients. The connection of treatment with the dominant values and beliefs in the community both inculcates and reinforces the patient's faith in the shaman's procedures. Many primitive people have little opportunity to develop reality-testing skills, being exposed from infancy to a system of beliefs that supports the shaman's authority and mode of treatment. Consequently, the shaman is able to foster the hope and the expectation of relief by emphasizing faith in himself, his method, and his religious orientation—all grounded in community norms and socially approved perspectives (Kiev 1972:123).

Witch Doctors and Psychiatrists: Points of Similarity

In many ways, the shaman or witch doctor is not unlike the modern-day psychiatrist. E. Fuller Torrey, for one, in his book *The Mind Game* (1973) suggested many similarities in the two types of healers. These similarities, organized under four general categories, indicate that both witch doctors and psychiatrists (1) provide a shared worldview to the patient that makes possible the naming of pathological factors in terms understood within his or her respective culture; (2) have a *personal* relationship with the patient that makes the therapist's personality characteristics significant to the healing process (despite the attempt by some psychiatrists to keep their personality removed from therapy); (3) engender hope in the patient and raise the expectation of being cured through the therapist's reputation and the atmosphere of the therapeutic setting; and (4) share techniques of psychotherapy. In regard to the latter, witch doctors, like psychiatrists, use drug therapy, shock therapy (for example, cold water, electric eels, drug-induced convulsions), confession, suggestion, hypnosis, dream interpretation, conditioning, and group and milieu therapies.[2] In their own cultures, Torrey points out that witch doctors have been known to obtain sometimes striking success. "If prostitution is the oldest profession," states Torrey (1973:202), "then psychotherapy must be the second oldest."

Greeks and Romans

Like many other attributes of Western civilization and intellectual development, modern concepts of mental illness originated with the ancient Greeks and Romans. The Greeks, in particular, are noted for formulating a rational approach toward understanding the dynamics of nature and society. They replaced concepts of the supernatural with a secular orientation that viewed natural phenomena as explainable through natural cause-and-effect relationships. One of the most influential Greeks in this regard was Hippocrates, who provided many of the principles underlying modern medical practice. Whether there actually was a Hippocrates, who is thought to have lived around 4000 B.C., is not known. Nevertheless, the Hippocratic method, which demands a rational and systematic mode of treating patients, is credited to him. This method, based upon thorough observation of symptoms and a logical plan of treatment according to proven procedures, is central to contemporary medical practice.

As for mental illness, Hippocrates is believed to have introduced a radical change in the concept of madness by insisting that diseases of the mind were no different from other diseases. In other words, mental illness was not the result of divine, sacred, or supernatural influences. Instead, mental illness was due to *natural causes* that affected the mind and produced delusions, melancholia, and so forth. Although Hippocrates was ahead of his time, he was clearly mistaken in attributing the cause of abnormal behavior to an imbalance in the interaction of the four so-called *humors*—blood, phlegm, black bile, and yellow bile—within the body. An excess of black bile was consistently men-

---

[2]An incident that serves as an amusing comparison of the similarities between witch doctors and psychiatrists was reported by psychiatrist Alexander Leighton during a stay in Nigeria:

> On one occasion a healer said to me, through an interpreter: "This man came here three months ago full of delusions and hallucinations; now he is free of them." I said, "What do these words 'hallucination' and 'delusion' mean? I don't understand." I asked this question thinking, of course, of the problems of cultural relativity in a culture where practices such as witchcraft, which in the West would be considered delusional, are accepted. The native healer scratched his head and looked a bit puzzled at this question and then he said: "Well, when this man came here he was standing right where you see him now and thought he was in Abeokuta" (which is about thirty miles away), "he thought I was his uncle and he thought God was speaking to him from the clouds. Now I don't know what you call that in the United States, but here we consider that these are hallucinations and delusions!" (CIBA Foundation Symposium 1965:23)

tioned by Hippocrates as the cause of mental illness; the recommended treatment was the administration of a purgative (black hellebore) to induce elimination of the disorder through the bowels (Mora 1985). Also, vapors, baths, and a change in diet were sometimes prescribed.

The greatest of the Roman physicians was Galen, who lived from A.D. 130 to 200. Galen was greatly influenced by Hippocrates' notion of the four humors, and he reinforced the Hippocratic view by holding that the health of the soul was dependent upon the proper equilibrium among its rational, irrational, and lustful parts. Furthermore, he argued that uterine discharges or the ejaculation of sperm was necessary if mental harmony was to exist and tension was to be avoided. Galen was a strong advocate of active sexuality for the promotion of mental health.

The Romans' most significant contributions to contemporary psychiatric practice were in three areas: the philosophy of Cicero, the humane attitude toward mental patients furthered by the physician Soranus, and the consideration of mental illness as a concept in Roman law. Cicero, who lived from 106 to 43 B.C., advanced the idea that strong emotions could cause bodily ailments. He disagreed, for example, with Hippocrates' notion of black bile as the cause of melancholia and suggested instead that psychological factors like emotional disturbances were the cause of this problem. Most important, he claimed that physical and mental illnesses were fundamentally different and that human beings, although not necessarily responsible for their physical ailments, were indeed responsible for the disorders of their minds. According to this view, all behavior, either normal or abnormal, was the responsibility of the individual, and abnormal behavior was due to the individual's "neglect of reason." As Franz Alexander and Sheldon Selesnick (1966:73) noted: "This thought is fundamental to modern psychotherapy, for when a person accepts and understands the psychological sources of his mental disturbance, he becomes capable of changing the circumstances that led to his problem."

Soranus, a leading Roman physician whose life overlapped the first and second centuries after the death of Christ, maintained that the personal relationship between the physician and the patient was of paramount importance in curing mental illness. He argued strongly that physicians needed to be supportive in helping mentally ill persons work out their insanity. Soranus is particularly known for his humanitarian treatment of the mentally ill. He insisted that caretakers of the mentally deranged be sympathetic, that mental patients be housed in peaceful surroundings, and that, whenever possible, mental patients should read, discuss what they read, and even participate in dramatic plays to offset depression. But, as Mora (1985) observes, probably very few people in ancient Rome could afford the treatment recommended by Soranus. Most treatment was limited to drugs, spells, and religious pilgrimages.

Roman law also redefined insanity as a condition that could decrease an individual's responsibility for having committed a criminal act. The defendant's state of mind, however, was determined by a judge, not a physician.

Those persons presumed to be mentally ill were typically remanded to the custody of their relatives or a guardian who was charged with the responsibility for their control, safety, and well-being. Other laws were introduced that defined the ability of the mentally ill to marry, be divorced, testify in court, and make wills concerning the disposition of their property.

The Middle Ages, Renaissance, and Post-Renaissance

The progressive ideas of the Greeks and Romans were stifled with the fall of Rome in A.D. 476. The next five hundred years were particularly chaotic, as wars, plagues, and famines disrupted the social order. At that time, the Roman Catholic Church became the center for learning and for preserving intellectual knowledge as Western Europe became dominated by the military power of various barbarian tribes, mostly of Germanic origin. The uncertainty of the period generated great insecurity as many people merged primitive beliefs with Christian theology to explain the nature of human existence. Norman Cantor, a medieval historian, describes the situation as follows:

> The leadership which was so badly needed by the disorganized Western society of the sixth century could come initially only from the church, which had in its ranks almost all the literate men in Europe and the strongest institutions of the age. The church, however, had also suffered severely from the Germanic invasions. The bishops identified their interests with those of the lay nobility and in fact were often relatives of kings and the more powerful aristocrats; the secular clergy in general was ignorant, corrupt, and unable to deal with the problem of Christianizing a society which remained intensely heathen in spite of formal conversion of masses of Germanic warriors to Christianity. The grossest heathen superstitions were grafted onto Latin Christianity: the religiosity of the sixth and seventh centuries was infected with devils, magic, the crudest kind of relic worship, the importation of local nature dieties into Christianity in the guise of saints; and a general debasement of the Latin faith by religious primitivism. . . . By the beginning of the 7th century church discipline in Gaul was in a state of chaos, and the problem was the most basic one of preserving the sufficient rudiments of literacy to perpetuate the liturgy at doctrines of Latin Christianity. . . .
> The Latin church was preserved from extinction, and European civilization with it, by the two ecclesiastical institutions which alone had the strength and efficiency to withstand the impress of the surrounding barbarism: the regular clergy (that is, the monks) and the Papacy.[3]

The consequence of this belief system for the mentally ill was a return to the notion that supernatural forces, namely, the Devil and witches, were responsible for afflictions of the mind. Many psychotics had delusions and hallucinations containing religious content, which reinforced this view. Exorcism was frequently practiced by the Catholic clergy after the example of Christ in the New Testament driving evil spirits out of the bodies of those suffering from

---

[3]Norman F. Cantor, *Medieval History,* 2nd ed. (New York: Macmillan, 1969), p. 161.

bizarre and irrational thinking. Beliefs linking the Devil with mental disorder became so entrenched in the Christian world that they persisted through the Middle Ages, the Renaissance in the fifteenth century, and even the sixteenth and seventeenth centuries. It was not until the eighteenth century that scientific thought and logic prevailed and demonology was rejected as the cause of mental illness.

True, the Renaissance marked the beginning of a European enlightenment that would provide an intellectual orientation based upon empirical knowledge and demonstrated scientific validity to which pagan beliefs would eventually succumb. But two other conditions helped to continue the idea that the Devil was behind abnormal behavior. First, the more often science was able to answer some questions, the more often other questions were raised that perpetuated the uncertainty. That is, the more people learned, the more they realized how little they knew about their world and the universe beyond; intellectual discoveries stimulated the demand for more intellectual inquiry. Because so much remained unknown, the ancient beliefs that had been acceptable explanations in the past continued to support people against the anxieties of the present. Centuries of superstition were very difficult to overcome. Second, there was a tacit agreement between the church and medical science that allowed the church jurisdiction over the investigation of the human mind. The church made little or no objection to medicine's interest in the human body as a weak and imperfect vessel intended to convey the soul in its earthly existence, but the study of the mind was another matter, since human reason was defined within the province of religion, not medicine. Thus, physicians largely devoted themselves to research on the physical functions of the body, leaving considerations of mental processes to theologians.

Witchcraft   The church defined those persons who did the Devil's work on earth as witches. Szasz (1970) notes that it was very easy to blame misfortune on witchcraft. Persons identified as witches were relatively powerless and readily available as scapegoats. And who were these witches? Generally, they were women and included heretics, nonbelievers, eccentrics, the mentally ill, and those who in some way were regarded as different or odd by other people. Some of these women may have simply been strong willed. Most were probably innocent victims.

Persons suspected of being witches were often arrested or were simply rounded up, tried by a court, and punished. The punishment was usually death. The so-called witch trials began in earnest in 1245 in France and reached their zenith between 1450 and 1670. A papal bull published in 1486 became the basic how-to-do-it manual for witch hunters. Written by a pair of Dominican monks named Henry Kramer and James Sprenger, the *Malleus Maleficarum,* or *The Hammer of Witches,* was the bible of the Inquisition. Some twenty-nine editions of this document were published up until 1669. Kramer and Sprenger insisted that there were such things as witches and that to question the existence of witches was even itself a sign of being a witch. By these means, they rather adroitly overcame any criticism of their theories.

The authors of the *Malleus Maleficarum* argued that it was women who were chiefly addicted to evil superstition. The reason for this assertion was that they believed that all witchcraft was derived from carnal lust, which, they maintained, was insatiable in women. Men, on the other hand, were generally protected from witchcraft because Jesus Christ was a man, and by his being born and suffering for humankind, males were saved from becoming witches. As Szasz (1970:8) comments, "In short, the *Malleus* is, among other things, a kind of religious-scientific theory of male superiority, justifying—indeed, demanding—the persecution of women as members of an inferior, sinful, and dangerous class of individuals." Historically, it has been very convenient for men to support the belief that women are inferior and need to be subjugated and cared for. The dictates of the *Malleus* clearly matched the ideas of many males.

To aid in suppressing witchcraft, the *Malleus* required physicians to verify its presence. An illness was considered to be either natural or demonic in origin. If the physician could find no illness, he was expected to find evidence of witchcraft. Obviously, this gave physicians a convenient means by which to explain away illnesses they could not understand. Witchcraft was, therefore, thought to be behind those illnesses whose onset was sudden, which could not be identified, or both.

The number of people who lost their lives through persecution for witchcraft during the witchcraft mania is not known. One estimate claims that at least two hundred thousand people were put to death in Germany and France; considerably fewer were killed in Spain, because of nationalistic and independent attitudes, and in England, where the pagan Anglo-Saxon law insisted that a person was innocent until proven guilty (Mora 1985). The persecution of witches spread even to the New World, where one of the final outbursts occurred among Protestants in Salem, Massachusetts, in 1692. In Salem, a group of young girls, demonstrating manifestly silly behavior, was labeled "bewitched" after a physician, failing to find any illness, claimed that the source of the problem was beyond medicine. The resulting witch trials, in a community where tension was rising between local farmers and merchants over town politics and the distribution of wealth, saw some nineteen alleged witches executed out of the twenty-five brought before the court.[4]

Those who lost their lives were mostly community outcasts or others with little social standing. However, as more and more persons of increasingly higher social status began to be accused and as the quality of the evidence correspondingly decreased, the trials came to an end. The final blow was the with-

---

[4]Mary Warren, one of the original group of "afflicted" girls in Salem, attempted to reverse her testimony and discredit that of the other girls during one of the trials. The judges refused to believe her denials, and she herself was eventually accused of witchcraft.

drawal of the support of Puritan clergymen like Cotton Mather, a noted demonologist of the day, who came to express serious doubts about the affair, after having been very influential in initially stimulating community reaction to witches.

The processes that ended witch trials in Salem were similar to those that ended them elsewhere. Eventually, the public became appalled at the excesses committed by the witch hunters, and as people of higher and higher social station were called out as witches, both the Catholic and Protestant churches and the local governments withdrew their support. Accusations had reached the point at which they were contrary to reason and unsupported by emerging scientific views.

Treatment of the mentally ill   Not all mentally deranged people were killed or persecuted as witches. Some mentally ill individuals during the Middle Ages and the Renaissance were simply regarded as "fools" and "village idiots." They were tolerated by their communities for purposes of amusement, sadism, or charity, or because they were harmless. Others were kept at home by their families, sometimes in chains; and still others were driven out of their homes and forced to wander over the countryside attempting to survive as best they could.

Some mentally ill people were supposedly placed in boats or ships, the so-called ships of fools, whose boatmen or sailors were bribed to put them ashore at a distant place. According to French sociologist Michel Foucault (1965), these ships of fools sparked the imagination of certain early Renaissance literary figures and artists, notably the writer Sebastian Brant and the painter Hieronymus Bosch, both of whom created highly symbolic works depicting cargoes of mad people adrift in search of their reason. Foucault says:

> Confined on the ship, from which there is no escape, the madman is delivered to the river with its thousand arms, the sea with its thousand roads, to that great uncertainty external to everything. He is a prisoner in the midst of what is the freest, the openest of routes: bound fast at the infinite crossroads. He is the Passenger *par excellence:* that is, the prisoner of the passage. And the land he will come to is unknown—as is, once he disembarks, the land from which he comes. He has his truth and his homeland only in that fruitless expanse between two countries that cannot belong to him.[5]

This theme also produced in the European literature of that period the symbol of the soul as a skiff or small boat, abandoned on the sea amid unreason, yet surrounded by mirages of knowledge—"a craft at the mercy of the sea's great madness, unless it throws out a solid anchor, faith, and raises its spiritual sails so that the breath of God may bring it to port" (Foucault 1965:12).

---

[5]Michel Foucault, *Madness and Civilization: A History of Insanity in the Age of Reason* (New York: Pantheon, 1965), p. 11.

Beginning in the late Middle Ages, many mental patients were institutionalized in custodial centers to remove them from the general population and to attempt to cure them through prayer or physical means such as bloodletting, emetics, and cathartics. It was generally believed that the only way to cure mental derangement was by the divine intercession of saints; therefore, religious practices were emphasized. Finally, in 1409 in Valencia, Spain, the first mental hospital was founded by a Catholic priest, Father Gilabert Jofré (1350–1417). The impetus behind Father Jofré's action was his reaction to witnessing a particular brutal street scene in which mentally ill persons were tormented and teased. Shortly thereafter, Spanish missionaries founded other mental hospitals in Spain and later, in 1567, in Mexico City.

The relatively tolerant attitude in Spain toward the mentally ill was most likely influenced by its proximity and cultural ties to the Arab world. The Arab countries of North Africa and the Middle East had taken a much more humane view of mental illness. The basis of this approach was the Moslem view that the insane are loved by God and are especially chosen to tell the truth. According to Mora (1985), as early as the twelfth century, travelers returning to Europe reported a high standard of humanitarian treatment for the insane at various Arab mental asylums. One description tells of fountains, gardens, and a relaxed atmosphere in which patients were treated with special diets, drugs, baths, and perfumes. Note is also made of concerts in which the musical instruments were tuned so as not to jar the patients' sensitivities. Rich and poor were apparently given access to the same facilities.

There were some humane trends discernible in Western Europe other than the work of the Catholic Church in supporting institutions to protect and care for the mentally ill. Johann Weyer (1515–1588), a Dutchman known as the first psychiatrist, strongly rejected the idea of witchcraft and the policies of those clergy who supported witch hunts. He insisted that patients should be treated with kindness and understanding. Therapy was to be derived only from the scientific investigation of a patient's complaints. Another significant physician was Paracelsus (1493–1541), a Swiss who argued that the insane were neither sinners nor criminals but sick people who needed medical help. The first conceptualization of unconscious motivation promoting anxiety is found in his writings. In Spain, Juan Luis Vives (1492–1540), who became the father of modern psychology, likewise spoke out against beliefs in demonology and claimed that mental patients should be treated peacefully if reason and sanity were to be returned. He believed, in opposition to theologians, that the mind should be studied and posited that emotions and instincts are central influences upon behavior. The work of individuals like Weyer, Paracelsus, Vives, and Cornelius Agrippa (1486–1535), a German scholar who defended women's rights and risked his life to save a woman accused of witchcraft, eventually led to the separation of psychology and psychiatry from theology. But their ideas had little immediate impact, and in some cases, especially that of Weyer, they were viewed as radicals and were deliberately ignored by their contemporaries.

Divine healing   The early Christian explanation of mental disorder, which implicated the Devil and sin, persists today among some churches. In a study by Gillian Allen and Roy Wallis (1976) of members of a small congregation of a Pentecostal church, the Assemblies of God, in a city in Scotland, it was found that "possession by evil spirits" is still used to explain not only mental illness but also certain other problems, such as dumbness, blindness, and epilepsy. These people believe that demons can be transferred from one person to another by touch and that exorcism by prayer can remove them. Although most church members agree that disease in general can be caused by the Devil, mental illness appears especially demonic in origin.

Accepting the Bible as the literal truth, the Assemblies of God officially support the belief in *divine healing*. This belief is derived from biblical passages indicating that (1) some people have the power to transmit the healing forces of the Holy Spirit or to exorcise demons and (2) healing can be obtained through faith in the same way as can salvation from sin. The healing procedure is described as follows:

> Prayer for healing in the Assembly of God occurs at the end of normal services when those who need healing or help and advice, are asked "to come out to the front." There the pastor and the elders perform the laying on of hands and sprinkling with holy oil and pray simultaneously: "Oh Lord, heal this woman! Yes, Lord. We know You can heal her." The occasional case of demon possession is dealt with in a similar way when the pastor or evangelist addresses the demon along these lines: "Get out, foul demon! In the name of Jesus, leave her!"[6]

Although the Pentecostal church utilizes divine healing as central to church dogma, it does not prohibit members from seeking professional medical care. Use of divine healing is preferred, however, because it offers the advantage of providing both spiritual and physical healing; it is also believed to work in many cases in which orthodox medical practice has failed. There are many stories among the members attesting to spectacular cures either through the specific effect of the emotional healing services or through the power of prayer in general. Yet because church members also believe that "God's methods are sometimes through men" and that "God put doctors in the world and gave them their skills," it is permissible to seek a physician's assistance. For serious illnesses in particular, divine healing is used in conjunction with professional medicine. Hence, church members simultaneously hold both religious and scientific beliefs about the causation and treatment of illness, without any apparent conflict. "In serious illnesses," state Allen and Wallis (1976:134–35), "members were not faced with the choice between breaking their religious principles by fetching the doctor and refusing medical treatment altogether." Unlike some faith healers who utilize emotionally charged healing rituals, or

---

[6]Gillian Allen and Roy Wallis, "Pentecostalists as a Medical Minority," in *Marginal Medicine*, ed. Roy Wallis and Peter Morley (New York: Free Press, 1976), p. 121.

believers in the unemotional approach of Christian Science, where the focus is exclusively upon faith and prayer, Pentecostalists are usually able to avoid the dilemma of whether to use *either* a religious *or* a medical curing process.

The Eighteenth Century: The Great Confinement and Reform

The Great Confinement   The eighteenth century marked the age of the *Great Confinement,* for it was during this century that numerous institutions, many of them called "hospitals," spread across Europe, intended to house and control persons considered to be social problems. Actually, this process began in the middle of the seventeenth century with the founding in 1656 of the *Hôpital Général* in Paris, but it reached its zenith in the eighteenth century when an entire network of such institutions was built across Western Europe. Economic recession, unemployment, higher prices, and losses of land had created a serious problem of vagrancy throughout Europe. Many vagrants, turning to begging on the streets of Europe's cities, became a great public nuisance. In recognition of this problem and in accordance with a new definition of social welfare as a community rather than a church responsibility, municipal and national authorities began to extend public assistance to the poor by offering them food and shelter. This policy was also in line with the new notion of enlightened absolutism in which the monarchs of Europe assumed responsibility for the safety and well-being of their subjects in return for absolute authority. Thus, for the first time, purely negative measures of exclusion (for example, the ships of fools) were replaced by the measure of confinement. The unemployed were no longer driven away or punished. Instead, they were cared for at the expense of the nation, but also at the cost of their liberty.

Consequently, an implicit system of obligation was set into motion between the poor and society at large. The poor had the right to be taken care of, but only by accepting confinement in society's "social warehouses" where the poor, including the sick, invalids, the aged, orphans, and the insane, were removed from the mainstream of social life. A legacy of this, existing even today in the United States, is that people with chronic health problems requiring long-term hospitalization—the insane, the incurable, and persons afflicted with highly infectious diseases—tend to be sent to public institutions, whereas private hospitals generally accept patients needing to be hospitalized for relatively shorter periods of time. Custodial care thus remains within the purview of the state. For the seriously mentally ill, of course, this means commitment to a state mental hospital.

Another legacy from this period is the emergence of the Protestant Ethic, grounded in Puritanism, which had an important impact upon the thinking of many Europeans and Americans in the seventeenth and eighteenth centuries and lingers today. The Protestant Ethic equates productive labor with goodness and morality; idleness and unemployment are viewed as sinful and immoral. The able-bodied poor who were confined to poorhouses and hospitals were required to work to contribute to their support, thereby becoming a source of cheap labor. The insane, however, as described by Foucault (1965), were distinguished by their inability to work and to follow the patterns of community life. Hence, madness became defined as a vice as well as an unfortunate circumstance. It joined idleness as a sin. Foucault suggests that the effect of confinement upon the mentally ill was a decisive event in that insanity was now ranked among the problems of the city, similar to poverty, unemployment, and a failure to commit one's self to the collective interest. The ethical value of labor, the obligation to work, and the meaning of poverty all combined to determine the fate of the insane.

For the mentally ill, the era of the Great Confinement was a time of hardship and brutality. Foucault notes that the insane were regarded as being little more than animals and that their animalness was considered protection from hunger, heat, cold, and pain. "It was common knowledge," says Foucault (1965:74), "until the end of the 18th century that the insane could support the miseries of existence indefinitely. There was no need to protect them; they had no need to be covered or warm." The insane were crowded into rooms or cells with little or no warmth even on the coldest days; most were chained to walls or beds. Some had no beds and slept on straw pallets in cells that were damp and perhaps rat infested. Some went about naked. Those who were violent were subjected to brutal punishment, because discipline was thought to be a sound method of promoting the return of reason.

Although the insane were locked away from society, they still were the objects of bizarre curiosity. On weekends, it was not uncommon for the mad to be displayed to visitors who would pay an admission price to view the human oddities. For example, it was reported in the House of Commons in London in 1815 that the Bethlehem Hospital for the insane took in about four hundred English pounds in admission fees. At a penny a visitor, this suggests that over ninety thousand people visited the hospital that year during its Sunday open houses. Not only did the general public get a chance to peer at the insane, but sometimes the insane were made to perform dances and acrobatics. "The only extenuation to be found at the end of the 18th century," Foucault (1965:69) states, "was that the mad were allowed to exhibit the mad, as if it were the responsibility of madness to testify to its own nature."

Reform: Chiarugi, Tuke, and Pinel   Toward the end of the eighteenth century, public outrage began developing as the abuses suffered by the mentally ill received widespread attention. An illustration of this reaction is reflected in the comments made by Daniel Defoe, an English journalist and author (Defoe wrote *Robinson Crusoe*), and his colleagues castigating unworthy husbands who attempt to shed their allegedly normal wives after becoming tired of them by placing them in mental institutions. Defoe complains:

If they are not mad when they go into these cursed Houses, they are soon made so by the barbarous Usage they there suffer, and any Woman of spirit who has the least Love for her Husband, or Concern for her family, cannot sit down tamely under a Confinement and Separation the most unaccountable and unreasonable. Is it not enough to make any one mad to be suddenly clap'd up, stripp'd, whipp'd, ill fed, and worse us'd? To have no Reason assign'd for such Treatment, no Crime alleg'd, or accusers to confront? And what is worse, no Soul to appeal to but merciless Creatures, who answer but in Laughter, Surliness, Contradiction, and too often Stripes? All conveniences for Writing are denied, no Messenger to be had to carry a Letter to any Relation or Friend; and if this tyrannical Inquisition, join'd with the reasonable Reflections, a woman of any common Understanding must necessarily make, be not sufficient to drive any Soul stark staring mad, though before they were never so much in their right Senses, I have no more to say.[7]

Reform, however, was on the way, and three individuals—Vincenzo Chiarugi, an Italian; William Tuke, an Englishman; and especially Philippe Pinel, a Frenchman—were instrumental in this regard. Chiarugi (1758–1820), a physician in Florence, argued that medical personnel had a moral duty to treat the mentally ill as individuals and to treat them tactfully and humanely. Chiarugi put his ideas into operation while directing a large mental hospital and also wrote a three-volume work on insanity. Unfortunately, his ideas were obscured by the turmoil, revolts, and wars taking place in and between the various Italian city-states at the time. William Tuke (1732–1819), a Quaker tea merchant living in England, was exceedingly more influential and established a mental asylum at York in 1792. Tuke's approach was strikingly radical for the day, because he advocated that mental patients be treated as guests, with kindness and respect. He organized a friendly and sympathetic environment on an estate called "the Retreat" where he housed about thirty patients. There were no chains, physical punishment, or direct physician influence. Work in the form of moderate physical exercise was thought to be very therapeutic. Observers from throughout Europe and the United States came to view Tuke's methods, and he achieved much humanitarian reform in England.

Slowly, small pockets of humane care for the mentally ill appeared in the Western world, but it remained for Philippe Pinel (1745–1826) to induce widespread change in the treatment of mental patients. Pinel, a shy, retiring French physician, had impressed his superiors while still a medical student by formulating a program of "moral treatment" for the insane. Pinel believed that mental health was dependent upon emotional stability, what he called a "balance of passions." He argued that mental patients would respond to kindness and sympathy under the firm guidance of the therapist as a father figure. If possible, patients should be allowed to work and participate in recreational activities

---

[7]Daniel Defoe, Sir John Fortesque-Aland, and John Conolly, "Observations on Psychiatric Confinement, 1728–1830," in *The Age of Madness,* ed. Thomas Szasz (Garden City, NY: Doubleday, Anchor Books, 1973), p. 8.

(for example, concerts, lectures, games) rather than be confined to cells or held in restraint by mechanical devices. The main causes of mental disorder were thought to be psychological (for example, passions, lust, excessive masturbation) or environmental (for example, too much freedom, economic uncertainty). As it evolved, moral treatment was essentially a program of re-education in which mental patients were to be taught how to behave normally within the context of sympathetic living conditions.

In August 1793, in the midst of the French Revolution, Pinel received his wish and was appointed as a physician to the insane asylum of Bicêtre for male patients. Persuading the warden to allow him to unchain the inmates, Pinel walked through the asylums, going from cell to cell freeing the patients. The first man unchained had not walked in forty years but somehow managed to hobble out of his cell to view the sky in a state of amazement.

> The second to be released was a drunkard who had been discharged from the French Guards, Chevigné by name. For ten years he had been in chains. His mind disordered, assaultive, and surly, he was considered incurable. Pinel went to him, took off the iron anklets and handcuffs. Behold a revelation! The vicious sot stood up, and with a courtly flourish bowed to Pinel. He became a model of good conduct and in time was released.[8]

Pinel ordered beatings and other forms of physical abuse halted; food was improved, and the patients were treated with a new drug: kindness. And apparently in many individual cases, there was great improvement. "Dazed lunatics, rubbing their eyes at their good fortune, talked for the first time in years, and became almost human again" (Bromberg 1975:97). Pinel's program thus called attention to the need for and possible benefits of reform in the care of the mentally ill. It was also an act of great personal courage on his part because it came when the French Revolution had turned on a course of terror. Citizens suspected of royalist rather than republican sympathies or whose actions could be judged as supporting the old regime were sent to be beheaded on the guillotine. Pinel's ideas, however, turned out to be extremely successful. His book, *Treatise on Insanity*, published in 1801, was likewise very popular, and his concept of moral treatment became the basis for French laws pertaining to mental health. He was appointed to a top medical school faculty position and honored by election to the membership of the Institute of France. For about twenty years, he enjoyed success and fame, but eventually he was affected by politics. Suspected of being a royalist for allegedly allowing certain priests and refugees wanted by the government to stay at the Bicêtre mental asylum, Pinel lost his teaching post and spent the remainder of his life living in relative poverty. Pinel's fate was aptly summarized by Walter Bromberg (1975:99): "Great as the man was, his times were greater."

---

[8]Walter Bromberg, *From Shaman to Psychotherapist* (Chicago: Henry Regnery, 1975), p. 96.

The Nineteenth Century: Emergence of the Medical Model

The decline of moral treatment   The nineteenth century began with the influence of Pinel's moral treatment in full bloom. Also influential, especially in England and in the United States because of their close cultural ties, were Tuke's methods as practiced at the York Retreat. In response, several mental asylums were founded in the United States between the turn of the century and the American Civil War. The most noted of these, initially, was the Worcester State Hospital in Worcester, Massachusetts. Here the philosophy of moral treatment was held as an example for the rest of the country, but the reader should not get the impression that all or even most mental patients received moral treatment. Generally, moral treatment was provided by private hospitals or by only the most progressive public asylums. In the United States, moral treatment was most prevalent in New England, and the patients were usually from upper- and middle-class families. Mentally ill persons who were poor or black often found themselves in jails or workhouses.

The dream of moral treatment for all the insane was not to be realized, for within a few decades its influence declined significantly. Four factors were largely responsible for this outcome. First, there was no truly cohesive program detailing a systematic approach to moral treatment. Thus, it was difficult to train others in its methods and to implement any type of standardization or coordination. This also impeded public recognition of its value. Second, mental asylums became overcrowded with people who not only were insane but also had related problems of criminality, alcoholism, vagrancy, and poverty. Most mental patients were not misguided souls from relatively affluent families. Instead, most were from the lower class and thus were held in low social esteem. This circumstance was common in the United States, where the inmates of mental institutions came to be considered unworthy tax burdens by many citizens. Resentment was bred by the notions of moral treatment, with its emphasis upon pleasant surroundings and recreation for socially objectionable people who had outraged the morals of the community. Particular targets were blacks and immigrants, especially the flood of Irish arriving on the East Coast whom some considered ill adapted to life in the United States (Mora 1985).

A third factor was the increasing popularity of the theory that madness was incurable, a theory that was due principally to contemporary ideas about heredity. This influence, largely European in origin but embraced in the United States, encouraged a pessimistic outlook that little or nothing could be done to return mental patients to society in any normal capacity. Social Darwinism, with its advocacy of the survival of the fittest, further contributed to doubts about helping the insane. With a view primarily toward reducing costs, there was a great expansion of *large* mental hospitals, whose role was to become essentially custodial.

Ironically, this process was helped by Dorothea Dix (1820–1887), a New England schoolteacher who devoted her life to reforming conditions for the mentally ill. During a visit to a Massachusetts jail in 1841, she was outraged by the sight of the mentally ill being housed with criminals, and so she visited every jail and poorhouse in Massachusetts over the following two years. Her next step was to send a report to the Massachusetts legislature describing the plight of the insane. This report caused a sensation, not only in Massachusetts, but nationwide. She subsequently devoted her life to traveling throughout the country inspecting mental institutions and demanding increased financial support from state governments. She personally founded or enlarged some thirty-two mental hospitals and saw to it that physicians were added to the staffs of many of those institutions. In addition, she got the mentally ill out of jails and poorhouses and into asylums.

One of those hospitals helped by Miss Dix was the Worcester State Hospital, formerly a model of moral treatment. What had happened at Worcester was typical of many other places. The low status and bizarre behavior of the inmates promoted contemptuous attitudes toward them on the part of both the staff and the community. The overwhelming number of patients and the limited amount of funds available to run the hospital thus combined with the low social value of the inmates to influence the administration to discontinue maintaining an environment for moral treatment. Instead, they adopted custodial procedures that were more cost effective (Grob 1966). Hence, Worcester adopted a custodial orientation, as did other institutions. The use of mental hospitals to house the aged poor in particular remained common in state and county mental hospitals until well into the twentieth century (Sutton 1991).

Finally, there was the advent of a fourth factor, the influence of psychiatrists who viewed mental disorder as primarily a disease brought on by organic causes. Benjamin Rush (1745–1813), the father of American psychiatry, maintained, for example, that abnormal behavior was derived from brain disease that had its locus in the brain's blood vessels. At the Worcester State Hospital, staff psychiatrists emphasized similar ideas as part of their claim to professional legitimacy in medicine (Grob 1966). They saw themselves as "scientists" working in the same manner as other medical doctors. Although moral treatment recognized both organic and psychological causes of mental disorder, psychiatric ideology tended to negate measures like moral treatment because they featured the therapeutic value of the environment. Instead, purely medical techniques were to be used in treating mental patients.

The overall result was the demise of moral treatment, which may not have been the most effective approach for some patients, but had brought improvement to others; and its philosophy had meant humane care for all.

The medical model   Physicians of the nineteenth century were not the first to argue that abnormal mental behavior was the result of mental disease, not the manifestation of witchcraft and sin. Such arguments had been growing louder since the sixteenth century, but the 1800s saw the emergence of a scientific framework supporting the concept as it never had before. This was a period of tremendous advancement for medicine as research discoveries led to highly significant improvements in medical knowledge, procedures, and technology. Louis Pasteur, Robert Koch, and others engaged in bacteriological research leading to the conceptualization of the germ theory of disease established the premise that every disease had a specific pathogenic cause whose treatment could best be accomplished within a biomedical mode. This approach, as is well known, was highly successful in producing cures for acute communicable diseases. In view of this success, it was perhaps inevitable that physicians as psychiatrists would come to view mental disorder in a similar fashion, as an extension of the germ theory. Consequently, organic dysfunctions of the brain were credited as the primary etiology of mental disorder. The most influential textbook of this period, for instance, was written by a leading German psychiatrist, Wilhelm Griesinger (1817–1868), and was entitled *Pathology and Theory of Mental Diseases.* The title clearly indicates the approach of its author, for Griesinger claimed that mental illness was brought on by biochemical changes in the nervous system caused by disease. By the mid-1850s, as Mora (1985) notes, almost all American psychiatrists had come to believe that psychological problems had physiological causes. This viewpoint also became accepted by the American public.

Postmortem examinations now were primary methods of attempting to discover the origins of mental disorder. Research moved away from living patients to morgues and clinical laboratories as the emphasis turned to brain dissection. Neurology became an important ally of psychiatry as diseases of the nervous system gained acceptance as causes of insanity. Psychiatry, however, struggled with organic definitions of mental disorders, since it was unable to produce scientific verification of the disease approach. Syphilis was one disease under investigation that produced a psychosis that could be verified as having an organic pathology, and that was treatable by biomedical means. Except for a few other mental disorders related to such conditions as cerebral atherosclerosis, chronic intoxication, vitamin deficiency, and outright physical injury to the brain, there was a lack of direct evidence to sustain the medical model. Nevertheless, bolstered by success in treating *physical* diseases of the body, the medical model remained the most widely accepted explanation of mental disorder during the late 1800s.

The Twentieth Century: The Age of Therapies

The twentieth century has been unlike any other century preceding it in the variety of concepts of mental illness. Some ideas of the past remain, such as beliefs based upon superstition or notions of the role of the Devil. Other ideas, however, compete for attention and money. Those ideas range from sophisticated biochemical research to psychoanalysis, behavior modification, and community psychiatry, to self-help procedures embodied in techniques like biofeedback and transcendental meditation. All in all, there are at least two hundred therapies and numerous pseudotherapies available in contemporary Western society, all intended to counteract psychological stress and behavioral abnormality. Professionals, paraprofessionals, and laypeople are involved in treating mental problems.

The most influential developments in mental health during the twentieth century are the work of Sigmund Freud, the extensive use of psychoactive drugs, and the community mental health movement.

Sigmund Freud   Freud (1856–1939), an Austrian physician who began practice as a neurologist, established a theoretical basis for much of modern psychiatry. He emphasized psychological concepts of learning, motivation, and personality over purely organic approaches. Most important, he directed attention to the role of instincts and the unconscious in shaping behavior. Freud was a controversial figure, and even some of his supporters and students disagreed with him and broke away to form their own approaches. Yet he was extremely influential—particularly in the United States, where many psychiatrists were receptive to new ideas. At that time, psychiatry had become a relatively static branch of clinical medicine mired in the search for organic causes of mental disorders. Freud had the effect of breathing new life back into psychiatry with the formulation of the psychoanalytic approach, which was highly popular with white middle- and upper-class Americans in the 1940s and 1950s. In psychoanalysis, patients reconstructed their childhood experiences and life events over a period of time. This process was directed toward resolving present conflicts by uncovering the source of mental discomfort in the formative years of the patient's life. Behind this technique was Freud's belief that human behavior was determined by unconscious influences shaping conscious thoughts and actions. Freud, accordingly, developed an elaborate theory of instincts, personality structure, stages of psychosexual development, and ego defense mechanisms, as well as delving into dreams, group psychology, religion, and other matters.

Psychoactive drugs: The new medical model   By the 1960s, however, the optimism that had been generated by Freud had begun to run its course. Psychoanalysis was time-consuming, expensive, and not particularly effective with seriously deranged patients like schizophrenics and others lacking ego strength and an adequate sense of reality. Its greatest gains had been with patients suffering from anxiety. But as psychiatry was again becoming stalled, it was rescued by the second twentieth-century revolution in mental health, the discovery and use of psychoactive drugs to treat the mentally ill. Although the attempt to justify the medical model through theories of organic brain disease had failed, success came through the biochemical approaches.

Research in France in 1952 had shown that chlorpromazine was effective in treating psychotic patients. Chlorpromazine was first used in the United States in 1954, and by 1977 other phenothiazines had been developed for treating schizophrenia and manic states; drugs like iproniazid and, later, imipramine were used for depression. The results were astounding, and the number of resident patients in mental hospitals decreased significantly from 1956 onward.

To recognize what has happened, we need to review briefly the situation in most mental hospitals since the mid-1800s. Following the reforms of Dorothea Dix, mental hospitals in the United States had grown progressively larger and were generally constructed away from large population centers in order to remove the insane farther away from society. Overcrowding continued to foster trends toward custodial care as hospital staffs became increasingly limited in their capabilities to contend with large numbers of patients. Beginning in 1860, there was a decline in discharges for mental hospitals as patients began to remain hospitalized for longer periods. Discharge rates and lengths of hospitalization stabilized somewhat in the 1920s, but from 1945 to 1955 there was an average annual increase of some thirteen thousand patients. As Oakley Ray (1978:251) observes, "The year 1955 was the high-water of residents in mental hospitals. If the 1945 to 1955 rate of increase had continued, there would have been over 850,000 patients in state mental hospitals by 1978." Philip Berger and his associates describe the situation in the 1950s before the introduction of drug therapies:

Pessimism toward severe mental illness was common because each year the number of patients admitted to hospitals increased, while very few were ever discharged. The patients' living areas were crowded and poorly furnished; schizophrenic patients with paranoid delusions crouched in corners in constant fear; catatonic patients were allowed to maintain the same rigid posture to the point of developing swollen legs and pressure sores; hallucinating patients paced the floor talking to their "voices" and unaware of what was going on around them. People sat year after year on benches or on the floor doing nothing, while their physical health deteriorated as well. Violent patients attacked staff members or other patients for reasons known only to themselves. Manic patients laughed, joked, and moved constantly for days at a time until they collapsed, exhausted. Combative patients were kept in rooms without furniture or strapped to beds that were bolted to the floor to prevent injury to themselves and others. Agitated patients were often placed in warm baths or tied in wet sheets in an effort to calm their frenzy.

The psychiatrists charged with the care and treatment of these patients were baffled by these disorders. Both cause and therapy were quite unknown and untaught in medical schools. Before World War II patients were in the care of physicians trained mainly in neurology, but by the postwar period, many had studied psychoanalytic psychotherapy as well; but neither neurological diagnosis nor psychoanalytic psychotherapy had any substantial effect in the treatment of chronic schizophrenia or severe mania. Regardless of their training, psychiatrists functioned mainly as administrators and custodians.[9]

The decline in the number of resident state and county mental hospital patients between 1950 and 1992 is shown in Table 1–1. In 1950 there were 512,501 patients housed in state and county mental hospitals, a figure that had

---

[9]Philip B. Berger, Beatrix Hamburg, and David Hamburg, "Mental Health: Progress and Problems," in *Doing Better and Feeling Worse: Health in the United States,* ed. John H. Knowles (New York: Norton, 1977), pp. 263–64.

Table 1–1 Number of resident patients, total admissions, net releases, and deaths; state and county mental hospitals, United States, 1950–1992

YEAR	NUMBER OF HOSPITALS	RESIDENT PATIENTS AT END OF YEAR	ADMISSIONS	NET RELEASES	DEATHS
1950	322	512,501	152,286	99,659	41,280
1955	275	558,922	178,003	126,498	44,384
1956[a]	278	551,390	185,597	145,313	48,236
1960	280	535,540	234,791	192,818	49,748
1965	290	475,202	316,664	288,397	43,964
1970	315	337,619	384,511	386,937	30,804
1975	313	193,436	376,156	384,520	13,401
1980	276	132,164	370,344[b]	366,766	6,800
1985	286	109,939	335,940[b]	N.A.	N.A.
1990	281	92,059	277,813[b]	N.A.	2,321
1992	275	83,320	254,932[b]	N.A.	N.A.

[a]First year of widespread use of psychopharmaceuticals in state and county mental hospitals.
[b]Includes admissions, readmissions, and returns from leave.
Source: National Institute of Mental Health data.

risen to 558,900 by 1955. In 1956, the first year of the widespread use of psychopharmaceuticals in state and local mental hospitals, the number of resident patients dropped to 551,390. This drop has continued, and in 1992 the number of resident mental patients had fallen to 83,320. Moreover, there has been a decline in the average length of stay. In 1955, the average time of hospitalization for mental patients was six months; by 1992, it had dropped to fifteen days.

Although not all the credit for the reduction in numbers of mental hospital resident patients is due to psychopharmaceuticals, certainly the use of psychoactive drugs has played a central role. Additionally, the use of drugs helped to promote feelings of optimism and innovation among hospital staff members and encouraged other new forms of therapy, such as family therapy, crisis intervention, and brief psychotherapy. Yet the use of psychoactive drugs does not result in a miracle cure for mental disorder, and enthusiasm for them should be tempered. These drugs do not cure; they assist in the *control* of abnormal behavior and make social life possible when it was not before. Unpleasant side effects, such as interference with thinking, nausea, and addiction, accompany the use of certain drugs. Hence, the use of psychoactive chemical compounds has both positive and negative results.

Community mental health   The third mental health revolution in the twentieth century in the United States has been the community mental health movement. With the release of large numbers of mental hospital patients back into the community, many of whom were not cured but merely sustained by drugs, some new measure was needed to assist these patients in maintaining themselves outside the hospital. In 1955, Congress authorized and funded the Joint Commission on Mental Illness and Health. The commission's final report, *Action for Mental Health,* published in 1961, described institutional mental health care as hopelessly custodial and recommended the establishment of local community mental health centers. In the United States, the 1960s were a time of social protest and demand for reform. Particular issues were civil rights and, later, American involvement in the Vietnam War; yet reform in the area of mental health was also included in those issues that attracted community support. Congress passed the Mental Retardation and Facilities and Community Mental Health Centers Construction Act in 1963 to support the establishment of easily accessible and locally controlled mental health centers. This law reflected the philosophy that the objective of modern treatment should be to support mental patients in their own communities as much as possible, so that such persons could lead relatively normal lives.

Advocates of community psychiatry cite four goals as the guiding principles of community mental health programs (Cohen 1974). First is the idea that the mental patient's entire social environment be viewed as a "therapeutic community" with treatment resources for mental health professionals. The second goal, clearly related to the first, is that some means must be found to use the patient's relationships with family and friends to improve therapy and to prevent recurrence of the mental disorder. The third goal is to develop and organize local community control over these centers so that center policies are community based and oriented. Fourth is the goal of reducing patient populations at state and local mental hospitals by providing prompt response and twenty-four-hour service.

The establishment of community mental health centers also has meant the emergence of a new kind of mental health worker—a layperson, living in the community, who can fill the gap between the mental health center client and the professional worker. The community mental health worker is supposed to be someone who can understand and work with people living in lower-class environments more effectively than middle-class professionals can. This broadening of community participation in mental health has recognized that many client problems are social rather than medical. These problems include unemployment, poverty, poor housing, lack of food and clothing, racial discrimination, law violations, child support, and other characteristics of low-income living.

The movement to extend mental health services into community settings was not just the result of new psychoactive drugs and the negative effects of housing people in mental institutions for extensive periods. A host of other influences were important as well. These included growing public support for a more enlightened and humane approach to treating mental patients; the extension of civil rights as a means to solve social problems to mental patients, thereby making it difficult to administer psychiatric care to people without their consent; and strong lobby efforts on the part of community psychiatry interest groups aimed at obtaining greater government funding and resources for community care. There was also the emergence of critical literature in psychiatry, particularly the work of R. D. Laing (1969) and Thomas Szasz (1970, 1974, 1987), who depicted mental illness as either a different type of reality or a myth, and mental hospitalization as a form of oppression.

By the 1980s, there were 691 community mental health centers in the United States treating noninstitutionalized patients. Although these clinics had some success in working with patients who could be helped best in the community and in providing prompt crisis intervention services, they have been handicapped by low levels of funding and overburdened by patients. Furthermore, a comprehensive system of facilities and services to support the work of the mental health clinics, to include halfway houses and support networks for patients, never fully materialized in many communities. Consequently, the community mental health movement has not shown widespread success and, in fact, has contributed to a new problem, which is the presence of mental patients living in the community who are ill equipped to deal with life outside an institution. Many of these patients do not live with their families for various reasons and tend to congregate in ghettos of the mentally ill where some live lonely, disorganized, frustrated lives in slum environments. Mental disorder remains a major social problem in the United States.

SUMMARY

This chapter has reviewed the economic and social cost of mental illness, defined mental disorder, and traced the changing concepts of madness through the ages. We have seen how ideas about the cause of mental illness have changed from those of evil spirits in preliterate times to contemporary views based largely upon psychoanalytic or medical perspectives. In the twentieth century, there have been three revolutions in the United States that have initiated highly influential patterns of treatment for the mentally ill: (1) psychoanalysis and the theories of Sigmund Freud, (2) the widespread use of psychoactive drugs to treat mental patients, and (3) the establishment of community mental health centers. Several problems still exist, however, and they will be the focal point of discussion in forthcoming chapters. Curiously enough, as the observant reader may have noticed, there is as yet no conclusive explanation of the causes of mental disorder nor an established cure—despite all the cost, effort, and attention that mental illness has generated throughout human history.

2

Types of Mental Disorders

Mental disorders take different forms with respect to the symptoms they produce and the effects they have upon the minds of mentally disturbed people. As background for the discussion in forthcoming chapters, this chapter will briefly review the various types of mental disorders and the manner in which they are classified in psychiatry. This discussion is not intended as a detailed, clinical portrayal of each disorder; instead, its purpose is to acquaint the reader generally with the different types of mental abnormalities.

The basis for classifying mental disorders in psychiatry is contained in the *Diagnostic and Statistical Manual of Mental Disorders,* fourth edition (DSM-IV), published in 1994 by the American Psychiatric Association. Earlier editions of the manual were criticized for the questionable scientific validity of the classification system (Kirk and Kutchins 1992). The categories of mental disorder listed in DSM-IV are based to a much greater extent on field trials, professional experience, and expert opinion than were any previous edition. Nevertheless, some categories—for example, "disorder of written expression" (bad writing) and "oppositional defiant disorder" (defiant acts by children, such as losing tempers or being annoying, angry, or spiteful)—would appear to be questionable mental disorders without evidence of other and more abnormal behavior. The problem, as DSM-IV (1994:xxi) observes, is that no definition of mental disorder adequately specifies its precise boundaries; therefore, no operational definition exists that covers all situations. Furthermore, many mental conditions are abstract concepts and difficult, if not impossible, to verify scientifically. Sometimes, too, it is difficult to separate mental from physical disorders. On balance, however, DSM-IV represents the best current thinking in American psychiatry about the diagnosis and classification of mental disorder and appears to be an improvement over previous editions.

DSM-IV assesses each disorder on the basis of five axes: (1) the symptoms or clinical psychiatric syndrome(s) being expressed; (2) the past history of personality disorders (for adults) or developmental disorders (for children and adolescents) as evidence of possible long-term disturbance; (3) the possibility of physical illnesses relevant to understanding or managing the distressed individual; (4) the severity of psychosocial stressors that may be significant in the development or exacerbation of the mental disorder; and (5) the highest level of adaptive functioning during the past year, especially the quality of the individual's social relations. DSM-IV also gives consideration to psychological, social, and cross-cultural variables in diagnosis. The major diagnostic categories in DSM-IV are shown in Figure 2–1 and will be discussed in the remainder of this chapter.

DISORDERS USUALLY FIRST DIAGNOSED IN INFANCY, CHILDHOOD, OR ADOLESCENCE

The disorders that are described in this category are those that begin in childhood or adolescence for which there are no other appropriate diagnoses listed elsewhere. These disorders include (1) *mental retardation* (subnormal intelligence) and problems with (2) *learning,* (3) *motor skills,* (4) *communication,* (5) *development,* (6) *attention* (attention-deficit/hyperactivity) and *behavior* (conduct, oppositional defiance, and disruption), (7) *eating,* (8) *tics,* (9) *elimination* (constipation, bed-wetting), and (10) *other disorders of infancy, childhood, or adolescence* (separation anxiety, selective mutism, reactive attachment, and stereotypic movement).

DELIRIUM, DEMENTIA, AND AMNESTIC AND OTHER COGNITIVE DISORDERS

The disorders listed in this section were classified as organic mental disorders in previous DSM editions, but the term "organic mental disorder" is not used in DSM-IV (1994:10) because "it incorrectly implies that the other mental disorders in the manual do not have a biological basis." The disorders in this section are caused by either a general medical condition or a substance (alcohol or drugs) or some combination thereof. *Delirium* is a disturbance in consciousness and cognition or thinking that develops over a short period of time

Figure 2-1 DSM-IV Classification

NOS = Not Otherwise Specified.

An *x* appearing in a diagnostic code indicates that a specific code number is required.

An ellipsis (. . .) is used in the names of certain disorders to indicate that the name of a specific mental disorder or general medical condition should be inserted when recording the name (e.g., 293.0 Delirium Due to Hypothyroidism).

If criteria are currently met, one of the following severity specifiers may be noted after the diagnosis:

Mild
Moderate
Severe

If criteria are no longer met, one of the following specifiers may be noted:

In Partial Remission
In Full Remission
Prior History

DISORDERS USUALLY FIRST DIAGNOSED IN INFANCY, CHILDHOOD, OR ADOLESCENCE
MENTAL RETARDATION
Note: *These are coded on Axis II.*
317   Mild Mental Retardation
318.0   Moderate Mental Retardation
318.1   Severe Mental Retardation
318.2   Profound Mental Retardation
319   Mental Retardation, Severity
         Unspecified

LEARNING DISORDERS
315.00   Reading Disorder
315.1   Mathematics Disorder
315.2   Disorder of Written Expression
315.9   Learning Disorder NOS

MOTOR SKILLS DISORDER
315.4   Developmental Coordination
         Disorder

COMMUNICATION DISORDERS
315.31   Expressive Language
         Disorder

315.31   Mixed Receptive-Expressive
         Language Disorder
315.39   Phonological Disorder
307.0   Stuttering
307.9   Communication Disorder NOS

PERVASIVE DEVELOPMENTAL DISORDERS
299.00   Autistic Disorder
299.80   Rett's Disorder
299.10   Childhood Disintegrative
         Disorder
299.80   Asperger's Disorder
299.80   Pervasive Developmental
         Disorder NOS

ATTENTION-DEFICIT AND DISRUPTIVE
BEHAVIOR DISORDERS
314.xx   Attention-Deficit/Hyperactivity
         Disorder
  .01   Combined Type
  .00   Predominantly Inattentive Type
  .01   Predominantly Hyperactive-
           Impulsive Type
314.9   Attention-Deficit/Hyperactivity
         Disorder NOS
312.8   Conduct Disorder
         Specify type: Childhood-Onset
         Type/Adolescent-Onset Type
313.81   Oppositional Defiant Disorder
312.9   Disruptive Behavior Disorder
         NOS

FEEDING AND EATING DISORDERS OF
INFANCY OR EARLY CHILDHOOD
307.52   Pica
307.53   Rumination Disorder
307.59   Feeding Disorder of Infancy or
         Early Childhood

TIC DISORDERS
307.23   Tourette's Disorder
307.22   Chronic Motor or Vocal Tic
         Disorder
307.21   Transient Tic Disorder
         Specify if: Single Episode/Recurrent
307.20   Tic Disorder NOS

ELIMINATION DISORDERS
——.–   Encopresis
787.6   With Constipation and Overflow
           Incontinence

307.7   Without Constipation and Overflow
             Incontinence
307.6   Enuresis (Not Due to a General
             Medical Condition)
             Specify type: Nocturnal Only/Diurnal
             Only/Nocturnal and Diurnal

OTHER DISORDERS OF INFANCY, CHILDHOOD,OR ADOLESCENCE

309.21   Separation Anxiety Disorder
             Specify if: Early Onset
313.23   Selective Mutism
313.89   Reactive Attachment Disorder of
             Infancy or Early Childhood
             Specify type: Inhibited Type/Disinhibited
             Type
307.3   Stereotypic Movement Disorder
             Specify if: With Self-Injurious Behavior

313.9   Disorder of Infancy, Childhood,
             or Adolescence NOS

DELIRIUM, DEMENTIA, AND AMNESTIC AND OTHER COGNITIVE DISORDERS

DELIRIUM

293.0   Delirium Due to . . . *[Indicate the
             General Medical Condition]*
——.–   Substance Intoxication Delirium
             *(refer to Substance-Related Disorders for
             substance-specific codes)*
——.–   Substance Withdrawal Delirium
             *(refer to Substance-Related Disorders for
             substance-specific codes)*
——.–   Delirium Due to Multiple Etiologies
             (code each of the specific etiologies)
780.09   Delirium NOS

DEMENTIA

290.xx   Dementia of the Alzheimer's
             Type, With Early Onset *(also code
             331.0 Alzheimer's disease on Axis III)*
   .10   Uncomplicated
   .11   With Delirium
   .12   With Delusions
   .13   With Depressed Mood
             Specify if: With Behavioral Disturbance
290.xx   Dementia of the Alzheimer's
             Type, With Late Onset *(also code
             331.0 Alzheimer's disease on Axis III)*
   .0   Uncomplicated
   .3   With Delirium
   .20   With Delusions
   .21   With Depressed Mood
             Specify if: With Behavioral Disturbance

290.xx   Vascular Dementia
   .40   Uncomplicated
   .41   With Delirium
   .42   With Delusions
   .43   With Depressed Mood
             Specify if: With Behavioral Disturbance
294.9   Dementia Due to HIV Disease
             *(also code 043.1 HIV infection
             affecting central nervous system on
             Axis III)*
294.1   Dementia Due to Head Trauma
             *(also code 854.00 head injury on
             Axis III)*
294.1   Dementia Due to Parkinson's
             Disease *(also code 332.0 Parkinson's
             disease on Axis III)*
294.1   Dementia Due to Huntington's
             Disease *(also code 333.4 Huntington's
             disease on Axis III)*
290.10   Dementia Due to Pick's Disease
             *(also code 331.1 Pick's disease on
             Axis III)*
290.10   Dementia Due to Creutzfeldt-
             Jakob Disease *(also code 046.1
             Creutzfeldt-Jakob disease on
             Axis III)*
294.1   Dementia Due to . . . *[Indicate
             the General Medical Condition
             not listed above] (also code the
             general medical condition on
             Axis III)*
——.–   Substance-Induced Persisting
             Dementia *(refer to Substance-
             Related Disorders for substance-specific
             codes)*
——.–   Dementia Due to Multiple
             Etiologies *(code each of the specific
             etiologies)*
294.8   Dementia NOS

AMNESTIC DISORDERS

294.0   Amnestic Disorder Due to . . .
             *[Indicate the General Medical
             Condition]*
             Specify if: Transient/Chronic
——.–   Substance-Induced Persisting
             Amnestic Disorder *(refer to Substance-
             Related Disorders for substance-specific
             codes)*
294.8   Amnestic Disorder NOS

OTHER COGNITIVE DISORDERS

294.9   Cognitive Disorder NOS

*MENTAL DISORDERS DUE TO A GENERAL
MEDICAL CONDITION NOT ELSEWHERE
CLASSIFIED*

293.89   Catatonic Disorder Due to . . .
          *[Indicate the General Medical
          Condition]*

310.1   Personality Change Due to . . .
          [Indicate the General Medical Condition]
          Specify type: Labile Type/Disinhibited
          Type/Aggressive Type/Apathetic
          Type/Paranoid Type/Other
          Type/Combined Type/Unspecified Type

293.9   Mental Disorder NOS Due to . . .
          *[Indicate the General Medical
          Condition]*

SUBSTANCE-RELATED DISORDERS
[a]*The following specifiers may be applied to
Substance Dependence:*
          With Physiological Dependence/Without Physiological
          Dependence

          Early Full Remission/Early Partial Remission
          Sustained Full Remission/Sustained Partial Remission
          On Agonist Therapy/In a Controlled Environment

*The following specifiers apply to Substance-Induced
Disorders as noted:*
          [I]With Onset During Intoxication/[W]With Onset During
          Withdrawal

ALCOHOL-RELATED DISORDERS

Alcohol Use Disorders
303.90   Alcohol Dependence[a]
305.00   Alcohol Abuse

Alcohol-Induced Disorders
303.00   Alcohol Intoxication
291.8   Alcohol Withdrawal
          Specify if: With Perceptual Disturbances
291.0   Alcohol Intoxication Delirium
291.0   Alcohol Withdrawal Delirium
291.2   Alcohol-Induced Persisting
          Dementia
291.1   Alcohol-Induced Persisting
          Amnestic Disorder
291.x   Alcohol-Induced Psychotic
          Disorder
    .5   With Delusions[I,W]
    .3   With Hallucinations[I,W]
291.8   Alcohol-Induced Mood
          Disorder[I,W]
291.8   Alcohol-Induced Anxiety
          Disorder[I,W]
291.8   Alcohol-Induced Sexual Dysfunction[I]

291.8   Alcohol-Induced Sleep
          Disorder[I,W]

291.9   Alcohol-Related Disorder NOS

AMPHETAMINE (OR AMPHETAMINE-LIKE)-
RELATED DISORDERS

Amphetamine Use Disorders
304.40   Amphetamine Dependence[a]
305.70   Amphetamine Abuse

Amphetamine-Induced Disorders
292.89   Amphetamine Intoxication
          Specify if: With Perceptual Disturbances
292.0   Amphetamine Withdrawal
292.81   Amphetamine Intoxication
          Delirium
292.xx   Amphetamine-Induced
          Psychotic Disorder
    .11   With Delusions[I]
    .12   With Hallucinations[I]
292.84   Amphetamine-Induced Mood
          Disorder[I,W]
292.89   Amphetamine-Induced Anxiety
          Disorder[I]
292.89   Amphetamine-Induced Sexual
          Dysfunction[I]
292.89   Amphetamine-Induced Sleep
          Disorder[I,W]

292.9   Amphetamine-Related Disorder
          NOS

CAFFEINE-RELATED DISORDERS

Caffeine-Induced Disorders
305.90   Caffeine Intoxication
292.89   Caffeine-Induced Anxiety Disorder[I]
292.89   Caffeine-Induced Sleep Disorder[I]

292.9   Caffeine-Related Disorder NOS

CANNABIS-RELATED DISORDERS

Cannabis Use Disorders
304.30   Cannabis Dependence[a]
305.20   Cannabis Abuse

Cannabis-Induced Disorders
292.89   Cannabis Intoxication
          Specify if: With Perceptual Disturbances
292.81   Cannabis Intoxication Delirium
292.xx   Cannabis-Induced
          Psychotic Disorder

.11   With Delusions[I]
.12   With Hallucinations[I]
292.89   Cannabis-Induced Anxiety
Disorder[I]

292.9   Cannabis-Related Disorder
NOS

COCAINE-RELATED DISORDERS
Cocaine Use Disorders
304.20   Cocaine Dependence[a]
305.60   Cocaine Abuse

Cocaine-Induced Disorders
292.89   Cocaine Intoxication
    Specify if: With Perceptual Disturbances
292.0   Cocaine Withdrawal
292.81   Cocaine Intoxication Delirium
292.xx   Cocaine-Induced Psychotic
Disorder
.11   With Delusions[I]
.12   With Hallucinations[I]
292.84   Cocaine-Induced Mood
Disorder[I,W]
292.89   Cocaine-Induced Anxiety
Disorder[I,W]
292.89   Cocaine-Induced Sexual
Dysfunction[I]
292.89   Cocaine-Induced Sleep
Disorder[I,W]

292.9   Cocaine-Related Disorder NOS

HALLUCINOGEN-RELATED DISORDERS
Hallucinogen Use Disorders
304.50   Hallucinogen Dependence[a]
305.30   Hallucinogen Abuse

Hallucinogen-Induced Disorders
292.89   Hallucinogen Intoxication
292.89   Hallucinogen Persisting
Perception Disorder (Flashbacks)
292.81   Hallucinogen Intoxication
Delirium
292.xx   Hallucinogen-Induced Psychotic
Disorder
.11   With Delusions[I]
.12   With Hallucinations[I]
292.84   Hallucinogen-Induced Mood
Disorder[I]
292.89   Hallucinogen-Induced Anxiety
Disorder[I]

292.9   Hallucinogen-Related Disorder NOS

INHALANT-RELATED DISORDERS
Inhalant Use Disorders
304.60   Inhalant Dependence[a]
305.90   Inhalant Abuse

Inhalant-Induced Disorders
292.89   Inhalant Intoxication
292.81   Inhalant Intoxication Delirium
292.82   Inhalant-Induced Persisting
Dementia
292.xx   Inhalant-Induced Psychotic
Disorder
.11   With Delusions[I]
.12   With Hallucinations[I]
292.84   Inhalant-Induced Mood Disorder[I]
292.89   Inhalant-Induced Anxiety
Disorder[I]

292.9   Inhalant-Related Disorder NOS

NICOTINE-RELATED DISORDERS
Nicotine Use Disorder
305.10   Nicotine Dependence[a]

Nicotine-Induced Disorder
292.0   Nicotine Withdrawal

292.9   Nicotine-Related Disorder NOS

OPIOID-RELATED DISORDERS
Opioid Use Disorders
304.00   Opioid Dependence[a]
305.50   Opioid Abuse

Opioid-Induced Disorders
292.89   Opioid Intoxication
    Specify if: With Perceptual Disturbances
292.0   Opioid Withdrawal
292.81   Opioid Intoxication Delirium
292.xx   Opioid-Induced Psychotic
Disorder
.11   With Delusions[I]
.12   With Hallucinations[I]
292.84   Opioid-Induced Mood Disorder[I]
292.89   Opioid-Induced Sexual
Dysfunction[I]
292.89   Opioid-Induced Sleep Disorder[I,W]

292.9   Opioid-Related Disorder NOS

PHENCYCLIDINE (OR PHENCYCLIDINE-LIKE)-RELATED DISORDERS

Phencyclidine Use Disorders
304.90   Phencyclidine Dependence[a]
305.90   Phencyclidine Abuse

Phencyclidine-Induced Disorders
292.89   Phencyclidine Intoxication
   Specify if: With Perceptual Disturbances
292.81   Phencyclidine Intoxication
   Delirium
292.xx   Phencyclidine-Induced Psychotic
   Disorder
 .11 With Delusions[I]
 .12 With Hallucinations[I]
292.84   Phencyclidine-Induced Mood
   Disorder[I]
292.89   Phencyclidine-Induced Anxiety
   Disorder[I]

292.9   Phencyclidine-Related Disorder
   NOS

SEDATIVE-, HYPNOTIC-, OR ANXIOLYTIC-RELATED DISORDERS

Sedative, Hypnotic, or Anxiolytic Use Disorders
304.10   Sedative, Hypnotic, or Anxiolytic
   Dependence[a]
305.40   Sedative, Hypnotic, or Anxiolytic
   Abuse

Sedative-, Hypnotic-, or Anxiolytic-Induced Disorders
292.89   Sedative, Hypnotic, or Anxiolytic
   Intoxication
292.0   Sedative, Hypnotic, or Anxiolytic
   Withdrawal
   Specify if: With Perceptual Disturbances
292.81   Sedative, Hypnotic, or Anxiolytic
   Intoxication Delirium
292.81   Sedative, Hypnotic, or Anxiolytic
   Withdrawal Delirium
292.82   Sedative-, Hypnotic-, or
   Anxiolytic-Induced Persisting
   Dementia
292.83   Sedative-, Hypnotic-, or
   Anxiolytic-Induced Persisting
   Amnestic Disorder
292.xx   Sedative-, Hypnotic-, or
   Anxiolytic-Induced Psychotic
   Disorder

 .11 With Delusions[I,W]
 .12 With Hallucinations[I,W]
292.84   Sedative-, Hypnotic-, or
   Anxiolytic-Induced Mood
   Disorder[I,W]
292.89   Sedative-, Hypnotic-, or
   Anxiolytic-Induced Anxiety
   Disorder[W]
292.89   Sedative-, Hypnotic-, or
   Anxiolytic-Induced Sexual
   Dysfunction[I]
292.89   Sedative-, Hypnotic-, or
   Anxiolytic-Induced Sleep Disorder[I,W]

292.9   Sedative-, Hypnotic-, or Anxiolytic-
   Related Disorder NOS

POLYSUBSTANCE-RELATED DISORDER
304.80   Polysubstance Dependence[a]

OTHER (OR UNKNOWN) SUBSTANCE-RELATED DISORDERS

Other (or Unknown) Substance Use Disorders
304.90   Other (or Unknown) Substance
   Dependence[a]
305.90   Other (or Unknown) Substance
   Abuse

Other (or Unknown) Substance-Induced Disorders
292.89   Other (or Unknown) Substance
   Intoxication
   Specify if: With Perceptual Disturbances
292.0   Other (or Unknown) Substance
   Withdrawal
   Specify if: With Perceptual Disturbances
292.81   Other (or Unknown) Substance-
   Induced Delirium
292.82   Other (or Unknown) Substance-
   Induced Persisting Dementia
292.83   Other (or Unknown) Substance-
   Induced Persisting Amnestic
   Disorder
292.xx   Other (or Unknown) Substance-
   Induced Psychotic Disorder
 .11 With Delusions[I,W]
 .12 With Hallucinations[I,W]
292.84   Other (or Unknown) Substance-
   Induced Mood Disorder[I,W]
292.89   Other (or Unknown) Substance-
   Induced Anxiety Disorder[I,W]

292.89   Other (or Unknown) Substance-
         Induced Sexual Dysfunction[I]
292.89   Other (or Unknown) Substance-
         Induced Sleep Disorder[I,W]

292.9   Other (or Unknown) Substance-
         Related Disorder NOS

*SCHIZOPHRENIA AND OTHER PSYCHOTIC
DISORDERS*

295.xx   Schizophrenia
*The following Classification of Longitudinal
Course applies to all subtypes of Schizophrenia:*
         Episodic With Interepisode Residual Symptoms
           (*specify if:* With Prominent Negative
           Symptoms)/Episodic With No Interepisode
           Residual Symptoms/Continuous (*specify if:* With
           Prominent Negative Symptoms)
         Single Episode In Partial Remission (*specify if:*
           With Prominent Negative Symptoms)/Single
           Episode In Full Remission
         Other or Unspecified Pattern

   .30   Paranoid Type
   .10   Disorganized Type
   .20   Catatonic Type
   .90   Undifferentiated Type
   .60   Residual Type
295.40   Schizophreniform Disorder
         Specify if: Without Good Prognostic
         Features/With Good Prognostic
         Features
295.70   Schizoaffective Disorder
         Specify type: Bipolar Type/Depressive
         Type
297.1   Delusional Disorder
         Specify type: Erotomanic
         Type/Grandiose Type/Jealous
         Type/Persecutory Type/Somatic
         Type/Mixed Type/Unspecified Type
298.8   Brief Psychotic Disorder
         Specify if: With Marked Stressor(s)/Without
         Marked Stressor(s)/With Postpartum
         Onset
297.3   Shared Psychotic Disorder
293.xx   Psychotic Disorder Due to . . .
         *[Indicate the General Medical
         Condition]*
   .81   With Delusions
   .82   With Hallucinations
——.–   Substance-Induced Psychotic
         Disorder *(refer to Substance
         Related Disorders for substance-
         specific codes)*
         Specify if: With Onset During
         Intoxication/With Onset During Withdrawal
298.9   Psychotic Disorder NOS

MOOD DISORDERS
*Code current state of Major Depressive Disorder or
Bipolar I Disorder in fifth digit:*
         1 = Mild
         2 = Moderate
         3 = Severe Without Psychotic Features
         4 = Severe With Psychotic Features
           Specify: Mood-Congruent Psychotic
           Features/Mood-Incongruent Psychotic Features
         5 = In Partial Remission
         6 = In Full Remission
         0 = Unspecified

*The following specifiers apply (for current or most
recent episode) to mood disorders as noted:*
         [a]Severity/Psychotic/Remission
         Specifiers/[b]Chronic/[c]With Catatonic Features/[d]With
         Melancholic Features/[e]With Atypical Features/[f]With
         Postpartum Onset

*The following specifiers apply to mood disorders as
noted:*
         [g]With or Without Full Interepisode Recovery/
         [h]With Seasonal Pattern/[i]With Rapid Cycling

DEPRESSIVE DISORDERS
296.xx   Major Depressive Disorder,
   .2x   Single Episode[a,b,c,d,e,f]
   .3x   Recurrent[a,b,c,d,e,f,g,h]
300.4   Dysthymic Disorder
         Specify if: Early Onset/Late Onset
         Specify: With Atypical Features
311   Depressive Disorder NOS

BIPOLAR DISORDERS
296.xx   Bipolar I Disorder,
   .0x   Single Manic Episode[a,c,f]
              Specify if: Mixed
   .40   Most Recent Episode
              Hypomanic[g,h,i]
   .4x   Most Recent Episode
              Manic[a,c,f,g,h,i]
   .6x   Most Recent Episode
              Mixed[a,c,f,g,h,i]
   .5x   Most Recent Episode
              Depressed[a,b,c,d,e,f,g,h,i]
   .7   Most Recent Episode
              Unspecified[g,h,i]
296.89   Bipolar II Disorder[a,b,c,d,e,f,g,h,i]
         Specify (current or most recent episode):
         Hypomanic/Depressed
301.13   Cyclothymic Disorder
296.80   Bipolar Disorder NOS

293.83   Mood Disorder Due to . . .
         *[Indicate the General Medical
         Condition]*

Specify type: With Depressive
Features/With Major Depressive-Like
Episode/With Manic Features/With Mixed
Features

—.— **Substance-Induced Mood Disorder** *(refer to Substance-Related Disorders for substance-specific codes)*
Specify type: With Depressive
Features/With Manic Features/With Mixed
Features
Specify if: With Onset During
Intoxication/With Onset During Withdrawal

296.90 **Mood Disorder NOS**

ANXIETY DISORDERS
300.01 Panic Disorder Without Agoraphobia
300.21 Panic Disorder With Agoraphobia
300.22 Agoraphobia Without History of Panic Disorder
300.29 Specific Phobia
Specify type: Animal Type/Natural
Environment Type/Blood-Injection-Injury
Type/Situational Type/Other Type
300.23 Social Phobia
Specify if: Generalized
300.3 Obsessive-Compulsive Disorder
Specify if: With Poor Insight
309.81 Posttraumatic Stress Disorder
Specify if: Acute/Chronic
Specify if: With Delayed Onset
308.3 Acute Stress Disorder
300.02 Generalized Anxiety Disorder
293.89 Anxiety Disorder Due to . . .
[Indicate the General Medical Condition]
Specify if: With Generalized Anxiety/With
Panic Attacks/With Obsessive-Compulsive
Symptoms
—.— **Substance-Induced Anxiety Disorder** *(refer to Substance-Related Disorders for substance-specific codes)*
Specify if: With Generalized Anxiety/With
Panic Attacks/With Obsessive-Compulsive
Symptoms/With Phobic Symptoms
Specify if: With Onset During
Intoxication/With Onset During Withdrawal
300.00 Anxiety Disorder NOS

SOMATOFORM DISORDERS
300.81 Somatization Disorder
300.81 Undifferentiated Somatoform Disorder
300.11 Conversion Disorder

Specify type: With Motor Symptom or
Deficit/With Sensory Symptom or
Deficit/With Seizures or Convulsions/
With Mixed Presentation
307.xx Pain Disorder
.80 Associated With Psychological Factors
.89 Associated With Both Psychological Factors and a General Medical Condition
Specify if: Acute/Chronic
300.7 Hypochondriasis
Specify if: With Poor Insight
300.7 Body Dysmorphic Disorder
300.81 Somatoform Disorder NOS

FACTITIOUS DISORDERS
300.xx Factitious Disorder
.16 With Predominantly Psychological Signs and Symptoms
.19 With Predominantly Physical Signs and Symptoms
.19 With Combined Psychological and Physical Signs and Symptoms
300.19 Factitious Disorder NOS

DISSOCIATIVE DISORDERS
300.12 Dissociative Amnesia
300.13 Dissociative Fugue
300.14 Dissociative Identity Disorder
300.6 Depersonalization Disorder
300.15 Dissociative Disorder NOS

SEXUAL AND GENDER IDENTITY DISORDERS

SEXUAL DYSFUNCTIONS
The following specifiers apply to all primary Sexual Dysfunctions:
Lifelong Type/Acquired Type/Generalized
Type/Situational Type Due to Psychological
Factors/Due to Combined Factors

Sexual Desire Disorders
302.71 Hypoactive Sexual Desire Disorder
302.79 Sexual Aversion Disorder

Sexual Arousal Disorders
302.72 Female Sexual Arousal Disorder
302.72 Male Erectile Disorder

Orgasmic Disorders
302.73   Female Orgasmic Disorder
302.74   Male Orgasmic Disorder
302.75   Premature Ejaculation

Sexual Pain Disorders
302.76   Dyspareunia (Not Due to a
          General Medical Condition)
306.51   Vaginismus (Not Due to a
          General Medical Condition)

Sexual Dysfunction Due to a General
Medical Condition
625.8   Female Hypoactive Sexual Desire
          Disorder Due to . . . *[Indicate the
          General Medical Condition]*
608.89   Male Hypoactive Sexual Desire
          Disorder Due to . . . *[Indicate the
          General Medical Condition]*
607.84   Male Erectile Disorder Due to . . .
          *[Indicate the General Medical
          Condition]*
625.0   Female Dyspareunia Due to . . .
          *[Indicate the General Medical
          Condition]*
608.89   Male Dyspareunia Due to . . .
          *[Indicate the General Medical
          Condition]*
625.8   Other Female Sexual Dysfunction
          Due to . . . *[Indicate the General
          Medical Condition]*
608.89   Other Male Sexual Dysfunction
          Due to . . . *[Indicate the General
          Medical Condition]*
——.–   Substance-Induced Sexual
          Dysfunction *(refer to Substance-Related
          Disorders for substance-specific codes)*
          Specify if: With Impaired Desire/With
          Impaired Arousal/With Impaired
          Orgasm/With Sexual Pain
          Specify if: With Onset During Intoxication

302.70   Sexual Dysfunction NOS

Paraphilias
302.4   Exhibitionism
302.81   Fetishism
302.89   Frotteurism
302.2   Pedophilia
          Specify if: Sexually Attracted to
          Males/Sexually Attracted to
          Females/Sexually Attracted to Both
          Specify if: Limited to Incest
          Specify type: Exclusive Type/Nonexclusive Type

302.83   Sexual Masochism
302.84   Sexual Sadism
302.3   Transvestic Fetishism
          Specify if: With Gender Dysphoria
302.82   Voyeurism
302.9   Paraphilia NOS

GENDER IDENTITY DISORDERS
302.xx   Gender Identity Disorder
   .6   in Children
   .85   in Adolescents or Adults
          Specify if: Sexually Attracted to
          Males/Sexually Attracted to
          Females/Sexually Attracted to
          Both/Sexually Attracted to Neither
302.6   Gender Identity Disorder NOS

302.9   Sexual Disorder NOS

EATING DISORDERS
307.1   Anorexia Nervosa
          Specify type: Restricting Type;
          Binge-Eating/Purging Type
307.51   Bulimia Nervosa
          Specify type: Purging Type/Nonpurging
          Type
307.50   Eating Disorder NOS

SLEEP DISORDERS
PRIMARY SLEEP DISORDERS

Dyssomnias
307.42   Primary Insomnia
307.44   Primary Hypersomnia
          Specify if: Recurrent
347   Narcolepsy
780.59   Breathing-Related Sleep Disorder
307.45   Circadian Rhythm Sleep Disorder
          Specify type: Delayed Sleep Phase
          Type/Jet Lag Type/Shift Work
          Type/Unspecified Type
307.47   Dyssomnia NOS

Parasomnias
307.47   Nightmare Disorder
307.46   Sleep Terror Disorder
307.46   Sleepwalking Disorder
307.47   Parasomnia NOS

SLEEP DISORDERS RELATED TO ANOTHER
MENTAL DISORDER
307.42   Insomnia Related to . . .
          [Indicate the Axis I or Axis II Disorder]
307.44   Hypersomnia Related to . . .
          [Indicate the Axis I or Axis II Disorder]

OTHER SLEEP DISORDERS

780.xx   Sleep Disorder Due to . . .
[Indicate the General Medical Condition]

   .52   Insomnia Type
   .54   Hypersomnia Type
   .59   Parasomnia Type
   .59   Mixed Type

——.–   Substance-Induced Sleep Disorder *(refer to Substance-Related Disorders for substance-specific codes)*
Specify type: Insomnia Type/Hypersomnia Type/Parasomnia Type/Mixed Type
Specify if: With Onset During Intoxication/With Onset During Withdrawal

IMPULSE-CONTROL DISORDERS NOT ELSEWHERE CLASSIFIED

312.34   Intermittent Explosive Disorder
312.32   Kleptomania
312.33   Pyromania
312.31   Pathological Gambling
312.39   Trichotillomania
312.30   Impulse-Control Disorder NOS

ADJUSTMENT DISORDERS

309.xx   Adjustment Disorder
   .0   With Depressed Mood
   .24   With Anxiety
   .28   With Mixed Anxiety and Depressed Mood
   .3   With Disturbance of Conduct
   .4   With Mixed Disturbance of Emotions and Conduct
   .9   Unspecified
Specify if: Acute/Chronic

PERSONALITY DISORDERS

Note: *These are Coded on Axis II.*

301.0   Paranoid Personality Disorder
301.20   Schizoid Personality Disorder
301.22   Schizotypal Personality Disorder
301.7   Antisocial Personality Disorder
301.83   Borderline Personality Disorder
301.50   Histrionic Personality Disorder
301.81   Narcissistic Personality Disorder
301.82   Avoidant Personality Disorder
301.6   Dependent Personality Disorder
301.4   Obsessive-Compulsive Personality Disorder
301.9   Personality Disorder NOS

OTHER CONDITIONS THAT MAY BE A FOCUS OF CLINICAL ATTENTION

PSYCHOLOGICAL FACTORS AFFECTING MEDICAL CONDITION

316   *. . . [Specified Psychological Factor]* Affecting . . . *[Indicate the General Medical Condition] Choose name based on nature of factors:*

Mental Disorder Affecting Medical Condition
Psychological Symptoms Affecting Medical Condition
Personality Traits or Coping Style Affecting Medical Condition
Maladaptive Health Behaviors Affecting Medical Condition
Stress-Related Physiological Response Affecting Medical Condition
Other or Unspecified Psychological Factors Affecting Medical Condition

Reprinted with permission from *Diagnostic and Statistical Manual of Mental Disorders,* 4th ed., Washington, DC, American Psychiatric Association, 1994.

and includes problems like impaired awareness, focus, and perception. The origin of the problem is often injury or substance abuse.

    Dementia is associated with aging. A major form of dementia is Alzheimer's disease, which is the deterioration of previously acquired intellectual abilities to the extent that usual social behavior is severely affected. The most prominent symptom is loss of memory, although there may also be impairment in judgment and control of impulses. Another symptom may be personality change in which an individual begins to act markedly different from his or her typical self. The person may become unusually compulsive, cantankerous, uncooperative, paranoid, or perhaps withdrawn from others. It is estimated that between 2 and 4 percent of the population over age sixty-five have Alzheimer's disease, and the prevalence rises with increasing age, particularly after seventy-five years of age. Other forms of dementia are caused by other diseases, HIV, head injury or trauma, and substance abuse. *Amnestic disorders* are disturbances in memory caused not by aging but by a medical condition or the persistent effects of alcohol or drugs.

MENTAL DISORDERS DUE TO A GENERAL MEDICAL CONDITION NOT ELSEWHERE CLASSIFIED

The disorders in this section are all psychosocial problems caused by a general medical condition and include problems such as a *catatonic* state (physical immobility or excessive mobility) or *personality change.*

SUBSTANCE-RELATED DISORDERS

Substance-related disorders are caused by alcohol or drug abuse, the side effects of a medication, or exposure to toxins like lead, aluminum, rat poison, and carbon monoxide. *Substance-related disorders* produce behavior considered maladaptive or undesirable in most cultures and impairment in social or occupational functioning, inability to control use of a drug, and development of severe withdrawal symptoms after cessation of use.

Substance-related disorders are divided into two groups: substance use disorders (characterized by dependence and abuse) and substance-induced disorders (intoxication and withdrawal symptoms). "Substance use" refers to behavior related to the taking of substances, and "substance-induced" pertains to the direct effects of the substance on the nervous system. The substances that most commonly produce these effects are alcohol, amphetamines, caffeine, cannabis, cocaine, hallucinogens, inhalants, nicotine, opioids (heroin), phencyclidine (PCP), sedatives, and polysubstances (repeated use of at least three different substances, not including caffeine or nicotine). The inclusion of nicotine and caffeine (both widely used and usually not thought of as producing a substance-induced disorder) is based on the behavioral problems that some people (not all) have in withdrawing from tobacco use and caffeine intoxication. The latter is very rare and requires a history of excessive caffeine ingestion.

For a substance to be regarded as abused, there must have been at least one month of use with corresponding social complications, like disturbed relations with other people or problems with work or school. Moreover, a definition of abuse also requires that there be either a psychological dependence on the substance or a pathological pattern of use. Pathological patterns consist of being intoxicated for long periods (for example, throughout the day), using a substance nearly every day for at least a month, or having two or more episodes of complications (blackouts, hallucinations, and so on) as a result of intoxication.

As for dependence, the requirements for substance abuse must be met as well as additional conditions of tolerance *or* withdrawal. To show tolerance, a person requires increasing amounts of the substance to achieve or maintain the desired effect; simply continuing a regular dosage has a diminished effect. The other condition denoting dependence is the presence of withdrawal symptoms (usually absent with the use of cannabis or hallucinogens).

Alcohol is the most abused substance in the world. In the United States, nine million people are estimated to be alcoholics, and about one-third of all arrests involve drunkenness. The greatest amounts of alcohol are consumed by young white males in late adolescence and early adulthood, and alcoholism tends to appear after about five to fifteen years of heavy drinking. The demarcation between a heavy drinker and an alcoholic is not clear, but a primary factor in being an alcoholic is addiction to or dependence on alcohol. Most researchers agree that physical withdrawal symptoms (tremor of hands, tongue, and eyelids; nausea; malaise; anxiety; and depressed mood or irritability) are integral to such dependence, and alcohol is often consumed to relieve or avoid the symptoms.

To summarize the research and various accounts of drinking behavior given by alcoholics themselves, it would seem that the alcoholic is a person who (1) lacks the emotional stamina to refrain from drinking, (2) has a strong mental and physical craving for alcohol, (3) suffers from severe mental and physical withdrawal symptoms when deprived of alcohol, (4) shows signs of physical and emotional deterioration, and (5) can be characterized by a relinquishment of all other interests to a preoccupation with obtaining and consuming alcohol. Consider, for example, an alcoholic named Nick:

> Nick's hangovers were spectacular. As he said, the first sensation is blinding pain. It's like what I imagine a brain tumor would feel like. Your head hurts so bad that you cannot even open your eyes. I go to the bathroom and swallow some aspirin but they always make me throw up. I go back to bed and wait till I get sick then I rush to the john and have the "dry heaves" for nearly an hour. . . . Then I go back to sleep but I don't sleep long because I have nightmares, and wake up dying of thirst. A bloody Mary in the morning is the only solution. When I get one I nearly choke on it, but in about five minutes my head comes back to my shoulders and my eyes start to focus again.[1]

The extent of drug abuse in American society is not known, but it ranks as one of the nation's most important social problems. Marijuana (cánnabis) is the most popular and controversial of the illicit drugs. There is a lack of confirmed evidence showing that it causes physical addiction or influences people to behave in a manner incompatible with their basic personality. However, marijuana has a potential for abuse (through social complications, pathological patterns of use) and psychological dependence. Cocaine is currently the

---

[1]Elton McNeil, *The Quiet Furies* (Englewood Cliffs, NJ: Prentice Hall, 1967), p. 130.

second most popular drug, and twenty million Americans are estimated to have tried it. There is general agreement that a person can become psychologically dependent on cocaine, but disagreement exists as to whether cocaine is physically addicting. An overdose of the drug, however, can quickly lead to death or other serious complications, such as seizures. Although the use of marijuana and cocaine remains strong among young adults, there is evidence of a decline in such use by high school students because of social disapproval and, in the case of cocaine, the perceived risks in ingesting the drug (Bachman, Johnston, and O'Malley 1990; O'Malley, Bachman, and Johnston 1988).

Drugs like heroin and other opioids are clearly physically addictive. Chronic, intensive users of such drugs lead lives that are profoundly disrupted and degraded by the process of procuring and using them. Opioid dependence produces an inability to reduce or stop drug use; results in impairments in social functioning, including loss of friends and job; and creates legal problems owing to possession, purchase, or sale of drugs, committing crimes to acquire the money for drugs, or antisocial behavior while under their influence. Prolonged use can result in damage to the central nervous system and other medical complications. Males are more likely to abuse drugs than females, which is seen in the higher proportion of males than females with substance-related disorders.

SCHIZOPHRENIA

Schizophrenia is the most commonly diagnosed mental disorder requiring hospitalization in the United States. Out of 245,932 admissions to state and county mental hospitals in 1992, 118,852 (32.1 percent) were diagnosed as schizophrenic. About 1 percent of the entire U.S. population, over two million people, are schizophrenic or have schizophrenic tendencies, according to some estimates. Even though diagnoses of schizophrenia may be inflated by error ("I have seen them [psychiatrists] apply it to people as freely and meaninglessly as one might apply it to cattle," reports one observer),[2] there appears to be *enough* "real" schizophrenia to constitute a major psychiatric condition.

Schizophrenia can be characterized as a disturbance in mood, thinking, and behavior, manifested by distortions of reality that include delusions and hallucinations. The disorder always includes a disorganization of a previous level of functioning that represents a significant impairment of behavior. The disorganization is typically expressed through one or more psychotic symptoms that include distortions in language (usually incoherence), thought content (delusions), perception (hallucinations), affective expression (emotions), sense of self (loss of ego), volition (disturbance in self-initiated activity), rela-

---

[2]Otto Friedrich, *Going Crazy: An Inquiry into Madness in Our Time* (New York: Simon & Schuster, 1975), p. 21.

tionship to the external world (withdrawal from reality), or perhaps motor behavior (catatonic states). Illustrations of these symptoms can be found in accounts of schizophrenics' experiences. Consider, for example, the situation of Renee, a young French woman trying to work as a secretary while suffering from delusions. The delusions were in the form of orders that seemed to enter her head. The orders were given by something she called the "System," which she believed was trying to take over her mind. Renee reported:

> At the same time I received orders from the System. I did not hear the orders as voices; yet while they were as imperious as if uttered in a loud voice. While, for example, I was preparing to do some typing, suddenly, without any warning, a force, which was not an impulse, but rather resembled a command, ordered me to burn my right hand or the building in which I was. With all my strength I resisted the order. I telephoned Mama to tell her about it. Her voice, urging me to listen to her and not to the System, reassured me. If the System was to become too demanding, I was to run to her. This calmed me considerably, but unfortunately only for a moment.
>
> . . . In the midst of this horror and turbulence, I nonetheless carried on my work as a secretary. But with what a hardship! Adding to the torment, strident noises, piercing cries began to hammer in my head. Their unexpectedness made me jump. Nonetheless, I did not hear them as I heard real cries uttered by real people. The noises localized on the right side, drove me to stop up my ears. But I readily distinguished them from the noises of reality. I heard them without hearing them and recognized that they arose within me.
>
> I knew that more and more I would let myself be controlled by the System, that I would sink down in the Land of Enlightenment or the Land of Commandment, as I also called it.[3]

Eventually, Renee did give in to her delusions and placed her right hand into a bed of hot coals as the orders demanded, and she was subsequently hospitalized for burns and mental treatment. Renee's delusions are typical of schizophrenia in that such delusions often feature passivity and some imagined outside influence directing the schizophrenic's thoughts and actions.

An example of schizophrenic hallucinations can be found in the experience of a young college student under pressure to earn good grades and yet support a wife on very little money. After turning in a thesis so that he could graduate with honors, he went to a friend's apartment where he felt "a strange rush" go through his body like "an electric shock." It happened again the next day and he began to experience difficulty sleeping, knowing something was wrong with him and yet being very curious about the ideas that he was having. He felt as though he were going mad and investigating madness at the same time. One night he imagined that his wife was dead (he thought he had killed her), and he spent the night covering her with his body. He stated:

---

[3]Marguerite Sechehaye, "Autobiography of a Schizophrenic Girl," in *The Inner World of Mental Illness,* ed. B. Kaplan (New York: Harper & Row, 1964), pp. 170–71.

I had more or less stayed in bed during those two days, trying to sleep, unable to sleep. A friend of mine came by, and we went to his place for drinks and I was— I was just like on coals—I didn't know what to say any more. Then, in some effort to shock them, I went over to my wife and tore open her blouse, and I said, "Look at her! She's decomposed under that!" Because I was convinced that she was dead, that she was a walking ghost.

Going crazy is a symbolic experience. Reality is still there but you keep interpreting it. Everything becomes symbolic. The symbols chase each other. The fact that you're wearing that striped tie could mean rivers to me, the Rhine, or the Niger. The ticking of a clock can be the chimes of the universe. My venetian blinds changed color as I watched them during the night, and this became to me eons—I was going through cycles of life that were much larger than day or night, they were eons. Then at one point I had a vision of being celebrated in an age beyond, in which people no longer had hair or windows. Everything was terribly white. Narrow streets. A kind of brushed-up, futuristic brave new world. And I was famous, with my name on streets, for having been the founder of this age. . . .[4]

The next day, while visiting the father of his friend, he sensed that madness radiated around him in some kind of glow and that the sight of him would kill his friend's father. He ran away, howling. But in his mind he was not howling; rather, it was *something else* inside him that was making the cries. At that point, he was placed under psychiatric observation and committed to a mental hospital.

Another characteristic commonly found among schizophrenics is withdrawal from other people. The wife of Sam P., another schizophrenic, explains how Sam became increasingly isolated from her:

What hurt me most was the feeling I began to get more and more of the time that I was losing contact with him. It was as if he were drifting away from me and I didn't know what to do about it. I would talk to him for a while, but when I looked at him, I would realize he wasn't listening. He was off somewhere lost in thought and never heard a word I said. Then he began to do scary things and creepy things. I would wake up in the middle of the night and he would be gone. Once I found him sitting on the grass in the middle of the backyard at 4 A.M. and he didn't seem to know where he was or what was going on.[5]

Sam's bizarre behavior continued. Once he was brought home by the police after being found knocking on the door of a bank during the night; another time he woke up in bed and began to crow like a rooster. Finally, he was arrested at 3 A.M. in a small town some forty miles away from home after driving at eighty-five miles an hour. He told the police he was trying "to get up escape velocity for a trip to Mars." He was sent directly from jail to a mental hospital, where he was openly agitated and hallucinogenic. For a while, he was convinced that he was Robin Hood:

---

[4]Friedrich, *Going Crazy,* pp. 141–42.
[5]McNeil, *Quiet Furies,* p. 177.

He had not notified anyone of his sudden shift in identity and it was discovered only when he leaped from a perch atop a door on the back of an unsuspecting attendant who had just entered the room. After a brief scramble, Sam informed the hospital authorities that Robin Hood also jumped out of trees whenever the king's men approached and that the attendant looked very much like the Sheriff of Nottingham.[6]

DSM-IV lists five subtypes of schizophrenia: (1) *paranoid*, a condition of persecutory or grandiose delusions or hallucinations; (2) *disorganized*, a condition of extreme social impairment; (3) *catatonic*, characterized by marked psychomotor disturbances (such as stupor, rigidity, purposeless excitement, or posturing); (4) *undifferentiated*, characterized by prominent psychotic symptoms that cannot be classified as any of the above subtypes or cannot meet the criteria for more than one subtype; and (5) *residual*, a category for persons who have had a past episode of schizophrenia as evidenced by persisting signs but who are currently not overly psychotic.

A diagnosis of schizophrenia requires that signs of the disorder have been present for at least a six-month period, are not the result of an organic mental disorder, and include an active phase of prominent psychotic symptoms. Usually, the onset of the disorder is during adolescence or early adulthood; it rarely appears in childhood or middle and old age.

The cause of schizophrenia is unknown. The strongest evidence is from genetic studies, particularly those studies of children of schizophrenic parents who are raised in foster homes by normal adults. These children have ten times the incidence of schizophrenia seen in the normal population and about the same incidence of schizophrenia for children raised by their own schizophrenic parents. The genetic mechanisms that may be involved in the transmission of schizophrenia from parents to children have not been identified. Another theory suggests that biochemical abnormalities bring on the disorder. This approach is based upon findings that demonstrate that certain psychoactive drugs are able to control schizophrenic symptoms. Large doses of sympathomimetic drugs can also produce schizophrenic symptoms in normal persons. Furthermore, in the genetic transmission of schizophrenia, the factors in that transmission are certainly biochemical, that is, nucleic acid sequences (Snyder 1977). But again, there is no solid evidence to pinpoint the exact role of biochemistry in schizophrenia.

Sociocultural factors may also be significant. The onset of schizophrenia is sometimes related to the presence of a precipitating situation. The essential difference between the schizophrenic and nonschizophrenic lower-class Puerto Ricans in a study by Lloyd Rogler and August Hollingshead (1965) was that before the overt appearance of schizophrenic symptoms, those who became schizophrenic were engulfed by a series of insoluble and mutually reinforcing

---

[6]Ibid., p. 178.

problems. As for the examples of schizophrenic symptoms given in this section, Renee had had a very unhappy childhood; the college student had had difficulty in earning good grades and supporting his wife; and Sam P. had failed in business. If certain people are therefore predisposed genetically toward schizophrenia, stressful life events may in fact elicit the disorder (Grebb and Cancro 1989). Nevertheless, the exact etiology of schizophrenia remains unidentified. Most likely, the cause is exceedingly complex and possibly involves some combination of genetic, biochemical, and sociocultural factors.

MOOD DISORDERS

Although schizophrenia may be the most commonly diagnosed class of mental disorders for persons hospitalized in state and county mental institutions, schizophrenia is not the most common form of severe mental disorder in American society. Instead, that dubious distinction falls to the *mood disorders,* especially depression, but also mania and manic-depressive disorders, which collectively represent the largest category of incapacitating mental dysfunctions in the nation. At least 2.5 percent of the U.S. population can expect to suffer from a mood disorder at some point in their lives, but the actual percentage is probably several times higher. Something like one out of every five adults becomes significantly depressed in his or her life.

The basic feature of mood disorders is a fundamental disturbance in mood. The term "mood" in this context refers to a condition of prolonged emotion consisting of either depression or elation. As shown in Figure 2–1, the mood disorders are divided into depressive and bipolar disorders.

Depressive Disorders

DSM-IV states that the essential feature of a *depressive disorder* is a period of at least two weeks during which a person experiences either a depressed mood or loss of interest or pleasure in nearly all activities. The individual must experience at least four additional symptoms: changes in appetite or weight, sleep, or psychomotor activity; decreased energy; feelings of worthlessness or guilt; difficulty thinking, concentrating, or making decisions; or recurrent thoughts of death or suicide ideas, plans, or attempts. In a major depressive episode, DSM-IV points out, the individual typically describes his or her mood as depressed, sad, hopeless, discouraged, or "down in the dumps." The depressed person may no longer care about anything or be able to enjoy former pleasures. The following account is an example of a woman in her late forties who is suffering from a major depressive episode:

> For her, being ill means waking before it is light, a clutching gnawing vague pain inside, the beginnings of a dull headache, and a feeling of terror. Before she is

properly awake, she worries that she has overslept, will miss the train, be late for work, has adequate clothes for the weather, will it snow; then, awake, she feels alone, utterly alone, utterly useless, utterly without value, facing a meaningless day that will be a constant battle with which to cope. The ache feels so bad she thinks she cannot get out of bed; it seems that no one cares whether she lives or dies; she cannot read, she cannot write letters, her bedroom is in a state of shocking disorganization but it does not seem worthwhile to tidy it.

. . . She is utterly self-absorbed. She cannot discuss anything but her pain and her fears, and when other things are discussed around her, she retreats into the stubborn, accusing silence that embarrasses everyone else. She pours her story out to everyone who will listen, and for a time, most people do, sympathetically and kindly. But her demands are consuming, terribly consuming, not only of time, but of energy and emotion, and people find that they are neglecting things they ought or want to do. Once started, she cannot be stopped: words, problems, judgments, fears, categorical statements, frightened appeals hurtle on.[7]

What causes mood disorders like depression is not known. Such disorders appear to cluster within family groups, thereby strongly suggesting the presence of a genetic component. But other factors also seem significant. Studies of mood disorders have often shown a relationship to stressful life events, particularly for depression. Stressful life events, however, are not the whole story, since practically everyone experiences them and most people do not develop mood disorders. Depressive symptoms are much more common among women than among men.

Bipolar Disorders

The *bipolar disorders* are a combination of manic and depressive episodes, with depression being the more prominent. It is equally common among men and women and usually occurs before age thirty. In the manic bipolar episode, the predominant mood is one of excessive elation, excessive anger, or both. The person is likely to have extremely grandiose ideas about his or her abilities, speech is likely to be rapid and loud, and irritability is apparent when the person is thwarted in some manner. Hyperactivity is also a usual feature of the manic episode. The bipolar depressive episode is more common, and here the predominant mood is depression or a pervasive loss of interest or enjoyment.

Other Mood Disorders

This group of disorders is not as severe as the major mood disorders. A person with one of these disorders is not, as a rule, incapacitated. There are two types of disorders in this category: (1) the *cyclothymic disorder,* characterized by both manic and depressive symptoms that are not serious enough to

---

[7]Joseph Mendels, *Concepts of Depression* (New York: Wiley, 1970), pp. 3–4.

constitute a major disorder; and (2) the *dysthymic disorder,* a less severe form of depression. These disorders are also more common among women than among men.

ANXIETY DISORDERS

As the classification indicates, these disorders represent conditions in which some form of anxiety is the main characteristic. Many of those disorders that in the past were classified as neuroses are included in this section. *Anxiety disorders* are relatively common, with 2 to 4 percent of the U.S. population estimated to have had an anxiety disorder at some point in their lives. The anxiety disorders include panic disorders, phobias, and obsessive-compulsive, posttraumatic stress, acute stress, generalized anxiety, and substance-induced anxiety disorders. Anxiety disorders are more common among women than among men.

Panic disorders consist of recurrent attacks of anxiety or panic. These attacks are characterized by the sudden onset of extreme misapprehension, fear, and terror usually associated with feelings of doom. The person may experience physical discomfort such as choking, chest pains, dizziness, vertigo, sweating, faintness, palpitations, and trembling. The attacks usually last minutes but can last longer (perhaps a few hours) for some people. This disorder, too, is more common among women and tends to run in families. Often, a person with a panic disorder will develop an anticipatory fear of helplessness and become reluctant to leave home, never knowing when a panic attack might occur.

Anxiety disorders also include *phobias.* A phobia is an irrational fear of a specific object, activity, or situation. This fear is usually recognized by the individual as unrealistic with respect to any actual danger posed by whatever is feared, yet the person goes to great lengths to avoid the feared object or situation, regardless. The avoidance behavior appears to be very compelling for the person subject to the phobia. The subtypes of phobias are (1) *agoraphobia* (fear of leaving home, closed or open spaces, and so on); (2) *social phobia* (fear of public speaking, eating in public, using public lavatories, and so on); and (3) *specific phobia* (fear and avoidance behavior other than agoraphobia or social phobia). The most common specific phobias are those of animals (especially snakes and other reptiles, insects, and rodents). Women are more likely than men to have a phobic disorder. An example of agoraphobia is found in this report of a young British woman (she eventually had a normal recovery):

> Mrs. J. H., a housewife of twenty-six with a son of four and a baby daughter of eighteen months, had begun to suspect that her husband might be interested in one of the girls at his work. He was coming home late, was occasionally absent for hours at a time over weekends ostensibly to pick up a little extra money by odd jobs, and displayed less tenderness to her during the past eighteen months than

she had grown to expect. She developed symptoms of general anxiety and tension, which rapidly focused themselves upon an inability to go more than a few hundred yards from her house without becoming faint and fearing that she might fall down unconscious in the street.

Eventually she reached the stage at which she could no longer take the children out, do the shopping, or care for the house. Neighbours did what they could to help, and her husband was undecided about what line to take with her. One morning she began to feel panic-stricken, and feared she might drop dead in the house. She got a neighbour to ring her husband's place of employment, and to call a doctor. He returned precipitately from work to find her in bed, with a very high pulse rate, gasping for breath, and convinced that she was soon to die.[8]

The principal characteristics of an *obsessive-compulsive disorder* are recurrent *obsessions* (repetitive ideas and thoughts) and *compulsions* (repetitive irrational acts) that are recognized by the individual as foreign to his or her personality. Common examples of obsessions are thoughts of doubts, violence, and contamination. Common forms of compulsions include repetitive hand washing, counting, checking, and touching. Efforts to resist a compulsion promote so much anxiety that it can be relieved immediately only by acting out the compulsion; eventually, the individual may just quit resisting the compulsions and give in to them. For instance, someone might take up to four hours to have a bath because the bathing must be accomplished in a set, precise, and unchanging routine.

The disorder typically begins in adolescence or early childhood and is more common to certain families than to others. It is not known if there are any differences by sex. Often, the discomfort experienced by obsessive-compulsive persons is not elicited so much by tangible situations as by the anxiety surrounding the possible consequences of the situation. As one psychiatrist reports, "A patient I treated for compulsive rituals centering around contamination from dogs was made more uncomfortable by being in a room where a dog *might* have been than by actually encountering a dog" (Marks 1979:101).

Posttraumatic stress disorders stem from direct exposure to, witnessing, or learning about an extremely traumatic event, such as wartime combat, violent personal assault, terrorist attack, being taken hostage, being a prisoner of war, a severe automobile accident, or a natural disaster like a flood, earthquake, or tornado. The event must involve the threat of death or serious injury to the individual or someone else's actual death or injury. The person's response must involve intense fear, helplessness, or horror. The characteristic symptoms are a persistent reexperiencing of the traumatic event, typically through recollection, dreams, and nightmares. Individuals with posttraumatic stress disorders may have painful guilt feelings about surviving when others did not.

---

[8]David Stafford-Clark and Andrew C. Smith, *Psychiatry for Students*, 5th ed. (London: Allen and Unwin, 1978), pp. 132–33.

Acute stress disorders are anxiety symptoms that develop within a month after exposure to an extremely traumatic event, such as those associated with posttraumatic stress disorders. Acute stress disorders differ from the posttraumatic version, however, in that the person has a general absence of emotional responsiveness. He or she finds it difficult or impossible to derive pleasure from previously enjoyable activities, experiences the world as unreal or dreamlike, and has difficulty recalling specific details of the traumatic event.

The *generalized anxiety disorder* consists of a chronic (at least six months) anxiety that does not resemble the other anxiety disorders. Instead, the person must experience anxiety in at least three of the following four areas: (1) motor tension (shakes, muscular aches), (2) autonomic hyperactivity (heart pounding, sweating, dizziness), (3) apprehensive expectation (fear, worry), and (4) vigilance and scanning (being on guard). The anxiety is not due to a specific stressor that would cause the anxiety to disappear if the stressor were removed.

Substance-induced anxiety disorders are anxiety symptoms caused by the direct physiological effects of drug abuse. These effects include prominent anxiety, panic attacks, or obsessions and compulsions and cannot be accounted for by an anxiety disorder that is not substance-induced.

SOMATOFORM DISORDERS

Somatoform disorders are symptoms of physical illness for which there are no demonstrable physical causes but that are apparently due to psychological factors. The main difference between somatoform disorders and factitious disorders is that the somatoform disorders are *not* under a person's voluntary control. The principal subtypes of somatoform disorders are (1) the *somatization disorder,* recurrent and multiple bodily complaints for which medical attention is sought; (2) *conversion disorder,* loss or alteration of physical functioning because of a psychological conflict or need; (3) *pain disorder,* complaint of pain in the absence of physical evidence; (4) *hypochondriasis,* anxiety about physical functioning; and (5) *body dysmorphic disorder,* preoccupation with a defect in appearance. These disorders are more common among women than among men.

FACTITIOUS DISORDERS

Factitious disorders are characterized by physical or psychological symptoms that are intentionally produced or faked so that the person will appear sick. Individuals with these disorders tend to present their history with a dramatic flair but are vague and inconsistent when questioned about details. When confronted with evidence that their symptoms are factitious, they typically deny the allegations or have themselves discharged to seek care elsewhere.

DISSOCIATIVE DISORDERS

Dissociative disorders are a sudden and temporary loss of motor behavior, consciousness, or identity. Females tend to have these disorders more than males do. There are five types of dissociative disorders. First, there is *dissociative amnesia,* which consists of memory loss in the absence of an organic mental disorder. The memory loss may be localized (the most common type), in which there is a failure to recall all events during a particular period of time. Less common is selective amnesia, in which there is a failure to recall some but not all events during a specific period. Least common are generalized amnesia, in which a person forgets his or her entire life, and continuous amnesia, in which a person is unable to remember events up to a particular time, including the present. The various forms of amnesia generally occur suddenly and usually follow exposure to some exceedingly severe stress.

Second is *dissociative fugue,* which consists of leaving home or work and assuming a new identity without being able to recall one's prior life. Third is *dissociative identity disorder* (formerly *multiple personality*). This condition is the domination of a person by one of two or more distinct personalities at any one time. Each personality has its own complex pattern of memories, behavior, and social relationships that determine the person's behavior when that personality is dominant. Transition from one personality to another is often stressful. Usually, the person cannot remember his or her other personalities, only the one that is dominant at the time. The dissociative identity disorder is very rare and is typically seen in adolescent and young adult females.

Fourth is the *depersonalization disorder.* This disorder consists of an alteration in one's sense of self, so that feelings about one's own self-reality are temporarily lost (that is, feeling dreamlike, mechanical, seeing one's self from a distance). Fifth is the *dissociative disorder not otherwise specified,* which does not meet the criteria for the specific dissociative disorders listed above. Examples of this condition are trancelike states without depersonalization.

SEXUAL AND GENDER IDENTITY DISORDERS

This category of disorders consists of disorders that cause sexual dysfunctions and problems in gender identity. As shown in Figure 2–1, these disorders are organized into (1) sexual dysfunctions, (2) paraphilias, and (3) gender identity disorders.

Sexual Dysfunctions

The principal problem inherent in *sexual dysfunctions* is an inhibition in the psychophysiological changes that occur in the complete sexual response cycle. This cycle consists of (1) fantasies about or a psychological interest in or desire for sexual activity, (2) sexual excitement, (3) orgasm, and (4) resolution or general relaxation after intercourse. Resolution is usually not of pathological significance. Sexual dysfunctions include (1) *sexual desire disorders,* consisting of hypoactive sexual desire (the deficiency or absence of sexual desire) or sexual aversion disorders; (2) *sexual arousal disorders,* involving an inadequate lubrication-swelling response for females or erection inability for males; (3) *orgasmic disorders,* consisting of persistent delay or absence of orgasm in males and females after normal sexual excitement and premature male ejaculation; (4) *sexual pain disorders,* characterized by genital pain associated with sexual intercourse and vaginismus for females; and (5) *sexual dysfunction due to a general medical condition,* which is a sexual dysfunction caused by a physiological problem. These disorders must cause the individual marked distress and interpersonal difficulty to qualify as sexual dysfunctions.

Paraphilias

The *paraphilias* are persistent, intense sexually arousing fantasies, urges, or behaviors that are associated with either (1) nonhuman objects, (2) suffering or humiliation, or (3) children or other nonconsenting partners. The specific paraphilias are (1) *exhibitionism* (sexual excitement obtained by exposing one's genitals to an unsuspecting stranger; seems to occur only in males exposing themselves to females); (2) *fetishism* (use of nonliving objects as the preferred or exclusive method of obtaining sexual arousal); (3) *frotteurism* (touching and rubbing against a nonconsenting person; behavior usually occurs in crowds); (4) *pedophilia* (sexual activity with children); (5) *sexual masochism* (sexual excitement caused by one's own suffering—being humiliated, beaten, bound, or otherwise made to suffer); (6) *sexual sadism* (sexual excitement caused by making someone else suffer); (7) *transvestic fetishism* (wherein a heterosexual male cross-dresses as a female and masturbates while imagining himself to be both the male and the female subject of his sexual fantasy); (8) *voyeurism* (looking or "peeping" at naked or disrobing individuals, usually strangers, for sexual excitement); and (9) *paraphilia not otherwise specified,* such as telephone scatologia (lewdness over the telephone) and zoophilia (sex with animals). Paraphilias are most likely to occur in men.

Gender Identity Disorders

Gender identity disorders consist of strong and persistent cross-gender identification and desire to be the other sex. There must be evidence of continued discomfort about one's assigned sex or a sense of inappropriateness about it. Additionally, there must be evidence of clinically significant distress in social, occupational, or other important areas of functioning. DSM-IV indicates that the prevalence of gender identity disorders is unknown; however, studies from smaller countries in Europe suggest that approximately 1 per 30,000 adult males and 1 per 100,000 adult females seek sex-change surgery.

EATING DISORDERS

Eating disorders consist of severe disturbances in eating behavior, primarily *anorexia nervosa* (refusal to maintain a minimally normal body weight) and *bulimia nervosa* (binge eating followed by food elimination behavior, such as self-induced vomiting). These disorders are prevalent in industrialized societies where there is an abundance of food and are common to women.

SLEEP DISORDERS

Sleep disorders are organized into two general categories: *dyssomnias* (abnormalities in the amount, quality, and timing of sleep) and *parasomnias* (abnormal behavioral or physiological events associated with sleep, such as breathing-related conditions, nightmares, sleep terror, and sleepwalking).

IMPULSE-CONTROL DISORDERS NOT ELSEWHERE CLASSIFIED

Impulse-control disorders not elsewhere classified refers to disorders that involve an inability to control impulses, such as *intermittent explosive disorder* (failure to resist aggressive impulses), *kleptomania* (impulse to steal objects not needed for personal use), *pyromania* (setting fires for pleasure, gratification, or relief of tension), *pathological gambling,* and *trichotillomania* (pulling out one's hair for pleasure, gratification, or relief from tension).

ADJUSTMENT DISORDERS

Adjustment disorders pertain to the impairment of social or occupational functioning that exceeds the normal or expected reaction to stress that is characteristic of most people. The severity of the adjustment disorder may not be directly predictable from the severity of the stressful life event. The person may overreact to a situation in which the stress would normally be considered insignificant or moderate. The different types of adjustment disorders are associated with anxious or depressed moods, mixed moods, disturbance of conduct (fighting, vandalism), and mixed emotions and disturbance of conduct.

PERSONALITY DISORDERS

Personality disorders represent a major category of abnormal behavior dysfunctions. These disorders are more common among men and are widespread. They seldom result in hospitalization in a mental institution. Their essential features are deeply ingrained, inflexible, maladaptive patterns of behavior that pertain to perceiving and thinking about the social environment and one's own self in relation to that environment in such a way that behavior is impaired and the person, in some cases, feels subjective distress. The personality disorders are manifested as particular types of personality traits and are expressed in not one but a variety of social and personal situations. They first appear during adolescence and continue throughout most of the adult life, although they tend to become less obvious in middle and old age.

DSM-IV groups the personality disorders into three "clusters" that share characteristics. The first cluster contains the paranoid, schizoid, and schizotypal personality disorders, whose presence causes a person to appear odd or eccentric. The second cluster includes histrionic, narcissistic, antisocial, and borderline personality disorders. Persons with these disorders seem overly dramatic, emotional, or erratic. And third are the avoidant, dependent, compulsive, and passive-aggressive personality disorders, in which individuals usually appear fearful or anxious. There is also a residual category for personality disorders not otherwise specified.

Paranoid, Schizoid, and Schizotypal Personality Disorders

The *paranoid personality disorder* is the pervasive and long-standing suspicion and distrust of other people. Persons with this disorder are highly sensitive and easily slighted; they often seem to look for evidence that confirms their paranoid ideas and prejudices. However, in contrast to persons who are not mentally disordered, they completely reject evidence that their views are incorrect, regardless of the weight of the evidence, and may even become suspicious of those who challenge or discount their paranoid ideas. They are often argumentative, excitable, and "make mountains out of mole hills." They find it very difficult to relax and enjoy other people. The *schizoid personality disorder* fits someone who is excessively introverted and lacks the capacity to form social relationships. These people appear equally indifferent to praise or criticism; they are withdrawn and seclusive and pursue solitary interests. They appear as "loners" with little desire for social involvement. The *schizotypal personality disorders* are oddities in thinking, perception, communication, and behavior. They are not severe enough to be schizophrenia; rather, they are deep-seated peculiarities that lack a basis in reality.

Antisocial, Borderline, Histrionic, and Narcissistic Personality Disorders

The *antisocial personality disorder* is found among individuals with a history of consistent antisocial behavior in which the rights of others are ignored. Early childhood signs are lying, fighting, truancy, and resisting authority. In adolescence, aggressive sexual behavior, excessive drinking, and the use of illicit drugs are typically added. In adulthood, there is fighting, criminal activity, sexual promiscuity, and vagrancy. Even though the person may appear to have normal mental health, there are signs of personal distress (for example, tension, depression). About 3 percent of all American males (less than 1 percent of females) are estimated to have an antisocial personality disorder. As for the *borderline personality*, it represents a situation in which a person is unstable in several areas, namely, interpersonal relationships, behavior, mood, and self-concept. Frequently, the person is impulsive and unpredictable, possibly even to the point of self-damage, such as risking physical injury, excessive drinking or drug use, overspending, bouts of sexual promiscuity, shoplifting, overeating, gambling, and the like.

Avoidant, Dependent, and Obsessive-Compulsive Personality Disorders

A person with an *avoidant personality disorder* is extremely sensitive to being rejected by others. Therefore, this person is very reluctant to enter into relationships unless there is some assurance beforehand of uncritical acceptance. Such individuals are devastated at the slightest form of disapproval; hence, they avoid others. The essential difference between an introverted personality disorder and the avoidant personality disorder (both involve social isolation) is that in the avoidant disorder there remains a strong yearning for approval and affection. This disorder, unlike the others previously discussed, is more common among women.

The *dependent personality disorder* is also more prevalent among women. It consists of exceptional dependence on others to the point of even abdicating responsibility for major areas of one's life. Such persons invariably lack self-confidence.

The basic feature of an *obsessive-compulsive disorder* is a preoccupation with orderliness, perfection, and control at the expense of flexibility, openness, and efficiency. People with this disorder may become so involved in making every detail of a project perfect that they never finish it. They display excessive devotion to work and productivity to the exclusion of leisure and friendships. DSM-IV (1994:669) states that "the emphasis is on perfect performance." There is also a strong tendency on the part of a person with this disorder to insist that everyone do things only as he or she does them and to become preoccupied with trivial details. Decision making may be avoided because of an unrealistic fear of making a mistake. This disorder is more common among males.

SUMMARY

This chapter completes an outline of the DSM-IV to acquaint the reader with the system of classification of mental disorders as currently employed in psychiatry. The most prevalent disorders in American society are those classified as substance-related disorders, schizophrenia, mood disorders, anxiety disorders, and personality disorders. The exact causes of these disorders are not known, but social factors seem highly significant in diagnosis.

3

Mental Disorder: Concepts of Causes and Cures

Sociological views pertaining to the collective aspects of mental disorder are part of a larger body of literature that features the work of psychiatrists and psychologists whose role is to ascertain for individual patients the possible causes and cures of abnormal behavior. Because mental disorder is a highly complex phenomenon, most likely involving a variety of causal factors, it is necessary to consider the approaches of relevant disciplines if a comprehensive understanding of insanity is to be achieved. Therefore, it is the purpose of this chapter to review briefly some of the theoretical models that have been formulated to explain the causes and treatment of mental disorders. It is the intent here to review not all models but only those that are the most influential at present. These models are (1) medical, (2) psychoanalytic, (3) social learning or behavior modification, (4) social stress, and (5) antipsychiatric.

It should be noted at the outset that there is no single model able to provide a definitive explanation of insanity, because there is simply too much that remains unknown about the causes of madness. Models are abstractions organized to place facts, events, and theories into an orderly framework for discussion and possible scientific verification; they provide a direction for research. And for the applied disciplines of psychiatry and clinical psychology, they are invariably a basis for therapy because they have been found to obtain results for certain patients—even though the exact mental processes affected by the treatment are not fully understood.

THE MEDICAL MODEL

The medical model views mental disorder as a disease or a diseaselike entity that can be treated through medical means. That is, the medical model attributes mental abnormalities to physiological, biochemical, or genetic causes and attempts to treat these abnormalities by way of medically grounded procedures such as psychopharmacology (drug therapy), electroshock therapy (EST), or psychosurgery (brain surgery). In this particular context, a person who is mentally ill is regarded as sick in much the same manner as if that person were physically ill. The medical model holds that abnormal behavior is symptomatic of an underlying psychic disturbance; therefore, its approach is to discover and treat the cause of that disturbance with a strategy similar to that of finding and curing a bacteriological infection.

As discussed in Chapter 1, the origins of this approach stem from the efforts of physicians during the Renaissance and post-Renaissance to combat the notion, prevalent during the Middle Ages, that mental disorder was caused by demons, spirits, and other supernatural forces. By the end of the seventeenth century, the medical profession had generally been successful in separating the social responsibility for treating mental disorder from theology and placing it within the field of medicine. Physicians thus looked to the study of human anatomy for evidence that madness was caused by pathological organic processes within the body, but with a few exceptions (for example, syphilis of the brain), such evidence was not forthcoming. Nevertheless, by the end of the nineteenth century, the idea had become widely accepted by both the medical profession and the general public that mental disorders were caused by mental diseases. In the twentieth century, however, it became clear that most mental disorders could not be attributed to physiological factors. As Robert Spitzer and Paul Wilson (1975:826–27) observe, most psychiatric conditions do not meet the four presumed criteria for a physiological dysfunction, which are (1) having a specific etiology (such as a germ), (2) being qualitatively different from some aspect of normal functioning, (3) showing a demonstrable physical change, and (4) being internal processes that when once initiated, proceed somewhat independently of environmental conditions outside the body.

Yet the medical model not only has persisted in psychiatry but also has become increasingly influential. It dominates the present-day search for solutions to mental disorder. Why? Basically there are three reasons. First, all psychiatrists are trained as medical doctors and are thereby socialized into a medical perspective. The medical profession, not surprisingly, regards medical training as the optimal preparation for working with mentally disturbed persons. Hence, the medical model is able to maintain a pervasive influence upon the practice of psychiatry because psychiatrists are trained to view health problems as medical problems.

Second, as Spitzer and Wilson point out, critics of the medical model often fail to realize that some physical disorders, such as essential hypertension, endocrine disorders, and vitamin deficiencies, likewise do not meet all the criteria for physiological dysfunctions. But these disorders are still treatable through medical means and unquestionably fall within the purview of a medical problem. Consequently, Spitzer and Wilson argue that the appropriateness of the medical model cannot always be derived from the requirements of logic but should be based upon how well the model works in actual practice. Even if it works poorly, they insist that it should not be abandoned until another model is developed that can be shown to work more effectively in treating patients. Their solution is to extend the definition of mental disorder to include those conditions of human suffering and disability that respond to medical treatments.

In this view, psychiatric problems are not necessarily "diseases"; instead, they are "disorders" treatable in a medical mode. This broader definition thus allows the medical practitioner to assume responsibility for a somewhat greater range of problems, providing that suffering or disability is present and a medical treatment is available. The danger inherent in such an approach, however, is that the definition of suitable disorders becomes too broad and extends beyond medicine's demonstrable capacity to "cure," a situation that Thomas Szasz (1974) warns is likely to occur if the medicalization of social problems continues in its current direction. Such a trend is indicative of the medical model's strength.

Third, there is growing enthusiasm among many psychiatrists about the effectiveness of psychoactive drugs in treating certain mental disorders and significantly reducing the inmate population of American mental hospitals. There was a period in the 1960s and early 1970s when some psychiatrists began to move away from the medical model toward a closer relationship with psychologists and sociologists. The idea was for psychiatry to develop a more humanistic approach by focusing its resources more on the treatment of major social problems like drug addiction, delinquency, and crime. This situation is now reversed, as a number of psychiatrists appear to want to "get back to medicine" as full-fledged partners with other medical specialists in the search for drugs as "magic bullets" to eliminate or control health dysfunctions. Bolstered by recent biochemical discoveries, a current view in psychiatry is that the discipline is entering a new era, possibly making psychiatry one of the most scientifically precise of all medical specialties and ending its traditional dependence upon subjective judgments of and insights into the human mind. Whether this new psychiatric era has arrived to the extent that some anticipate remains speculation at this time, but the research has been impressive enough to provoke among psychiatrists tremendous interest in psychopharmacology. It is no exaggeration, for instance, to state that the community mental health movement would not be able to function without the drug treatments that allow patients to sustain themselves in the community. Besides psychopharmacology, the remainder of this section on the medical model will briefly discuss behavioral genetics, electroshock therapy, and psychosurgery to provide an overview of those theories based upon procedures that are strictly medical.

Psychopharmacology

The concept of a biochemical cause of insanity goes back to the time of the ancient Greeks and is historically derived from a belief that "poisons" generated within the body are somehow able to affect the mind. At the beginning of the twentieth century, this idea was strengthened by findings demonstrating how syphilis was able to produce infection in the brain and cause manifestly bizarre behavior. Subsequent strategies to locate abnormal biochemical substances in the blood and urine of schizophrenic patients were generally unsuccessful, but there was a major breakthrough in 1952. Two French psychiatrists, Jean Delay and Pierre Deniker, injected chlorpromazine into their patients and soon found that it would activate withdrawn schizophrenics and bring their characteristically flat manner into a relatively normal state. Later, in large controlled studies conducted in the United States, it was confirmed that chlorpromazine produced significant improvements in thought disorder, withdrawal, blunted affect, and autistic behavior.

The focus of biochemical research dealing with behavioral abnormalities has been on the neuronal activity in the central nervous system. This activity consists of signals carried via chemical agents (neurotransmitters) between one neuron and another. How such activity affects behavior is not certain, but the assumption is that the action of the neurotransmitters is very important in mental disorder. It may be that too much or too little of these chemical substances at particular receptor sites produces or fails to produce certain chemical responses that shape behavior. Neurotransmitters may work like keys in a lock; some fit correctly into receptor sites specifically designed to accept them, and others prevent insertion of the correct key. Or receptor sites may have a selective affinity for some compounds of a given type and a similar affinity for antagonistic compounds, which leads to the displacement of one or another substance (Snyder 1980). Or perhaps some other process is involved. At any rate, chlorpromazine and other drugs of the phenothiazine group are apparently able to block the action of dopamine, a neurotransmitter, whose hyperactivity is thought to be significant in the production of paranoid delusions and auditory hallucinations. An excessive amount of dopamine in brain receptor sites may also be involved in mania, and a deficiency in norepinephrine, another neurotransmitter, might produce depression (Maas 1979).

Even though the biochemical mechanisms that cause the effects brought on by psychoactive drugs are not fully understood, the effects of these drugs are of sufficient clarity that they can be prescribed for certain disorders. In other words, physicians may not know how they work, but they do know that in some cases they are effective. Thus, specific psychoactive drugs can be used for specific disorders. For example, benzodiazepine compounds like chlordiazepoxide (Librium) and diazepam (Valium), propanediols like meprobame (Miltown, Equanil), or perhaps barbiturates (phenobarbital) or antihistamines (hydroxyzine) all belong to the so-called minor tranquilizer class of psychoactive drugs and are used in the treatment of anxiety. The major tranquilizers used in the treatment of schizophrenia are the phenothiazines like chlorpromazine (Thorazine) or the butyrophenones like haloperidol (Haldol). For the treatment of mood disorders, calling for either antidepressants or antimania drugs, tricyclic antidepressants such as imipramine (Tofranil, Presamine) and amitriptyline (Elavil) are widely used. Other mood-elevating drugs are the MAO (monoamine oxidase) inhibitors like tranylcypromine (Parnate). Among the new antidepressant drugs is fluoxetine (Prozac), which has more specific biochemical effects than most older medications for depression. Prozac brightens mood and lessens anxiety and has become a highly popular drug in the 1990s—although the long-term side effects are not known.

Several studies attest to the effectiveness of psychoactive drugs in controlling mental disorders (Davis 1985; Lickey and Gordon 1991; Simpson and May 1985; Snyder 1980). There is, however, important criticism both within and outside psychiatry about reliance on drugs for therapy (Fisher and Greenberg 1989). Valium, for example, although widely prescribed for anxiety, may do little more than help people sleep and can be habit forming; Thorazine, on the other hand, can control the hallucinations and agitation in schizophrenia, but not apathy. Clozaril (clozapine) helps reduce apathy and improve motivation in schizophrenics and does not produce long-term effects found in Thorazine, like muscle stiffening and spasms. Yet Clozaril is expensive—it requires continual blood testing and monitoring of patients, since it causes a blood abnormality that can be fatal in about 1 percent of all patients who take it. The alternative to the extensive reliance on drugs, as argued by psychologists, clinical social workers, and other psychotherapists who cannot prescribe them, is greater use of cognitive and behavioral psychotherapies. Nevertheless, beginning in the late 1970s, psychiatrists have shifted toward the increased use of drugs to treat schizophrenia, as well as anxiety and mood disorders—with generally effective results.

In regard to the effectiveness of drug therapy, it should be kept in mind that drugs do not cure mental disorder—they control it. They help mental patients act in a reasonably normal manner when they would act bizarrely otherwise. Unfortunately, the emphasis on control may retard the emphasis on cure. As Albert Bandura (1969:16) explains, the overpromotion of drug therapy has "led to heavy reliance upon physical and chemical intervention, unremitting search for drugs as quick remedies for interpersonal problems, and long-term neglect of social variables as influential determinants of deviant response patterns." Therefore, although psychoactive drugs may provide an effective short-term solution to many mental problems, they do not get to the source of those problems, nor do they change the social situations that precipitate insanity.

Behavioral Genetics

Another component of the medical model is genetics. Research in the area of behavioral genetics has produced strong evidence that genetic factors are important in the transmission of certain mental disorders, notably schizophrenia and mood disorders (depression, mania), from parent to child. This would explain why certain people are prone, for example, to schizophrenia and why schizophrenia tends to be prevalent in certain families and not in others (Gupta 1993; Heston 1977; Rainer 1985). In the late nineteenth century, almost as soon as schizophrenia was defined as a specific type of mental disorder, it was noticed that it "ran in families." Under the scientific standards of the time, this was taken as "proof" that schizophrenia was inherited or at least involved genetics. Indeed, a number of family studies conducted since the early decades of the twentieth century supported this assumption by showing that the closer an individual's genetic relationship was to a known schizophrenic, the greater his or her chance was of developing the disorder. Among identical (monozygotic) twins, if one twin is schizophrenic, the other twin has about a 50 percent chance of likewise becoming (or being) schizophrenic. Fraternal (dizygotic) twins, ordinary siblings, and parents show a lower degree of genetic affinity (concordance) for schizophrenia, nieces and nephews still lower, and so on. The lowest degree of concordance is, of course, for people who are unrelated. The child of two severely affected schizophrenics would have a 50 percent or greater chance of developing the disorder, but the risk would drop to 25 percent for the child of two mildly schizophrenic parents. If only one parent is schizophrenic and the other is normal, the chances of avoiding schizophrenia altogether are the same as for the normal population (Heston 1977).

As for mood disorders, the concordance for monozygotic twins is even higher—around 70 percent; so if one twin has an affective disorder, there are seven chances in ten that the other twin will suffer similarly (Gershon 1979). This is the highest concordance rate for any mental disorder. For first-degree relatives like dizygotic twins, siblings, and so forth, the concordance rate drops significantly to about 15 percent and continues to decline accordingly.

The exact genetic factors involved in mental disorder are not known at present; some hypotheses favor the notion that abnormal behavior is related to a single dominant gene, and another view is that several predisposing genes are implicated. What apparently is not in dispute is that the mechanism of transmission is biochemical. What passes from parents to offspring are probably compounds (nucleic-acid sequences) that control the biosynthesis of other compounds (proteins); consequently, inherited abnormalities of either physiology or behavior imply an abnormality in the body's protein complement (Snyder 1977:133). Additionally, the relationship between heredity and the role of environment is not clear. It seems that there is a strong environmental component with regard to mental disorders like schizophrenia; thus, genetic transmission is not the entire answer. The best overall explanation is that some people are genetically "primed" for certain mental disorders as a result of heredity; whether the disorder actually develops, however, is most likely contingent upon environmental factors that "trigger" the predisposition toward mental illness. But it is also not known what environmental factors activate a mental disorder in a genetically susceptible person. A highly plausible theory of schizophrenia is that given a genetic predisposition, stressful life events or circumstances elicit the disorder (Weiner 1985). In sum, it is generally believed that for some people genetics play a significant role in the onset of mental disorder—although we do not know what it is, how it works, or what proportion of mentally ill people become that way because of the interaction between heredity and the environment.

Electroshock Therapy

Electroshock therapy (EST), sometimes referred to as electroconvulsive therapy (ECT), is a controversial method of therapeutic treatment. In fact, there is probably no procedure in medicine that is more surrounded by myths than EST is (Fink 1978; Lickey and Gordon 1991). Developed in Italy in 1938, EST gained a reputation in the mass media and among some psychiatrists as well for being a particularly harsh form of punishment for unruly mental patients and perhaps even damaging to the brain. The procedure, greatly improved since the 1940s, consists of placing electrodes around the brain and administering an electric current (ranging from 70 to 170 volts) for 0.75 to 1.25 seconds. The immediate effect on the brain is to produce a condition similar to a seizure. The most likely locus of action is the hypothalamus, the origin of the autonomic nervous system, which is thought to be involved in the expression of emotion. What actually happens in the central nervous system is not known, but it appears that electroshock causes the release of norepinephrine in the brain, which acts as an antidepressant. The most immediate feature of the experience for the patient, however, is a loss of memory, which eventually returns. Yet the therapeutic value of EST reportedly lies not in memory loss, causing the patient temporarily to "forget his or her problems," but in the organic changes in brain chemistry induced by the treatment (Fink 1978).

Despite our lack of knowledge about the exact brain processes affected by EST, advocates of the method point to the striking success it has with patients suffering from endogenous depression (Fink 1978; Kalinowsky 1975; Lickey and Gordon 1991; Weiner 1989). The effect of EST on endogenous depression, a type of depression that is associated with physiological dysfunctions (for example, loss of weight, insomnia, decreased bodily secretions) and that develops *without* relation to a specific life event (for example, death of a loved one), "is one of the most spectacular therapeutic responses in medicine" (Kalinowsky 1975:1973). The response is very rapid and is suggested for patients who are potentially suicidal, thus needing prompt treatment. EST is likewise regarded as the most effective method of treating catatonic schizophrenia because of the difficulty in breaching the patient's catatonic state through the use of psychotherapy or drugs. EST is also thought to be generally effective for psychotic depression and manic-depressive disorders. It is not considered particularly effective for depressions brought on by anxiety or for drug-induced psychoses or personality disorders.

Unfortunately, there are no controlled studies that demonstrate how EST affects the mind, and it is this lack of information that contributes most to the myths about electroshock. All we know is that the procedure produces a significant improvement in certain patients, especially those with endogenous depression, and does somehow alter the functioning of the brain. Thus, we are left with only speculation. We do not even know conclusively if EST causes brain damage. Nevertheless, EST remains a common form of treatment available in mental hospitals and is strongly supported by many psychiatrists who believe that it has a proper place in the treatment of mental disorder.

Psychosurgery

A treatment even more controversial than EST is psychosurgery, which is seldom employed and is generally considered a last resort for seemingly desperate cases. Psychosurgery first achieved prominence in 1936 in Portugal and was used in the United States to treat some fifty thousand mental patients during the 1940s and early 1950s. The decline in its use is generally recognized as resulting from the widespread use of psychoactive drugs beginning in the mid-1950s, the continuing social stigma attached to recipients of the operation, and adverse public opinion about the procedure. Psychosurgery usually is surgical mutilation of the frontal lobe (prefrontal lobotomy) of the brain where the higher intellectual functioning (memory, abstract reasoning, and speech) of the human being takes place. The results of the surgery are permanent, and critics have argued that although such surgery has had a "calming" effect on patients and has enabled some of them to be discharged from mental hospitals, they are frequently left as "semivegetables" (Goldenberg 1977). Modern surgical approaches, however, have been found to not result in any cognitive loss, and the procedure remains an alternative therapy for totally incapacitated patients who fail to respond to any of the other currently available forms of treatment (Donnelly 1985).

Generally, psychosurgery is advocated for only those patients who are chronically violent toward themselves or others, but there is strong controversy over whether physicians have the legal right to perform the operation on a person who may not be able to understand the consequences. There is also serious concern that psychosurgery may be used for the social control of relatively helpless persons. Some states, such as California and Oregon, have strict regulations pertaining to psychosurgery. Although some psychiatrists maintain that psychosurgery can be beneficial to certain patients, most avoid the practice.

Assessment of the Medical Model

The purely medical approach to mental disorders has unquestionably resulted in positive gains for many patients, especially those patients subject to drug therapy who are now able to lead relatively normal lives outside a mental hospital. Moreover, research in the areas of brain chemistry and behavioral genetics has produced promising leads that may in time help explain the etiology of mental disorder. But the medical model fails on two very important counts. First, the model focuses almost exclusively on the control of disorders rather than on definitive cures. Thus, it operates primarily to return abnormal behavior to as normal a state as possible and to stabilize it at that point. It does not eliminate the cause; it attempts to relieve the symptoms. And in doing so, the medical model generally ignores factors in the external social environment that may have been responsible for the onset of the insanity in the first place.

Second, the medical model has not been able to explain the cause of mental disorder, even though it has formulated treatments for it. It is true, as the French physician René DuBos (1959) notes, that in a few cases the search for *the* cause has led to effective measures of control—but it does not necessarily follow that these measures produce information about the problem they correct. As illustration, DuBos (1959:102–3) states: "While drenching fire with water may help in putting out a blaze, few are the cases in which fire has its origin in a lack of water." A similar example is brought up by Solomon Snyder (1977), an American psychiatrist, in regard to the role of the neurotransmitter dopamine in schizophrenia. Although noting that schizophrenic symptoms can be ameliorated by administering biochemicals antagonistic to dopamine (like haloperidol), which act to "break" the dopaminergic pathways of the brain, Snyder observes that this by no means demonstrates that schizophrenia is caused by some defect in the release or reception of dopamine in the brain. "This somewhat paradoxical conclusion," comments Snyder (1977:139), "may perhaps be clarified by an electrical analogy: the fact that a dangerous short circuit can be abolished by tripping the appropriate circuit breaker does not mean that the short is in the breaker—it may be anywhere in the circuit." Schizophrenic abnormalities may involve brain systems well beyond dopamine synapses, but these systems can be affected by changes in dopamine transmission. Or it may be that dopamine is the causal factor in schizophrenia; no one knows for sure. Consequently, the medical model's reliance upon control of or relief from symptoms of mental disorder still leaves unanswered the question of *what* actually causes insanity.

In essence, the medical model needs to develop a more comprehensive approach to allow it to deal with the wider spectrum of mental disorders represented by factors external to the individual and to do so in such a way that promotes cure as well as relief.

THE PSYCHOANALYTIC MODEL

The psychoanalytic model of mental disorder is analogous to the medical model in that it also focuses attention on internal factors that affect the mental health of the human being. But there is a notable difference between the two models in that the psychoanalytic approach views abnormal behavior in psychological terms. In its concern with psychic rather than physiological and biochemical conditions, the psychoanalytic model views human beings as driven by powerful instinctual forces. Not only is the individual unable to control these forces, but he or she is even unaware of their existence.

The psychoanalytic model is based upon the work of Sigmund Freud (1856–1939), who spent most of his life in Vienna, and upon the work of others whom he influenced, such as Erik Erikson, Carl Jung, Alfred Adler, Adolf Meyer, Karen Horney, Otto Rank, and Wilhelm Reich—to name only a few of the important figures in psychoanalytic literature. The scope of this chapter does not permit an extensive discussion of the wide range of Freud's many theories, which psychoanalysts regard as *the* most comprehensive and profound explanation of human behavior and which many behavioral scientists view as interesting but theoretically incorrect (Grünbaum 1993). Despite conflicting assessments of Freud's work, the reader should be aware that the psychoanalytic approach has influenced the training in and practice of psychiatry to the extent that it constitutes a fundamental aspect of psychiatric terminology, ideology, and understanding of the human personality.

Freud's Concept of the Personality

Briefly stated, Freud viewed the human organism as a complicated energy system with all the energy needed to perform the work of the personality being obtained from instincts, which Freud defined as mental stimuli arising from within the organism itself. However, instincts are seen as a special type of stimulus because they do not have a single or momentary impact but are a constant force within the personality. The *id,* one of the three major components in Freud's structure of the personality, functions as the discharger of any energy or tension brought about by internal or external stimulation. It is guided by the primary process, which produces a memory image of the object needed to reduce tension. The id uses its energy for instinctual gratification in fulfilling the pleasure principle (avoiding pain and finding pleasure) through the means of reflex action—eating, having sex, realizing wishes.

The failure of the id to obtain satisfaction gives rise to the *ego,* the second major part of the personality, which represents the energizing of new processes of memory, judgment, perception, and reason that are intended to bring harmony to a person's psychological system by synchronizing the subjective inner world with the objective outer world of social reality. Freud initially viewed the ego as somewhat weaker than the id, describing it as "a man on horseback," who has to hold in check the superior strength of the horse (meaning the power of the id). But he subsequently saw the ego as having great power of its own. The ego is governed by the reality principle, whose function is to postpone the release of energy until the actual object has been located that will satisfy the need; the ego tolerates or opposes tension until it can be discharged by an appropriate form of behavior. Thus, to the primary process of memory is added the secondary process of finding the correct solution (reality) through thought and reason. Sometimes the solution is not found until various realities have been tested and discovered to provide suitable fulfillment. Hence, the ego is primarily a product of interaction with the external environment.

The third major aspect of the personality, the *superego,* can be described as the moral or judicial branch of the personality. Freud hypothesized that the superego evolves from the ego as the child assimilates the moral authority of his or her parents' own overt behavior or motives and the parents' aspirations for the child. The internalization of parental values in the child is accomplished through fear of punishment and desire for parental approval, which cause the child to control his or her own behavior in accordance with the wishes of the parents. The superego represents what is ideal rather than what is real, and its aim is to strive for perfection instead of reality (the function of the ego) or pleasure (the function of the id). Through its two subsystems, the ego-ideal and the conscience, the superego has the power both to reward and to punish the organism psychologically through feelings of pride (ego-ideal) or of guilt and inferiority (conscience).

Seen in its basic form, Freud's concept of the personality is a system of psychic energy consisting of the id striving for pleasure in order to satisfy fundamental instincts and the superego striving for perfection while leaving the ego to balance the two drives with a sense of reality. Obviously, the personality would be maladjusted should the ego fail and either the id or the superego become dominant. Thus, for Freud, the ego was the focal point of concern.

Stages of Psychosexual Development

A basic premise of psychoanalytic theory, depicted by Freud in his book *Moses and Monotheism* (1964:187), is that "the child is psychologically father to the adult." What Freud meant by this is that the events of infancy and childhood persist in the personality of a person throughout all subsequent life. The impairment of the behavior of adults is therefore systematically related to early childhood experiences, particularly the fate of sexually oriented urges for bodily pleasure allowed under the method of training selected by the parents. There are five stages in the Freudian concept of psychosexual development: (1) oral, (2) anal, (3) phallic, (4) latency, and (5) genital.

The *oral stage* consists of the oral-erotic and oral-sadistic periods. The oral-erotic period lasts from birth until about the age of eight months and is characterized as a time when the mouth, lips, tongue, skin, and sensory organs are the focus of libidinal (sexual) energy. The primary mode of obtaining pleasure is passive incorporation (receiving) and is expressed by sucking and swallowing. The greatest normal frustration during this period is the lack of continuous and exclusive availability of the mother to satisfy the infant's demands for oral gratification. The oral-erotic period is followed by the oral-sadistic period, occurring between six and eighteen months of age, in which the center of sexual energy is found in the jaws, teeth, skin, and related sensory organs. The mode of obtaining pleasure is active incorporation (seizing) and is expressed by biting and chewing. The main normal frustration at this time for the child is the appearance of a new baby in the family who competes for the mother's attention.

As a whole, the oral stage is a time when the infant is confronted with a developmental crisis of trust versus mistrust. During this period, the infant establishes the dispositions toward being more or less trusting or mistrusting of the external world and of his or her own capacity to cope with urges (self-trust) and to elicit the appropriate response from others (trust in others). Ego development is reflected in the gradual emergence of the infant's ability to distinguish between internal and external reality. The infant becomes aware that he or she must develop the capacity to signal needs to the outside world, and by being frustrated the infant learns to try to find the correct solution to meeting his or her own needs. Psychoanalytic theorists claim that excessive or insufficient oral gratification can result in libidinal fixations that cause pathological traits in adulthood, such as excessive narcissism, optimism, pessimism, demandingness, or dependency.

The *anal stage* consists of the anal-sadistic and anal-erotic periods. During the anal-sadistic period, which occurs between eight and twenty-four months of age, the anus and buttocks are the center of libidinal energy. Here the primary mode of obtaining pleasure is eliminative (the discharge of feces) in which elimination is thought to allow for the expression of aggressive wishes. The anal-erotic period comes next and takes place between the ages of one and three years. The anus and buttocks remain eroticized, but the primary mode of pleasure is retention, in which the emphasis is upon retaining bodily wastes and offering them as a gift to the parents (and such "gifts" are usually welcomed with approval by the parents if it signifies that the child is becoming toilet trained). The normal frustration during both the anal-sadistic and the anal-erotic periods pertains to the conflict with the parents over toilet training and the demand for self-control.

The anal stage presents the child with the developmental crisis of autonomy versus shame and doubt in which the child learns to develop self-control without a loss in self-pride (ego-ideal). Obsessive-compulsive anxieties are most usually described as typical of the anal stage. This applies to people who show excessive orderliness, stubbornness, frugality, possessiveness, and a "tendency to collect things." For persons whose defense mechanisms are less effective, the traits of excessive ambivalence, hostility, messiness, lewdness, and sado-masochistic tendencies are also thought to be representative of developmental difficulties during the anal stage.

The *phallic stage* of psychosexual development usually begins during the third year of life and continues to about the age of six. The sex organs now become the source of libidinal energy, and the object of that energy becomes the opposite-sexed parent in what Freud called the Oedipus complex. The Oedipus complex is the unconscious tendency of the child to be attracted to the opposite-sexed parent and to develop feelings of hostility toward the same-sexed parent. In this unconscious conflict, the penis is the sex organ of interest to children of both sexes. In normal circumstances, the boy renounces his desire for his mother because of the threat of castration by the father, who is his rival for the mother's affection. Freud believed that the narcissistic fear of injury to the penis on the part of boys was stronger than the erotic attachment to the mother. In relinquishing his erotic attachment to his mother, the boy begins to identify with his father and a masculine self-image.

For girls it is different, according to Freud, in that they, having already been castrated symbolically by virtue of not having a penis, turn their affections from their mother (who is held responsible for bringing the child into the world without adequate sexual equipment—the penis) toward their father, who has a penis. The unconscious hatred of the daughter for the mother is supposed to become even more pronounced when the daughter realizes that the mother, too, lacks the all-important penis. The Oedipus complex in the girl is supposed to be resolved when the daughter is gradually disappointed and frustrated by the father's failure to give her a penis or a child in place of the penis. Also, by loving the father, the daughter may develop an identification with the mother whom the father loves and for whom he does provide children. Typically, the girl will eventually renounce her erotic interest in her father and turn to a nonincestuous, opposite-sexed love object.

The successful resolution of the Oedipal crisis leads to the formation of the superego as the child internalizes the values governing his or her own sex's adult roles and sex roles. Failure to accomplish this task, according to Freud, leads to a wide variety of anxiety problems in adulthood.

The *latency stage* is a stage of relative inactivity for the sexual drives and lasts from the ages of five or six until about twelve or thirteen. During this stage, notions of sex roles and sex-role identity are further consolidated as the ego continues to mature and exercise greater control over instinctual desires. The interest of the child becomes directed more toward peers and peer-related activities that occur outside the family. The latency period has been generally regarded as a period that does not give rise to any special forms of emotional problems that, if present, were derived from earlier stages of development. But it has been realized that latency is a very important stage in that the child learns to obtain a sense of accomplishment and mastery over objects, thus developing a sense of social competency.

Finally, there is the *genital stage,* or adolescent phase, of psychosexual development, which extends from the ages of approximately eleven to thirteen until the adolescent reaches young adulthood at around eighteen to twenty. The physiological maturation of the adolescent's sex organs and his or her corresponding hormonal systems produces an intensification of drives, especially sexual, and reopens conflicts from previous stages of psychosexual development. Thus, the genital stage provides the adolescent with the opportunity to resolve past conflicts as part of achieving a mature adult identity and sexuality. The primary objectives of this stage are independence from parents and the establishment of a mature, nonincestuous, heterosexual relationship. Failure to achieve this objective thereby introduces a potential multitude of problems because the developmental task of adolescence during the genital stage is a reworking and resolution of past problems.

Mechanisms of Ego Defense

Freud's concept of ego defense is based upon the premise that throughout each stage of psychosexual development, the ego builds up appropriate defense mechanisms to defend against the conflicts, anxieties, and frustrations that disturb the individual's normal psychological functioning. The ego is responsible for this defense because, as the personality's center of narcissism or self-love, it attempts to escape from any situation that threatens its sense of well-being and integrity. Threats to the ego that summon the ego's defenses come from three sources: (1) the id as it tries to overwhelm the ego with pressure for instinctual gratification, (2) the superego as it attempts to punish the ego through feelings of guilt, and (3) the external danger that is perceived as being directed toward the ego. All ego defense mechanisms operate at an unconscious level and are activated on a more or less automatic basis; therefore, the individual is not even aware of their existence.

Some of the most common ego defense mechanisms described by psychoanalysts are

> *Sublimation:* A mature defense well within the limits of normality. Involves a situation in which an instinct is turned into a new and more socially acceptable channel of expression, such as aggression being channeled into sports or the strong desire for sex being converted into energy for professional achievement.
>
> *Repression:* A forgetting of events or internal impulses that would be painful if they became conscious. In *primary repression,* the ego exerts energy against an experienced event to prevent it from being remembered, as in the case of cir-

cumscribed amnesia in which incidents occurring during a certain period of time are forgotten because they are painful or traumatic. In *secondary repression,* the ego blocks objectionable ideas or feelings from reaching consciousness.

Projection: The denial of objectionable ideas within the individual and the projection of them outward toward other persons or objects in the external environment. A husband who consciously believes himself to be an adequate spouse, but who unconsciously believes himself to be inadequate, and instead accuses his wife of being inadequate would be engaging in projection.

Introjection: The opposite of projection in that a person incorporates into himself or herself the characteristics of another person or object. For example, a person internalizes the aggressive characteristics of a feared person so that anxiety about the aggression will be reduced and the formerly fearful person also will feel aggressive and strong.

Reaction Formation: A rigid attitude or character trait that allows the management of objectionable impulses by permitting expression of the impulse in an opposite form. An illustration of reaction formation would be a person who acts anxious to please other people but whose attitude is artificial and hides an underlying hostility.

Denial: A denial of external reality. An example is a person who refuses to recognize that he or she has harmed someone else and instead sees only good in the action that took place, despite the obvious nature of the harm.

Isolation: A situation in which memory and the effect of the memory are separated. For example, a person remembers a traumatic experience but does so without emotion.

Regression: A person who returns to an earlier stage of psychosexual development to seek the security of that stage and avoid the anxieties of later stages exhibits regression. For instance, an older child demands to be fed by a bottle when a new child comes into the family, thereby hoping to regain the attention that once belonged to the older child alone.

Rationalization: Substitution by the ego of an acceptable reason for an unacceptable one in attempting to justify a particular idea or action. It is an attempt to fool the superego and is a very common defense. For example, a student goes to a motion picture instead of studying for an examination and rationalizes that this behavior was best because it provided relaxation that will produce a better performance on the test.

Displacement: An effect of one object is transferred to another object in the interest of solving a conflict. A man is verbally abused by his employer and upon his return home verbally attacks his wife. Thus, the anger toward one object is displaced to another, safer object.

Psychoanalysis, Psychoanalytic Therapy, and Group Therapy

Freud's ideas, through his introduction of psychoanalysis, had a profound effect upon the practice of psychiatry. Psychoanalytic theory holds that emotional problems are likely to be revealed in one of four ways. The person (1) develops a personality disorder (displaces conflicts toward the external world), (2) becomes neurotic (develops excessive ego defenses), (3) develops a psychophysiologic disorder (tension is experienced within the body and eventually produces an organic pathology), or (4) becomes psychotic (the ego disintegrates with a loss of the ability to cope with reality). The forms of treatment used for the individual to eliminate or reduce the effects of these unconscious pressures on the personality are psychoanalysis and psychoanalytic therapy.

Psychoanalysis   Psychoanalysis is a one-to-one relationship between the therapist and the patient that utilizes free association as its primary technique. In free association, the patient is encouraged to say whatever comes to mind, while the analyst ensures that the sequence of the undirected thought remains unchanged and that the patient does not withhold any information, no matter how trivial or distressing. Psychoanalysis is a lengthy process and can take years to complete, but its proponents believe that sooner or later the patient will direct the underlying disorder toward the therapist in a process known as transference. Once that happens and the unconscious tendencies are revealed, the patient can be made aware of the source of the problem and counseled on ways to deal effectively with it.

Psychoanalysis is used most often with patients who are suffering from chronic anxiety and who have some ego strength. Besides being time-consuming, psychoanalysis is expensive and does not lend itself to the simultaneous treatment of large numbers of patients. Total therapy time can be as long as a thousand hours spent in hour-long sessions, four to five times a week or less for five to seven years or more. The total cost can range from $5,000 for a period of a few months to more than $100,000 for several years. Just how effective psychoanalysis is in treating patients is a subject of controversy. Patients with anxiety rooted in childhood experiences may benefit significantly from the treatment. But some critics contend that psychoanalysis is no more successful than other psychotherapeutic methods (Eysenck 1961). Psychoanalysis is not useful with patients who are schizophrenic, who have subnormal intelligence, or who reject intimate, personal, therapeutic relationships.

Psychoanalytic therapy   Psychoanalytic therapy is a modified form of psychoanalysis. The major difference is that psychoanalytic therapies focus on current conflicts instead of attempting to work through the entire history of a person's psychosexual development; however, before treatment, an extensive psychiatric diagnosis is obtained that is based upon as much information as possible about the patient's history. This therapy also requires a moderately superficial transference reaction and relies more upon interviewing and discussion than upon free association.

Group therapy   Another type of treatment influenced by the psychoanalytic model is group therapy, which has the advantage of treating several patients at one time. Group therapy is popular in the United States and consists of having selected participants meet with a trained therapist so that the participants may help one another confront problems and achieve personality change. Group therapy emphasizes the values of individualism within the context of a collective approach to problems, while at the same time allowing for the expression of deviant behavior. In traditional psychoanalytic group therapy, identification with the group is stressed, and the process of transference is subsequently utilized in a group context to elicit awareness of unconscious personality conflicts.

Assessment of the Psychoanalytic Model

One of the most striking criticisms of the psychoanalytic model is that it is based largely upon myth. Supporters of the psychoanalytic model are required to accept as dogma the unproven assumptions of Freudian thought in much the same way that persons living in the Middle Ages accepted on faith the idea that mental disorder was caused by the Devil. There is no actual evidence that the human personality has a tripartite structure consisting of an id, an ego, and a superego. A second major criticism of the psychoanalytic model is that it portrays human beings as being propelled by instincts, without taking into account the person's own free will. Some behavioral scientists argue, for instance, that the mind is not a structure but a process. This concept arises from the unique human ability to engage in reflexive thinking, an ability that makes possible the control and organization of conduct by the individual in relation to the environment. Third, most research does not support the view that "the child is psychologically father to the adult." There is no conclusive evidence linking personality problems of adults with specific experiences of pleasure or frustration during a particular developmental stage of childhood. Fourth, the psychoanalytic approach has been accused of underemphasizing the importance of cognitive development and overemphasizing emotional development. Alfred Lindesmith, Anselm Strauss, and Norman Denzin (1975:319) point out that the separation of emotional experience from cognition neglects "the fact that emotional experiences do not exist as pure states, but are shot through with cognitive elements." And the fifth major criticism of psychoanalytic theory is that it is vague, is difficult to test empirically, and does not lend itself to predictive assessments. For example, it does not offer any guidance to parents about what they can do in advance to protect their children from experiencing an inadequate psychosexual development.

Why, then, has the psychoanalytic perspective been so influential? There are two major reasons that account for its great success. First, no other theoretical approach has provided so many insights into the development and functioning of the human personality.[1] Even though the central propositions of

---

[1]For a comprehensive discussion of Freud's work, see Freud (1953–1966), Meissner (1985), Reif (1961), and Wong (1989). The few works that apply psychoanalytic theory to sociology include those of Bocock (1981), Elliot and Meltzer (1981), Parsons (1951), and Weinstein and Platt (1973).

psychoanalytic theory are not empirically verifiable, neither are many of the theories of the classic masters of sociological thought—Emile Durkheim, George Herbert Mead, Georg Simmel, and Max Weber, among others—or, ultimately, other branches of human behavior. "Freud is provocative," states Guy Swanson (1972:41), "because he provides a rich set of differentiations readily interpretable as variations in mind which, in turn, are particularly significant consequences of social organizations' impact on individuals." Furthermore, psychoanalytic theory explains some of the subtle features of human behavior that have been overlooked elsewhere in psychology and addresses the presence of unconscious influences upon the individual that is lacking in other theoretical analyses.

Second, psychoanalytic theory is important because it offers a model that is inseparable from physiological concepts and is therefore an ideal psychology for the physician. It provides the physician with an objective structure of the personality and a prescribed mode of treatment, as well as a classification system by which physicians can communicate about, attempt to treat, and comprehend mental disorders. In the absence of other models that can be shown to be more effective when *applied to the care and treatment of patients,* the quasi-medical psychoanalytic model and the medical model dominate the practice of psychiatry. However, as psychiatry moves into the twenty-first century, psychoanalysis is losing ground as a major therapeutic approach.

THE SOCIAL LEARNING MODEL

Another alternative to the medical and psychoanalytic models of mental disorder is the social learning model, based chiefly upon theories of learning and techniques of behavioral conditioning derived from the classical conditioning experiments of Ivan Pavlov (1849–1936) and Edward Thorndike (1874–1949). The underlying premise of this model is that behavior is learned but that it can also be unlearned and replaced with behavior that is more socially appropriate (Agras 1989; Bandura 1969; Bellack et al. 1990; Brady 1975). The therapeutic technique of the social learning model, known as behavior modification, emphasizes that treatment should be centered upon behavior that is externally observable and measurable. Preferred techniques include symptom desensitization (learning to approach feared situations or objects without anxiety), positive reinforcement (reward), aversive conditioning (punishment), extinction (eliminating a stimulus), conditioned avoidance (electric shocks or drugs paired with situational stimuli), and contingency contracting (agreeing with others to engage in certain behavior in return for a similar response).

However, behavior modification is subject to four limitations. First, there are serious questions as to whether human beings can actually be "conditioned" to the extent that they respond more or less automatically to the play of stimuli upon their cerebral functions. Second, even if such conditioning is possible, there are questions concerning the duration of the effects and their strength in real-world, nonclinical settings. Third, behavior modification may not be a totally sufficient form of therapy for many types of mental disorders in which the complexity of the disorder may require much more than just learning new behaviors. And fourth, behavior modification requires that patients be willing and able to learn, have a certain amount of willpower, and recognize and cope with reality at least somewhat consistently—which many mental patients may not be able to do.

Still, it can be argued that behavior modification does have certain strengths. It is based upon experimental psychology, which lends itself to research, and some studies have shown it to be an effective approach (Bandura 1969; Bellack et al. 1990), especially for short-term results and simple symptom configurations such as bed-wetting. This therapy may also be more appropriate for the treatment of poorer and less well educated persons, both because it is less expensive than psychoanalysis and because it does not demand a high degree of self-analysis and introspection. Just how effective behavior modification actually is has yet to be determined.

THE SOCIAL STRESS MODEL

A particularly active line of research, incorporating aspects of both medical and sociological concepts, is found in current investigations of the relationship between mental disorder and social stress. Usually, stress is thought to occur when individuals are faced with a situation for which their usual modes of behavior are inadequate and the consequences of not adapting to the situation are perceived as serious. Thus, we have a circumstance in which there is a gap between environmental demands and a person's capability to respond—possibly leading to a mental breakdown. The medical factors in this condition pertain to the possible predisposition of some individuals toward mental disorder when psychologically stressed because of genetic inheritance or some triggering of biochemical abnormalities. The social factors relevant to this condition rest on the fact that the majority of studies on stress indicate that most, if not all, stress is socially induced as a result of interaction between people (Moss 1973).

Accordingly, stress can be defined as an emotional-psychophysiological state of an organism that occurs in a situational context, involving stimuli that serve as cues to elicit fear or anxiety responses (Janis 1958). Stress can result in a psychophysiological reaction that causes changes in bodily tissues and promotes the onset of physical disorders such as heart disease, hypertension, peptic ulcer, muscular pain, and migraine headaches. The stress model in mental health research, in turn, is oriented more toward mental than physical dysfunctions, as would be expected—although both types of disorders may be present in a stressed individual (Kaplan 1985).

Yet to claim that stress is a likely factor in the promotion of mental disorder is not a particularly useful statement unless it can be shown what social events are most apt to be stressful and who is most likely to be affected by them. There is considerable evidence, for example, that many people can adjust to stressful situations and not suffer extensively, but other people simply fall apart and become susceptible to mental or physiological change (Moss 1973; Murphy 1961). Whether a stressful situation actually induces such change depends upon an individual's perception of the stress stimulus and the personal meaning that the stimulus holds for him or her. A person's reaction, for instance, may or may not correspond to the actual reality of the dangers that the stimulus represents; that is, a person may react appropriately, may overreact, or even may underreact. An individual's subjective interpretation of a social situation is the trigger that produces physiological and mental responses. Therefore, a considerable amount of attention in stress research focuses on the relative importance of life events and differences in the vulnerabilities of the people exposed to these events. First, let us consider what we know about reactions to extreme situations, like natural disasters and wars, and second, let us review the research on the more common stressful life events of ordinary day-to-day living.

Extreme Situations

Extreme situations like natural disasters would appear to be a likely starting point for research on stress and mental disorder because of the great anxiety people usually attach to being caught in such circumstances. But a common misconception about disasters is the notion of people fleeing in panic from the site of a potential disaster area. In reality, it is usually difficult to get people to evacuate their homes, even when damage or destruction is imminent (Tierney and Baisden 1979). Moreover, some people are attracted to potential disasters. For example, when the author lived in Hawaii, he found that a tidal wave alert would bring people to beach areas to watch the big wave come in rather than cause them to move to high ground. It was usually necessary for the police to clear the beaches of spectators. In the Midwest, some people may take risks to see a tornado. Trying to view a disaster and being a victim of one, however, are two entirely different matters. Past research has shown that extreme situations like earthquakes and tornados can induce stress (Dohrenwend 1973). Mass media reports commonly show or describe persons in large-scale disasters experiencing intense feelings of grief, loss, anguish, and despair. When tornado victims in rural Arkansas were interviewed shortly after a severe twister had touched down in their community, the great majority (about 90 percent) reported some form of acute emotional reaction (Fritz and Marks 1954).

Thus, there is sound reason for understanding the social and psychological consequences of disasters, especially from the standpoint of developing and implementing programs to assist disaster victims. According to a review by Kathleen Tierney and Barbara Baisden (1979:35) for the National Institute of Mental Health, most researchers tend to agree that "very few people become grossly psychotic in the face of major disasters and that incapacitating psychological reactions are unusual phenomena in catastrophes."

This is not to say that disaster victims generally escape all psychological trauma—quite the contrary. There is almost unanimous agreement that disasters do promote acute psychological stress, emotional difficulties, and anxiety related to coping with grief, property damage, financial loss, and adverse living conditions. And some disasters, notably the 1972 Buffalo Creek flood in West Virginia, which destroyed an entire community of five thousand people without warning, have been found to be responsible for long-lasting instances of depression, anxiety, emotional instability, apathy, insomnia, and a host of other related emotional problems (Erikson 1976; Titchener and Kapp 1976). At Buffalo Creek, the populace was supposedly so overwhelmed by the devastation (125 people were killed, and many others were injured or left homeless) that it generated a feeling of *collective helplessness* and overdependence on outside aid administered by an impersonal bureaucracy. Combined with the individual psychological impact of the disaster experience, this situation apparently further eroded what was left of community morale and solidarity (Tierney and Baisden 1979).

In contrast, a 1974 tornado in Xenia, Ohio (a suburb of Dayton), which left thirty-three people dead and over one thousand injured, and damaged over three thousand homes, did not generate serious, long-term psychiatric disorders (Taylor, Ross, and Quarantelli 1976). In Xenia, there was some warning, but most people did not think that a tornado would actually hit the town. After it happened, however, there was expression of optimism, mutual effort, and a strong sense of community solidarity. This situation was enhanced by both formal and informal helping networks organized to give psychological support to the victims. Particularly important, some local citizens' groups were formed to provide help on a personal and neighborly basis. Although there were some mental health problems, they were generally minor and short-term. Having successfully dealt with the challenges presented by the disaster, many of the victims felt emotionally and psychologically "healthier" after the tornado because they felt better able to cope with adversity (Tierney and Baisden 1979). Buffalo Creek lacked this collective sense of positiveness, and thus its residents suffered greater psychological damage.

In sum, Tierney and Baisden (1979:36) state that "while few researchers would claim that disasters create severe and chronic mental illness on a wide scale, victim populations *do* seem to undergo considerable stress and strain and *do* experience varying degrees of concern, worry, depression, and anxiety, together with numerous problems in living and adjustment in postdisaster." Groups of people with special needs in the aftermath of disasters are usually identified as the children and elderly. Older people, in particular, find it difficult to adjust to life after a disaster. Low-income groups also present special problems because they are often left without any material resources and become especially dependent on aid.

A pattern that emerges in studies of natural disasters and psychopathology is that the disaster experience, although severe, is usually short in duration, and the effects on mental health likewise tend to be short-term and usually self-limiting. The question thus arises about the possible effects of stress in extreme situations lasting long periods of time. Such situations are represented by the experiences of people exposed to the brutalities of Nazi concentration camps and the horrors of war. There is evidence that many concentration camp survivors have suffered persistent emotional problems and are particularly prone to physical illness and early death (Eitinger 1964, 1973). However, as Aaron Antonovsky (1979) notes, other concentration camp survivors have adjusted quite well to the effects of having been subjected to a most terrible experience and are now living lives that are essentially normal. Antonovsky states:

> More than a few women among the concentration camp survivors were well adapted, no matter how adaptation was measured. Despite having lived through the most inconceivably inhuman experience, followed by Displaced Persons camps, illegal immigration to Palestine, internment in Cyprus by the British, the Israeli War of Independence, a lengthy period of economic austerity, the Sinai War of 1956, and the Six Day War of 1967 (to mention only the highlights), some women were reasonably healthy and happy, had raised families, worked, had friends, and were involved in community activities.[2]

In other research on concentration camp survivors living in Montreal, Morton Weinfeld, John Sigal, and William Eaton (1981) found only modest or no significant differences between the respondents in mental stress. Weinfeld and his coworkers (1981:14) explained that their findings do not deny the reality of severe mental and physiological consequences or diminish the horror suffered by the survivors but, rather, "focus attention on the magnificent ability of human beings to rebuild shattered lives, careers, and families, even as they wrestle with the bitterest of memories." A more recent study of the children of concentration camp survivors living in Israel also did not find high rates of current psychiatric disorders (Schwartz, Dohrenwend, and Levav 1994).

When considering what differentiates people who are generally vulnerable to stress-related health problems, not just concentration camp survivors, from those who are not so vulnerable, Antonovsky argues that a strong sense of coherence is the key factor. Coherence, in his view, is a personal orientation that allows a person to view the world with feelings of confidence, faith in the predictability of events, and a notion that things will most likely work out reason-

---

[2]Aaron Antonovsky, *Health, Stress, and Coping* (San Francisco: Jossey-Bass, 1979), p. 7.

ably well. One achieves this sense of coherence as a result of life experiences in which one meets challenges, participates in shaping outcomes (usually satisfactorily), and copes with varying degrees of stimuli. Hence, the person has the resources to cope with unexpected situations if they arise. On the other hand, persons whose lives are so routine and completely predictable that their sense of coherence as defined above is weakened will find it difficult to handle unpleasant surprises and events. It is this latter person who is likely to be more susceptible to stress-induced health dysfunctions as he or she is overwhelmed by events. In other words, what Antonovsky is saying is that people who have the capability to come to terms with their situation rather than to be overcome by it are those who are most likely to emerge from an extreme situation in a healthy condition.[3]

A similar conclusion can be made about soldiers in combat. The environmental stresses faced by combat infantrymen are among the hardest faced by anyone in modern society (Rose 1956). They include the overt threat of death, loss of limbs, sight and sounds of dying men, battle noise, fatigue, loss of sleep, deprivation of family relationships, exposure to rain, mud, insects, heat, or cold, and so forth—all occasioned by deliberate exposure to the most extreme forms of violence intentionally directed at the soldier by the opposing side. Charles Moskos (1970) has compared combat with the Hobbesian analogy of primitive life: Both can be nasty, brutish, and short. According to the British military historian John Keegan (1976:297), "What battles have in common is human: the behaviour of men struggling to reconcile their instinct for self-preservation, their sense of honour and the achievement of some aim over which other men are ready to kill them." Yet somehow men generally seem to come to terms with the circumstances because most combat soldiers do not become psychiatric casualties. Two factors may be largely responsible. First is the existence of external group demands for discipline and efficiency under fire. Observing helicopter ambulance crews and Green Berets in Vietnam, Peter Bourne (1970), a psychiatrist, found these soldiers subjected to strong group pressures to be technically proficient, regardless of friendship ties. This finding was particularly true of the Green Berets, who urged their detachment leaders to prove themselves in combat in order to be worthy of their role. Although at times this social pressure added to the stress of the leaders, when the entire group faced an enemy threat there was unusual group cohesion and considerable conformity in the manner in which the threat was perceived and handled.

Second, Bourne suggests that there is a further psychological mobilization of an internal discipline in which the individual soldier employs a sense of personal invulnerability, the use of action to reduce tension, and a lack of personal introspection to perceive his environment in such a way that personal threat is reduced. Whether Bourne's findings are representative of other types of combat soldiers is subject to question because helicopter ambulance crews

---

[3]In regard to concentration camp survivors, however, Antonovsky believes their survival in the camps was due mostly to chance.

and Green Berets are highly self-selected volunteers for hazardous duty. Nevertheless, Bourne's study supports the conclusion of others (Kellett 1982; Rado 1949) that one of the most efficient techniques that allows soldiers generally to adjust to battle is to interpret combat not as a continued threat of personal injury or death but as a sequence of demands to be responded to by precise military performances. In failing to find significant physiological change (excretion of adrenal cortical steroids) occurring among most soldiers during life-endangering situations, Bourne suggests that the men allowed their behavior under stress to be modified by social and psychological influences that significantly affected physiological responses to objective threats from the environment.

When soldiers do break down emotionally in combat, data from World War II cite the loss of comrades as a particularly important factor. For instance, in a study of over twenty-five hundred American soldiers who had broken down during combat in Normandy, the expression of emotional stress and combat exhaustion in even previously normal soldiers seemed to occur when about 65 percent of their companions had been killed or wounded (Swank 1949). Primary group relations embodied in the squad or platoon were apparently very important sources of social support during World War II. The importance of the primary group in combat was that it set and emphasized group standards of behavior and sustained the individual in difficult situations. The group was able to enforce its standards by offering or withholding recognition, respect, and approval. The subjective reward of following group norms also enhanced the individual soldier's resources in dealing with combat. What motivated him to fight, according to an extensive study by Samuel Stouffer and his colleagues (1949), was to show other members of his group that he supported them so that he in turn would deserve their support in confrontations with the enemy.

However, it should be noted that most research agrees that the influence of primary group relationships tended to decline among American combat soldiers during the Korean and Vietnam wars because of the twelve-month rotation policy (Moskos 1970). A soldier's war began when he arrived in the war zone and ended a year later if he survived; thus, a time limit was placed on his exposure to stress and on whatever social relationships he formed. Primary group relations seemed to be restricted in Vietnam largely to actual combat situations, thereby limiting their overall effectiveness in influencing the soldier's behavior (Moskos 1970). Yet it is interesting to note that the United States had the lowest incidence ever of combat psychiatric casualties in Vietnam, some 12 cases per 1,000 troops medically evacuated per year (Bourne 1970; Jones and Johnson 1975).[4] This

---

[4] The rate of evacuation for psychoses in Vietnam was about 2 cases per 1,000 troops evacuated per year. Psychiatric casualties were actually quite low in Vietnam until 1971 and 1972, when drug abuse cases became increasingly prevalent and began to dominate the entire medical program (Jones and Johnson 1975).

is compared with rates of 101 cases per 1,000 troops evacuated per year in certain combat areas during World War II and 37 cases per 1,000 annually in Korea during 1950–52. The difference in Vietnam appeared to be due to the rotation policy, the availability of short rest-and-relaxation trips, the absence of large artillery barrages, the periodic safety of base camps, the general effectiveness of precombat training, rapid helicopter evacuation of the wounded, and psychiatric treatment (including the greater availability of psychoactive drugs). Most psychiatric casualties were treated in an atmosphere that emphasized a rapid return to duty (Jones and Johnson 1975).

What is obvious from this discussion of the effects of stress resulting from exposure to extreme situations on a person's mental condition is that such situations are relatively rare occurrences. They are unusual events in the lives of people living in societies at peace and not involved in internal strife or turmoil. In addition, whatever emotional difficulties are generated among persons subject to the stress of extreme situations tend to be temporary and disappear after a while. Many people are not emotionally affected at all, even though the circumstances are exceedingly stressful. Consequently, if there is a relationship between stress and mental disorder, it is necessary to focus on those life events that are common in the lives of most people—yet are so stressful that over time they affect the mental stability of those involved. As Bruce Dohrenwend (1975:384) points out, if stressful situations play a major role in causing mental disorder, the relevant events must be more ordinary and more frequent experiences in the lives of most people. These would be events like marriage, birth of a first child, death of a loved one, and loss of a job. Although such events are not extraordinary in a large population, they are extraordinary in the lives of the individuals who experience them.

Life Events

Life events research constitutes a significant area of inquiry in the attempt to understand what causes mental disorder. This approach does not focus on one particular life event (for example, exposure to combat) and then claim that it is more stressful than another life event (for example, unemployment). Rather, it is generally based on the assumption that it is the *accumulation* of several events in a person's life that eventually builds up to a stressful impact (Dohrenwend and Dohrenwend 1974; Dohrenwend 1975). Therefore, Bruce Dohrenwend (1975:384) observes that the central research questions pertaining to a stress model of mental disorder now become: "What kinds of events, in what combinations, over what periods of time, and under what circumstances are causally implicated in various types of psychiatric disorder?" At the present time, these questions are unresolved.

An important area of contention in life events research is, for example, the issue of whether any type of change in one's life, either pleasant or unpleasant, produces significant stress, or whether stress is largely a result of only unpleasant events. There is considerable evidence that supports the idea that any type of environmental change requiring the individual to adapt can produce a specific stress response (Selye 1956). Barbara Dohrenwend (1973), for one, concluded from her research on heads of families in the Washington Heights area of New York City that stressfulness is best conceived as emanating from life change itself rather than from just the undesirability of certain life events. In another study, George W. Brown and J. L. T. Birley (1968) compared a group of 50 schizophrenic patients suffering from either an onset or a relapse of schizophrenia with a control group of 377 normal persons. The primary difference between the two groups was that 60 percent of the mental patients, as opposed to 19 percent of the control group, had experienced at least one significant change in their lives during the three weeks preceding the study. This finding could not be explained away by the argument that mental patients tend to cause more problems (changes) because many of the events that the patients experienced were ones that the patients had no control over and whose outcome they were unable to affect. What is suggested by this finding is that schizophrenics tend to be excitable and easily aroused whether the event is positive or negative (Brown et al. 1966; Vaughn and Leff 1976).

Other research clearly comes down on the side of unpleasant events as being more important. Lloyd Rogler and August Hollingshead (1965) compared a matched set of twenty "well" families with twenty "sick" families (defined as having either the husband or the wife or both diagnosed as schizophrenic) of lower-class status in Puerto Rico. Based upon recall of life events by the subjects and others in the community, it was found that there were no significant differences in the family lives of the normals and the schizophrenics during childhood and adolescence. Members of both groups were exposed to the same conditions of poverty, family instability, and lower-class socialization. There was also a lack of difference in their respective adult lives, with the notable exception that for those persons who became schizophrenic, there was a recent and discernible period—*before the appearance of overt symptomatology*—during which they were engulfed by a series of insoluble and mutually reinforcing problems. Schizophrenia thus seemed to originate from being placed in an intolerable dilemma brought on by adverse life events largely stemming from intense family and sexual conflicts related to unemployment and restricted life opportunities.

Robert Lauer (1974) tested a "future shock" hypothesis on college students in a midwestern university regarding whether the rate or speed of change and the type of change, either positive or negative, were the most important variables in stress produced by change. Although stress was directly related to the perceived rate of change, his findings indicated that the effect of rapid change can be moderated by whether the change was perceived to be desirable. Rapid change and undesirability were the most stressful conditions. Still other research involving children and young adults in Manhattan (Gersten et al., 1974), male automobile drivers in Michigan (Vinokur and Selzer 1975), adult members of households in Sacramento, California (Mueller, Edwards, and Yarvis 1977), and New Haven, Connecticut (Ross and Mirowsky 1979), and married couples in the rural Midwest (Conger et al. 1993) find undesirability as the most stressful characteristic of life events. The New Haven study, conducted by Catherine Ross and John Mirowsky (1979), utilizing several different methods of weighting life events by how well they predict psychiatric symptomatology, found that the undesirability of events predicts psychiatric symptomatology better than change alone does. Employing multiple regression and controlling for undesirability, Ross and Mirowsky observed that the effects of desirable events, ambiguous events, change per se, and the number of events experienced were not significant. They conclude that undesirability is *the* characteristic of life events that is most associated with increased symptoms of mental disorder.

Moreover, research by George Brown and Tirril Harris (1978) on depression among women found that long-term depression results from negative circumstances, not positive ones. Widowhood is a particularly stressful life event, even though the vulnerability of men and women may differ (Umberson, Wortman, and Kessler 1992). Losing one's job is an undesirable life event that can also have potentially harmful effects on a person's physical and mental well-being (Hamilton, Broman, and Hoffman 1990; Kessler, House, and Turner 1987; Kessler, Turner, and House 1989). Reemployment, however, produces positive emotional effects, leading to the conclusion that the worst psychological effects of job loss can be minimized if opportunities exist for reemployment (Kessler et al. 1989).

A new area of research related to the pleasantness of an event focuses on whether the event is resolved. R. Jay Turner and William Avison (1992) define resolved events as those from which individuals are able to derive positive meaning for themselves or their futures and from which they obtain new skills and attitudes or positive self-images. They found that successful resolution of a life event significantly reduced the amount of stress associated with it, especially for persons with a low sense of mastery and members of lower socioeconomic groups. Resolution was not as important for high-status persons who typically bring a well-developed sense of personal mastery to their life events. The importance of resolution in reducing the stress of life events for some persons is seen in Peggy Thoits's (1994) study of a sample of adults in Indianapolis. Thoits focused on problems stemming from a person's job and love life. She found that people are often motivated to act in ways that deliberately reduce their stress. Negative psychological outcomes were attributable primarily to stressors that they were unable to resolve. Personal control over situations and the ability to successfully resolve problems may therefore be important in reducing the stress associated with life events.

Besides the type of change and the speed with which it occurs, the extent to which change affects a person's life may also be important. Libby Ruch (1977) investigated this and suggests that life change actually has three dimensions: (1) the degree of change evoked, (2) the desirability of change, and (3) the aspect of one's life that is affected (for example, personal, occupational). But Ruch found that the degree of change is more significant than either desirability or the area of life most affected. That is, the greater the change, the more likely stress will result. Although too much change may indeed be stressful, it may also be that too little change in a person's life induces stress (Wildman and Johnson 1977). It is not at all clear, however, that too much or too little change is a major stress factor in mental disorder. This is another area that needs to be clarified.

Research on the effect of life events also entails the severe problems of accurately measuring the presumed relationships between stress and particular life experiences. The most influential instrument at present is the Social Readjustment Rating Scale developed by T. H. Holmes and R. H. Rahe (1967). This scale is based on the assumption that change, no matter how good or how bad, demands a certain degree of adjustment on the part of an individual; the greater the adjustment, the greater the stress. Holmes and Rahe carried their analysis one step further and suggested that changes in life events occur in a cumulative pattern that can eventually build up to a stressful impact. Thus, the type of change does not matter so much; it is the extent to which change disrupts normal patterns of life that is important.

The Holmes and Rahe Social Readjustment Rating Scale, an adaptation of which is shown in Table 3-1, lists certain life events that are associated with varying amounts of disruption in the life of an average person. It was constructed by having hundreds of people of different social backgrounds rank the relative amount of adjustment accompanying a particular life experience. Death of a spouse is ranked highest, with a relative stress value of 100; marriage is ranked seventh, with a value of 50; retirement tenth with a value of 45; taking a vacation fortieth, with a value of 13; and so forth. Holmes and Rahe call each stress value a "life change" unit. They suggest that as the total value of life change units mounts, the probability of having a serious illness also increases, particularly if a person accumulates too many life change units in too short a time. If the individual accumulates two hundred or more life change units within the period of a year, Holmes and Rahe believe such a person will be at risk for a serious health disorder.

Although used extensively and found to measure the stress of life events about as well as or better than other scales (Dohrenwend et al. 1978; Ross and Mirowsky 1979), the Holmes and Rahe Social Readjustment Rating Scale nevertheless contains some flaws that need to be overcome in the future if the scale is going to continue as a major research tool. Some studies have found that the scale does not adequately account for differences between ethnic and cultural subgroups in the relative importance of various life events (Askenasy, Dohrenwend, and Dohrenwend 1977; Hough, Fairbank, and Garcia 1976; Rosenberg and Dohrenwend 1975). In other words, the Holmes and Rahe scale measures the quantity of change rather than the qualitative meaning of the event (Ruch

Table 3–1   Social readjustment rating scale

LIFE EVENT	MEAN VALUE
Death of spouse	100
Divorce	73
Marital separation	65
Jail term	63
Death of close family member	63
Personal injury or illness	53
Marriage	50
Fired at work	47
Marital reconciliation	45
Retirement	45
Change in health of family member	44
Pregnancy	40
Sex difficulties	39
Gain of new family member	39
Business readjustment	39
Change in financial state	38
Death of close friend	37
Change to different line of work	36
Change in number of arguments with spouse	35
Mortgage or loan for major purchase	31
Foreclosure of mortgage or loan	30
Change in responsibilities at work	29
Son or daughter leaving home	29
Trouble with in-laws	29
Outstanding personal achievement	28
Wife begins or stops work	26
Begin or end school	26
Change in living conditions	25
Revision of personal habits	24
Trouble with boss	23
Change in work hours or conditions	20
Change in residence	20
Change in schools	20
Change in recreation	19
Change in church activities	19
Change in social activities	18
Change in sleeping habits	16
Change in number of family get-togethers	15
Change in eating habits	15
Vacation	13
Christmas	12
Minor violations of the law	11

Source: T. H. Holmes and R. H. Rahe, "The Social Readjustment Rating Scale," *Journal of Psychosomatic Research* 11, Table 3–1 (1967), 213. Reprinted with permission of Pergamon Press, Ltd.

1977). Other research suggests that some life events, such as divorce, can be regarded as a *consequence* of stress instead of a *cause*. In addition to divorce, events like "major changes in sleeping habits," "major changes in arguments with spouse," "sexual difficulties," and "being fired from work" may be products of stress rather than causes (Holmes and Masuda 1974). This situation thus confounds the relationships being measured (Brown 1974; Dohrenwend 1974).

Another problem is that the scale does not account for intervening variables, such as social support, that for many individuals might modify the effects of life events. For example, in discussing the relationship between mental disorder and economic hardship, research reported by Susan Gore (1978) demonstrated how social support (being loved, cared for, and the like) assisted in maintaining the self-esteem of unemployed blue-collar workers in contrast to the unsupported, who had more severe psychological and health-related problems. Research by Nan Lin and his colleagues (1979) also addresses this problem. They found in a study of social support and stressful life events among a sample of Chinese Americans living in Washington, D.C., that both stressful life events and social support were significant in regard to psychiatric symptoms. But whereas stressful life events were positively associated with psychiatric symptoms, social support had a negative (fewer symptoms) and stronger relationship. This finding suggests that social support may exercise a very important influence upon psychiatric symptoms. Other studies indicate that the extent of one's integration into a social system significantly mediates the impact of life events (Antonovsky 1974; Kaplan, Robbins and Martin, 1983; Myers, Lindenthal, and Pepper 1975; Turner 1981; Wheaton 1985) and that members of a household provide support in times of crisis that helps prevent mental instability (Eaton 1978). Although interpersonal influence can be stressful in itself because of discrepancies, conflicting expectations, excessive demands to achieve or maintain a certain level of performance, or simply the volume of influence originating from several sources (Mettlin and Woelfel 1974), there is little doubt that supportive interpersonal influences can help reduce stressful feelings (Dean, Kolody, and Wood 1990; Flaherty and Richman 1989; Gore 1978, 1981, 1989; Jacobson 1986; Liem and Liem 1978; Lin and Ensel 1989; Lin et al. 1979; Lin, Woelful, and Light, 1985; Loscocco and Spitze 1990; Matt and Dean 1993; Schutt, Meschede, and Rierdan 1994; Wethington and Kessler 1986). In fact, it may be the lack of affective support that is the most important stress-inducing factor for some people (Brown, Birley, and Wing 1972).

It is obvious, therefore, that the stress model of behavior is in need of more extensive development. The relationship between stress and life events as a precipitating factor in causing or contributing to the onset of mental disorder is a highly complex phenomenon and not easily amenable to a simple cause-and-effect explanation. The process of explanation and prediction is confounded by the varying types of life events, subjective meanings attached to those events, forms of social support, personal and group vulnerabilities, and so forth, which need to be accounted for before a definitive model of social stress can be formulated. Although some researchers have argued that life events may not make a meaningful contribution to mental disorder (Gersten et al. 1977), there appears to be a general recognition in both sociology and psychiatry that subjective stress is highly significant. The research reported in this section attests to that. Moreover, some of the strongest support for a stress model of mental disorder comes from genetics, which has accumulated strong evidence of a genetic role in mental disorder but looks to social factors as instrumental in explaining the mechanisms that trigger genetic predispositions and help shape the existing variability (Grebb and Cancro 1989; Weiner 1985). Hence, the issue seems to be not so much whether social factors like life events are important but in what specific ways they are important.

THE ANTIPSYCHIATRIC MODEL

Another concept of mental disorder is the antipsychiatric view that rejects the notion that mental disorder qualifies as illness. The forerunner of this view was R. D. Laing (1967, 1969), a psychiatrist, who made the provocative suggestion that schizophrenia is a sane response to an insane world. That is, schizophrenia is primarily a reaction to a disturbing environment and seems practical from the schizophrenic's view. Therefore, it is Laing's position that schizophrenia is not a disease but a form of dissociation from intolerable social situations that affect what a person may say, do, or feel. In Laing's view, mental disorder is caused by social, political, and economic circumstances that influence an individual to dissociate himself or herself from the environment.

Szasz: The Myth of Mental Illness

Another psychiatrist who reinforced antipsychiatric views was Thomas Szasz, who claimed that mental illness is simply not an "illness" in any form. In his books *The Myth of Mental Illness* (1974) and *Insanity* (1987), Szasz argued the following: (1) Only symptoms with demonstrable physical lesions qualify as evidence of disease. (2) Physical symptoms are objective and independent of sociocultural norms, but mental symptoms are subjective and dependent upon sociocultural norms. (3) Mental symptoms result from problems in living. (4) Therefore, mental disorders are not diseases but are conflicts resulting from differing social values that the medical profession disguises as illnesses through the use of medical terminology. "Mental Illness," claims Szasz (1974:267), "is not something a person has but is something he does or is."

For example, Szasz says that a man's belief that he is Napoleon or is being persecuted by Communists cannot be explained by a defect or disease of the nervous system. Statements such as these are considered to be mental symptoms only if the observer (the audience) believes that the patient is not Napoleon or is not being persecuted by the Communists. Thus, the statement that X is a symptom of a mental disorder includes a social judgment. The observer must match the person's ideas and beliefs to those held by the observer and the rest of society. In other words, a person's behavior is judged by how well his or her actions "fit" a concept of normality held by a social audience. It is upon this basis, then, that Szasz insists that mental illness cannot be defined in a medical context. Mental illness should be defined within a social and ethical context, with psychiatrists recognizing that in actual practice they are dealing with problems in living rather than with illnesses.

There have been several critiques of Szasz's position, primarily by advocates of the medical model (Ausubel 1961; Reiss 1972; Spitzer and Wilson 1975). Generally, these critiques hold that mental symptoms do not have to result from physical lesions or obviously identifiable physiological pathologies to be defined as a disease. Subjective pain, for instance, is regarded as a disease state. Therefore, as previously noted, the medical model holds that mental symptoms, physiological or psychological, can be classified as disease if the personality is impaired and behavior is adversely affected. This view, of course, is based upon the broad perspective of disease that sees disease as being *dis-ease,* a condition of discomfort, pain, or suffering that can be relieved by medical means. Thus, in psychiatry, Szasz's concept of mental disorder as a problem in living rather than an illness or a disease state is seen as a radical position that is interesting but not terribly relevant to actual psychiatric practice. Szasz offers no particular form of therapy or ideas about how to treat insanity. Additionally, there is no evidence that conceptualizing mental disorder solely as interpersonal conflict is more useful in solving or managing abnormal behavior than an approach based upon the medical model (Spitzer and Wilson 1975).

However, among behavioral scientists and laypeople who object to an exclusive medical orientation toward mental disorder, and especially among sociologists who subscribe to the labeling theory approach, Szasz's work has been influential. Regardless of what causes mental disorder, its detection depends upon how well the person in question acts in his or her usual social role. Therefore, Szasz is correct when he argues that deciding if a person is mentally ill is a social judgment derived from comparing how well a person's behavior matches a standard of normality considered appropriate by others for the circumstances. But this view does not tell us what causes mental disorder or what to do about it.

Mental Disorder: Illness or Social Role?

The societal reaction perspective has been the source of a strong theoretical controversy between those who support the medical model and believe that mental disorder is an illness or a disease state and those like Szasz who insist that mental disorder is primarily a violation of norms and a rupture of social roles. This is an important issue because it has significant policy as well as theoretical implications and sets directions for research in the area. It also affects what people think about mental patients, how mental patients are treated, and what mental patients think of themselves. For example, John Marshall Townsend's (1975b) study of German and American mental patients suggests that beliefs about mental disorder influence patient perceptions and coping tactics and that it is quite possible that those beliefs affect the overt expression of symptoms as well. The American mental patients in Townsend's study tended to believe that mental disorders were induced by environmental factors and that the course of the disorder could be improved with personal effort and willpower on their part. The German mental patients demonstrated two views. One was that mental disorder was a reaction to an adverse psychological event and could be cured, and the other was that mental disorder was inherited and thus was a physical disease that could not be cured.

In a review, Townsend (1978) notes that the clinical universalists (those who assert that mental disorders are illnesses and fundamentally the same the world over) have accumulated much data from many different cultures that show that *schizophrenia seems to be found universally.* True, there are cultural variations in the *content* of symptoms. A schizophrenic in West Africa may suffer hallucinations pertinent to his or her life and culture as opposed to different hallucinations expressed by a Swede or an American in another environment. "This variation, notwithstanding," says Townsend (1978:68), "it appears that conditions resembling our categories of 'schizophrenia' . . . are recognized and considered aberrant in every society."

Jane Murphy's (1976) research on Eskimos in Alaska and the Yoruba tribe in Nigeria seems to bear out this point. Both societies had explicit labels for insanity that described mentally disturbed behavior as emanating from the mind of the disturbed individual. Although their expression was influenced by cultural beliefs, Murphy found a consistent pattern of symptoms composed of hallucinations, delusions, disorientations, and behavioral abnormalities pertaining to what is commonly recognized in Western culture as schizophrenia and that likewise appeared to identify the idea of "losing one's mind." Murphy (1976:1027) concluded: "Rather than being simply violations of the social norms of particular groups, as labeling theory suggests, symptoms of mental illness are manifestations of a type of affliction shared by virtually all mankind." Other research supports the contention that although mental disorders are likely to carry some local interpretation, there are no essential differences in mental conditions resembling schizophrenia between Western and non-Western cultures (CIBA Foundation Symposium 1965; Kiev 1972; Schmidt 1964). R. E. Kendell, a British psychiatrist, puts it this way:

> For the foreseeable future, the usefulness of the concept of schizophrenia is amply established by the universal occurrence of the behavioral and experien-

tial anomalies to which the term refers, irrespective of differences in language and culture; by the biological disadvantage associated with these anomalies, again irrespective of language and culture; by the evidence that these abnormalities are, at least in part, transmitted genetically; and by the influence on them of drugs which lack analogous effects on other people.[5]

Does all of this mean that the clinical universalists are right and that mental disorders are very definitely a form of illness that transcends social definitions? No, it does not. It has already been asserted that Szasz is correct in stating that deciding whether a person is mentally ill necessitates a social judgment and that this judgment is based upon how well that person acts out his or her social role. Besides the fact that the medical model is unable to explain what causes mental disorder, a central weakness in the clinical universalist position, as Townsend (1978) comments, is that their claims of universality are based upon cases of classic, unambiguous symptoms that most psychiatrists in any culture can agree on.

However, not all symptoms of mental disorder are unambiguous, and because there is no demonstrable organic pathology for most disorders, even psychiatric experts of similar cultural backgrounds disagree about diagnoses. A study often cited in this regard is that by R. E. Kendell and his associates (1971), who showed videotaped interviews of eight mental patients to over three hundred experienced American and British psychiatrists. Some patients were selected as typical cases, and others were deliberately chosen in the expectation that they might cause diagnostic disagreement. There was substantial diagnostic agreement on the three patients who exhibited textbook symptoms of schizophrenia. For three other patients with both schizophrenic and mood symptoms, a majority of both the American and the British psychiatrists diagnosed schizophrenia—although a large number of the British selected a mood disorder. On the last two patients there was serious disagreement. Most Americans selected schizophrenia, but most British decided on either a personality disorder or anxiety. For one of these patients, 69 percent of the Americans (92 out of 133) diagnosed schizophrenia, compared with only 2 percent (4 out of 194) of the British. Kendell and his associates suggested that the two groups of psychiatrists were *perceiving the abnormalities differently even though they observed the same behavior.* Other comparisons of American, British, and Canadian psychiatrists and of American psychiatrists in New York, Illinois, and California also found some important levels of disagreement (Kendell 1975; Sharpe et al. 1974).

Therefore, although schizophrenia may exist universally, its diagnosis remains a decision based upon subjective criteria. A term like "schizophrenia" does not refer to an obdurate clinical or social reality. It is an abstract concept

---

[5]R. E. Kendell, *The Role of Diagnosis in Psychiatry* (Oxford, Eng.: Blackwell Scientific Publications, 1975), pp. 22–23.

and does not exist in the material sense. Schizophrenia is a set of agreed-upon understandings and clinical assumptions that are affected by the judgment, training, and experience of those involved. Because objective scientific standards are lacking, clinical universality is difficult to prove in many cases.

What *brings* a person to a psychiatrist is emotional suffering and a problem in living based on social role expectations. What *happens* to that person before, during, and after treatment is social in nature. Research by Marvin Krohn and Ronald Akers (1977) showed that even when judgments of the nature and severity of psychiatric disorder were controlled, variables like social class, family influence, marital status, legal status, and challenges to psychiatric decisions determined whether patients were admitted to or discharged from mental hospitals. Hence, the hypothesis that social variables shape psychiatric decisions was supported. Even so, the mental state of the patients still provided cues to what should be done regarding hospitalization or release in the first place. Because it seems that both medical (genetic, biochemical) and social (environmental) factors are significant in causing and dealing with mental disorder, the question of whether mental disorders are diseases or problems in living is not particularly fruitful. Both concepts are useful and contribute to our understanding. The concepts should complement rather than compete with each other, excluding the merits of one at the expense of the other.

SUMMARY

This chapter has presented an overview of the various concepts of mental disorder based upon the competing perspectives of the medical, psychoanalytic, social learning, social stress, and antipsychiatric models. None of these models provides a satisfactory overall explanation of mental disorder, but if one model were to be selected for its potential significance for future psychiatric practice, it would likely be the medical model. This is so because the medical profession has high expectations for drug therapy and studies of brain chemistry. This trend seems likely, although such an approach ignores most psychological and sociological correlates of mental disorder and does not adequately deal with nonchemical causes or the external environments that provoke behavioral abnormalities. In the absence of definitive cures, the use of medical techniques like psychoactive drugs and electroshock therapy aims at the stabilization and reversal of symptoms to allow the patient to function as normally as possible. Medical procedures in this regard, however, are best viewed as a "holding" action in that they attempt to achieve and maintain a mental state that holds the patient in a relatively normal range of behavior in day-to-day social interaction. Sometimes, some form of counseling, psychoanalytically based psychotherapy, or behavior modification will be employed to reinforce stability and encourage the patient to gain psychological strength to reduce dependence on drugs. Nevertheless, there are those in psychiatry who insist that biochemistry is the key and that other measures will no longer be relevant once the brain's biochemical secrets have been determined. There are others who believe that the medical model is only one possible approach and that other methods may be more suitable for certain patients.

The psychoanalytic model will also remain influential, although less influential than in the past, because its definitions, terms, and conceptualizations still dominate the psychiatric perspective. A particular source of support for the psychoanalytic model is that most group therapies are based upon some form of psychoanalytic technique. The social learning model, with its emphasis upon behavior modification, seems to be particularly popular at present—especially among clinical psychologists. It deals with the present rather than with the past, since its techniques focus on unlearning abnormal behavior and on learning other behavior that is more personally and socially suitable. Thus, the advantage that the medical, psychoanalytic, and social learning models offer is both a concept of mental disorder and a particular method of treating mental dysfunctions through which a patient's symptoms can be alleviated.

As for the social stress model, it is a highly promising and very active arena of research. The focus here is primarily on the effects of stressful life events that occur routinely and eventually accumulate to trigger a stress-induced mental disorder. Many questions remain to be answered, however, in regard to the stress model, and any contribution to therapy remains to be fully articulated. The antipsychiatry model is an interesting but somewhat radical view that offers little insight for therapy administered on an individual basis. Its significance lies in helping us to understand how social and cultural standards of behavior help determine judgments about who is and who is not insane.

In sum, we have no scientifically verified theory of mental disorder that objectively explains what causes it, nor do we fully understand how various types of therapy actually work, even though they do seem to reduce the symptoms.

4

Mental Disorder as Deviant Behavior

Sociologists generally view mental disorder in terms of group or larger societal processes that have an impact upon people. Within that framework of analysis, mental disorders are perceived as *significant* deviations from what is usually considered "normal" behavior in a particular group or society. Although there are many ideas about deviance that are sociologically oriented, most sociological definitions describe deviance as any act or behavior that violates social norms.

The sociologist, therefore, views deviant behavior as conduct with distinctly social qualities. This view regards deviance as much more than simply a departure from a statistical norm or from a standard of characteristics. As Howard Becker (1973) has explained, a purely statistical view of deviance is far too limited a concept. It would take all the qualities of a certain group of people and lump them together to find a representative average. If most of those people were short, then being tall would be deviant; if most were right-handed, then being left-handed would be deviant, and so on. "Hunting with such a definition," says Becker (1973:5), "we return with a mixed bag—people who are excessively fat or thin, murderers, redheads, homosexuals, and traffic violators. The mixture contains some ordinarily thought of as deviants and others who have broken no rule at all."

Thus, the reason that the statistical definition of deviance is inadequate for understanding deviant behavior is that it leaves out *social judgments* about what is right and proper according to a prevailing social norm. Norms are expec-

tations of behavior shared by people in specific groups or in certain social settings, or they may be more general expectations of behavior common to a wide
variety of social situations. A norm has the effect of acting as an ideal standard
intended to guide, regulate, or control behavior in a fashion that is acceptable to
those concerned. Norms, accordingly, influence how people behave and do so
in a manner that goes beyond a mere statistical average of personal characteristics. This point is aptly illustrated in the following comparison made by O.
Meredith Wilson about the normative orientation of ninth-century Vikings:

> Led by men like Thorkill the Skull Splitter and Wolf the Unwashed, the Vikings
> were able to subdue much of the known world in the ninth and tenth centuries,
> not merely because they could mobilize their resources but because their social
> ideal or norm was indelibly fixed in the character of the people. The ultimate
> good was an act of war; and death itself, if one had a sword in hand or in the
> enemy's torso, became a triumphant fulfillment of life. Men so motivated made
> formidable opponents and could force differently motivated people into com-
> promise and submission. The nature of the Viking culture may illustrate the rela-
> tion between a normal that is normative and a normal that is average, for the
> total population is pulled toward the common cultural ideal character as iron fil-
> ings are toward a magnet. The normative ideal of their culture made the aver-
> age ninth century Viking's capacity for violence higher than was the capacity of
> the primitive Christians, whose norm was peace and who were counseled to turn
> the other cheek.[1]

Conformity to norms is usually rewarded by group acceptance and
approval of behavior, but deviation from norms can lead to disapproval, imprisonment, or some other form of group sanction imposed on the offender. What
would be the fate of a ninth-century Viking who disapproved of war? He would
be considered "abnormal" by their standards, and most likely he would be killed,
left friendless, or driven out of his village by those who were formerly his friends
and neighbors. Most norms, however, allow for some variation within a permissible range (that is, being a little intoxicated from alcohol at a party as opposed
to being completely drunk). Truly deviant behavior, in contrast, typically exceeds
the range of permissible behavior by being decidedly offensive. The usual
response to such behavior is an attempt to control or eliminate it. Hence,
deviant behavior can be regarded as behavior that (1) is different, (2) breaks
rules or violates norms, and (3) is exceedingly offensive.

Of course, not all deviant behavior is bad. Deviance in some creative fields
such as art, music, and literature leads to very valuable, exciting, and worthwhile
contributions to society. Consider, for instance, the reaction to Pablo Picasso,
possibly the greatest painter of the twentieth century, who shocked and outraged
even his closest friends and admirers when he unveiled his painting *Les Demoiselles d'Avignon* in 1907 while living in Paris. The painting was of five female

---

[1]O. Meredith Wilson, "The Normal as a Culture-Related Concept," in *Social Psychiatry: The
Range of Normal in Human Behavior*, Vol. 2, ed. J. Masserman (New York: Grune & Stratton,
1976), p. 22.

nudes whose forms were unified in an abstract but striking arrangement of angular planes and rounded wedges. This style violated trends that had dominated Western art since the Renaissance. It was too much for leading artists like Henri Matisse, who saw the *Demoiselles* as a deliberate insult to the modern art movement and vowed revenge against Picasso for the great embarrassment it provoked at the time. However, the painting was eventually acclaimed as the first "true" painting of the twentieth century and became an artistic breakthrough leading to the development of cubism, an important art form.

Most deviance is not rewarded so richly as Picasso's was. Most deviance, and the kind usually studied by sociologists, generally results in unpleasantness for the people involved. Sociologists focus primarily on those forms of deviance that require formal mechanisms of social control, such as police and mental institutions, and are an important threat to the well-being of society if allowed to continue unchecked. This would not necessarily include people who are merely obnoxious, eccentric, and disagreeable, but rather people who are criminals, alcoholics, drug addicts, suicidal, sexually perverted, and mentally ill.

To introduce the sociological perspectives on mental disorder, the remainder of this chapter will review those theoretical approaches to deviant behavior that are used most often to explain the relationship between society and madness. These approaches reflect two different levels of analyses. One level is the macro, or large-scale, approach, which is oriented toward understanding human behavior from the standpoint of society as a whole or the subsystems and social structures that constitute the major components of a large social system. The discussion in this section will revolve around *conflict* and *functionalist theories*. The other level of analysis is the micro, or small-scale, approach, which focuses upon the interaction among individuals as they participate in group life. This approach is oriented toward the form of behavior that takes place between married couples, within families, on mental hospital wards, and the like. The micro-level theories discussed in this section are *symbolic interaction*, with emphasis upon *labeling theory*, and *social learning theory*.

MACRO-LEVEL APPROACHES TO MENTALLY DEVIANT BEHAVIOR

The sociological literature on deviant behavior from a macro perspective features both functionalism and conflict theory. These theories attempt to explain how social conditions pressure people into deviant behavior.

Conflict Theory

Conflict theory traces its intellectual roots to Karl Marx (1818–1883), who argued that social relationships between people are determined by their relative positions in regard to the means of economic production common in their society. Those relationships are characterized historically as a class struggle between various groups of "haves" and "have-nots" until eventually a classless society, based upon economic, political, and social equality, evolves from the conflict. Class consciousness (an awareness of common interests with others in the same socioeconomic circumstances) is viewed by Marx as the key element in how a person interprets reality and organizes his or her behavior.

Marxist theory focuses on how particular social relationships and means of production, during specific historical periods, allowed the economically and politically powerful to shape the social order to their advantage. The poor, of course, would be disadvantaged; their social reality would tend to be alienating and conducive to deviance as defined by the power structure. In the meantime, the disadvantaged would remain in an exploited state. One possible effect of that exploitation could be mental illness.

For workers, scientific and technological advances under a capitalist system would not improve their lives. Workers would find themselves in an even more marginal economic position as new machinery and automation took the place of human labor. Those who remained employed would be subjected to greater stresses as they became tied to machine production and inflexible schedules capable of ruining their mental health. Modern capitalist production methods thus become a more subtle way of exploiting the mental state of workers as they are severely stressed on behalf of profits for their employers. Technological advancement is seen, accordingly, to promote polarization of society into the wealthy and the destitute.

However, stress, bad living conditions, slums, low incomes, economic and social exploitation, and unemployment by themselves would not constitute the entire Marxist explanation of mental disorder. Economic deprivation would be regarded as an oversimplification of a generally oppressive situation because the effect on the person would have to be considered within the wider context of the problems of capitalism. Marx maintained that self-consciousness is possible only in relation to the community and society as a whole. Capitalist culture, in contrast, is thought to isolate people because it depicts self-consciousness as the essence of being an individual. However, to be self-conscious in a capitalist mode is literally to be conscious of one's self and nothing more—which leaves individuals isolated and prone to alienation (Lichtman 1982). The most important factor in determining consciousness is work because it is the vehicle through which people come to realize themselves in relation to others. According to Vicente Navarro (1986:34), it is obvious that "in our consumer society today what *you have* depends on what *you do,* but even more important, that one's psychological framework—which determines one's level of expectations and behavior and patterns of interpersonal relations—is very much determined by one's work." But under capitalism, work is controlled by the upper class and organized to protect their socioeconomic advantage. This situation promotes alienation, and Marx maintained that the more alienated people are from their work, the less able they are to conceive of themselves as other than they presently are (Lichtman 1982). What is therefore important in understanding the cause of mental illness from a Marxist perspective is not problems in interpersonal situations but a sense of alienation from the general social environment. That alienation is based on feelings of despair associated with the exploitation of one's labor and disadvantaged position in life.

The application of Marxist theory to the study of mental disorder, however, has been extremely limited. Contemporary approaches to conflict theory in Western society have moved away from notions of class struggle and instead concentrate on the competition among interest groups like those representing labor, management, geographical regions, political parties, and professional and other organized pressure groups, including agencies within the government itself (Akers 1977; Akers and Hawkins 1975; Turner 1988). Laws and governmental regulations are viewed as outgrowths of power struggles among interest groups, not as reflections of consensus prevalent in the wider society. The more powerful a group is able to become in support of normative conditions, the more likely it is that it will escape being defined as deviant. Or in some cases, being powerful outside the normative system will allow a deviant group to escape some of the sanctions imposed by the wider society. In 1974, for instance, the strong political pressure exerted by organized groups of homosexuals influenced the American Psychiatric Association to remove homosexuality from its diagnostic categories of mental illness. In discussing this, Elliott Krause (1977:95) says, "What shows the social nature of the definition is that any definition which can be *lobbied against* politically can hardly be considered illness in the narrow sense."

Consequently, conflict theorists have tended to embrace Thomas Szasz's (1974, 1987) notion that mental illness is a myth and is, in fact, a problem in living as defined by the power structure. Szasz bases his argument upon the premise that the standards by which people are judged mentally ill are social, psychological, ethical, and legal—but not medical; a question of ethics thus arises in that it becomes debatable under these conditions whether psychiatrists represent their patients or the larger social order. A radical view along these lines is that psychiatry is not "unequivocally benign" but functions "simply as a mode of social control operating to preserve the social status quo" (Ehrenreich 1978:5).

Conflict theory is able to provide plausible explanations of slum-area and white-collar crime, including criminogenic acts committed by large business corporations and governments. It also illustrates the manner in which medicine in general and psychiatry in particular operate as mechanisms of social control and perpetuate their privileged positions in American society as major interest groups (witness how the American Medical Association has steadfastly opposed any legislation threatening the fee-for-service system of medical care). But this approach to mental illness appears to be too limiting. There is a distinct lack of empirical data detailing how conflict within society actually leads to mental disorder. It has not been demonstrated how murder, sex crimes, and certain forms of noncriminal deviance (such as most cases of mental illness) are directly related to conflicts among interest groups or social classes. Generally, the conflict perspective seems to assume that economic exploitation or struggles among interest groups produce alienating and unsettled social conditions without providing any precise accounting of how this takes place; the causal connection between social conflict and a particular person's insanity is left unspecified. When it comes to mental disorder, conflict theory remains undeveloped.

Functionalism

Like conflict theory, functionalism takes a broad approach to the study of human behavior. The functionalist theorist does not search for the causes of deviant behavior in the biology or psychology of individual persons; the functionalist looks for the sources of deviance in the relationship between individuals and social systems. This approach is based upon the view that society is held together in a cohesive range of equilibrium by harmonious patterns of shared norms and values. What makes social life possible is the *expectation* that people will behave in accordance with the norms and values common to their particular social system. This process is "functional" because it results in social harmony and counterbalances "dysfunctional" processes, such as crime and mental illness, that disrupt social order. The tendency of a society toward self-maintenance through equilibrium is very similar to the biological concept of homeostasis, in which the human body attempts to regulate physiological (internal) conditions within a relatively constant range to maintain adequate bodily functioning. A person may suffer from warts, indigestion, a broken leg, or perhaps even a benign cancer and still be *generally healthy*. Likewise, a social system is viewed in the functionalist perspective as maintaining social functioning by regulating its various parts within a relatively constant range. A social system may have problems with crime and mental illness but be "healthy" because of its overall capacity to function efficiently.

Because functionalist theorists perceive social systems as composed of various closely interconnected parts, they argue that changes, decisions, and definitions made in one part of the system inevitably affect, to some degree, all other parts of the system. Thus, a person's position within the social system subjects him or her to events and stresses originating in remote areas of the system. Behavior that is adaptive from one's own perspective and peculiar circumstances may be regarded as deviant by society at large; thus, one runs the risk of confrontation with those authorities, such as psychiatrists, the police, and the courts, charged with reducing dysfunctional social processes. The individual then has the choice of continuing the adaptive behavior (actually there may be little or no choice if one wants to survive) and being defined as deviant, or trying to change that behavior even though survival in the social system is based upon it. Many persons, not surprisingly, continue the disapproved behavior and are therefore pressured by the system into being deviant.

Emile Durkheim

The functionalist perspective in sociology is largely based upon the initial insight of the French sociologist Emile Durkheim (1858–1917), a major figure in the history and development of social thought. Durkheim began his scholarly career with strong opposition to two intellectual themes prevalent in the late 1800s: individualism and biologism. Some social theorists of the period, notably Herbert Spencer, viewed social reality as stemming from the individual and society mainly as a derivation of individuals, but Durkheim saw society as *the* basic reality and individuals personified only through their relation to the larger social order. It was society's norms, values, statuses, and roles that provided social reality for the individual, not the other way around.

Durkheim's opposition to biologism was also rooted in his belief in the preeminence of society. In this case, Durkheim objected to the early causal theories of deviance in sociology, which were essentially biological models of behavior. These models described something inherent in certain individuals as the source of deviant behavior, such as brain disease or the genetic inheritance of criminal traits. In rebuttal, Durkheim argued that biological concepts can never be fully sufficient explanations of human behavior. He believed that behavior can be understood only by accounting for those behavioral attributes that are clearly social, like roles, norms, status, and so forth. In Durkheim's view, individual behavior was largely determined by the social order, in that society existed as a distinct entity outside of and above the individual and so shaped the manner of individual responses.

That view is apparent in Durkheim's 1897 study, *Suicide* (1951), in which Durkheim suggested that suicide, despite its highly personal nature, is not entirely an act of free choice by the individual. Durkheim based that observation upon his analysis that the suicide rates for various countries in Western Europe are relatively constant, year after year. Therefore, something more than simply individual motives and circumstances appeared to be involved. He believed that suicide is a social fact, explainable by social causes. "Social facts," according to Durkheim (1950:13), were "every way of acting, fixed or not, capable of exercising on the individual an external constraint." Whether a person chooses to take his or her life is thus related to the constraints placed by society upon that person's behavior. Within this framework of analysis, Durkheim distinguished three principal types of suicide—all grounded in the relationship of the individual to society. These three types are (1) *egoistic* suicide, in which individuals become detached from society and, suddenly finding themselves left upon their own, are overwhelmed by the resulting stress; (2) *anomic* suicide, in which individuals suffer a sudden dislocation of the normative systems to which their own norms and values are no longer relevant, so the controls of society no longer restrain them from taking their lives; and (3) *altruistic* suicide, in which individuals feel themselves so strongly integrated into a demanding society that their only escape seems to be suicide.

Durkheim's typology of suicide suggests how a society might pressure individuals to kill themselves. Of the three types outlined by Durkheim, egoistic suicide has been deemed the most common in the United States (Shneidman 1975). It occurs when an individual has too few ties to the community. Often it is the result of stress brought on by the separation of a strongly integrated individual from his or her group. Durkheim used as an illustration of egoistic suicide the example of the military officer who is retired and left on his own without the group ties that typically regulated his behavior. Egoistic suicide is supposedly based upon the overstimulation of a person's intelligence by the realization that he or she has been deprived of collective activity and meaning. Stories of action-seeking individuals, like police officers, who commit suicide after retirement because they cannot adjust to their new life, occasionally appear in movies or on television and qualify as egoistic suicide. The determining factor in egoistic suicide, therefore, is the degree to which an individual is integrated into the social groups—religious, family, occupational, economic, and political—to which the person belonged. Durkheim found at the time of his study that Protestants (as compared with Catholics), single persons (as compared with married), persons in families without children (as compared with those with children), and so forth were more likely to commit suicide because of their lesser degrees of social integration and solidarity. Egoistic suicide is the form of suicide that stalks the "loner," who becomes alone by choice or by chance.

Anomic suicide is characterized by an overstimulation of emotions and a corresponding freedom from society's constraints. It is the result of sudden change that brings on a breakdown of values and norms by which an individual has lived his or her life. Sudden wealth or sudden poverty, for instance, could disrupt usual normative patterns for a person and induce a state of anomie or normlessness. It is not that the person has no norms but that his or her norms no longer seem to be appropriate. In this situation, a chronic lack of regulation results in a state of restlessness, unbounded ambition, or perhaps crisis, in which an individual's norms are no longer relevant. For example, during the Great Depression of the 1930s in the United States, there were instances of people killing themselves after losing vast sums of money when the stock market crashed. The onset of sudden poverty could have the effect of making usual normative controls meaningless and inducing anomic suicide.

Rose Coser (1976) studied the relationship between patient suicides and anomie among staff members of a mental hospital and noted a significant connection. Although it might be argued that mental patients are more likely than most other people to kill themselves because of their disturbed psychological condition, Coser found weakened staff relations were apparently an important factor in the patterns of suicide in the hospital under study. Anomie, however, was attributed to situations not among the patients on the wards but among the hospital staff. Yet it was the patients who committed suicide. Coser states:

The decision to study suicides of patients in relation to processes of staff interaction was prompted by my observation of a feeling of disturbance among psychiatric residents in the hospital. There were insinuations that recent suicides of patients were not unrelated to the quality of life among the staff, and there were specific complaints about the failure of a top-ranking psychiatrist to meet with the residents.

At one of my weekly visits to the hospital I noticed grave consternation because three suicides had occurred that month. A resident complained:

The residents are not important [here]. We are supposed to have weekly meetings with Dr. X. . . . The first-year residents haven't seen him yet; they came July 1st. . . . When three patients killed themselves in one week, then he came. The same resident approached me later that day to say:

You'll be interested to know that Dr. X has cancelled again. This is the fourth time. What we need is another suicide [smiles uncomfortably].[2]

Altogether there were twenty-one patient suicides over a six-year period. Although it might be farfetched, Coser notes, to speculate that patients committed suicide because a leader failed to meet with the residents, this was but one major indicator of a weakening of staff morale and social relations. Other problems were instability among the hospital administration with the departure of a key administrator and staff turnover among the residents themselves. Coser matched those events to show a correlation between the times when staff relations were weakest and the onset of waves of suicides among patients; when staff relations were stable, suicides likewise were down. Although it was possible that the suicides were the result of imitation once the first suicide took place, why did the suicides appear in clusters at particular times? Coser hypothesized it was because weakened staff relations communicated a sense of despair to the patients. If the relations between staff members are weak, Coser suggests, staff members are unable to obtain the support from one another needed to sustain their competence in working with patients. Hence, when patients lose confidence in the staff, they find it more difficult to believe they will get better or that life is worth living.

Finally, there is altruistic suicide, in which an individual kills himself or herself because society demands it. Although egoistic and anomic forms of suicide both are caused by "society's insufficient presence in individuals" (Durkheim 1951:256), altruistic suicide represents the strong presence of society mandating suicide because of the social circumstances. An example of altruistic suicide is the practice of *harakiri* in Japan, where certain social failures, wrongdoing, or loss of face by an individual is expected to be redressed by the individual's suicide. The ritual death by cutting into one's abdomen was derived from the *samurai* code of honor beginning in the twelfth century. It is a form of suicide deliberately intended to be extremely painful. Usually it was committed by those samurai who failed in some way or who sought to avoid

---

[2]Rose Laub Coser, "Suicide and the Relational System," *Journal of Health and Social Behavior* 17 (1976), 318–19.

dishonor such as capture in battle by an enemy, which was considered the greatest dishonor of all. According to the historian S. R. Turnbull (1977:47), "So horrible was the idea of harakiri that even the samurai modified it in later years to a purely nominal stabbing, while a friendly second cut off the victim's head." Nonetheless, the practice continued, since it had become part of a normative pattern of behavior for certain people (samurai) in certain circumstances (failure or defeat).

Durkheim's study of suicide contains some shortcomings. His typology of suicide, for example, does not explain all suicides and cannot be used to predict whether a certain individual is going to take his or her life. What Durkheim accomplished, however, was to point to the impact of society on the individual by noting that individuals commit suicide because the meaning and stability in their lives provided by the social order have been modified or weakened, or have disappeared. He contributes to our understanding of suicide by trying to explain how, according to sociological influences, society fosters intolerable emotion or unbearable despair in individuals, which in turn leads to suicide. Yet the significance of Durkheim's work in this regard extends well beyond the issue of suicide because this is only one of many possible ways a person might find to cope with social and psychological problems. The particular relevance of Durkheim's orientation to our discussion is his recognition that societal processes can create stressful situations in which people are forced to respond to conditions not of their own choosing.

Robert Merton and the Concept of Anomie

Robert Merton (1938), a contemporary American sociologist, devised one of the most influential theories of deviance in sociology based upon Durkheim's concept of anomie. Merton argued that anomie, a chronic lack of normative regulation according to Durkheim, could be a *normal* situation for some people because of society's pressure upon them to engage in nonconforming rather than conforming conduct. Merton suggested that societies contain both a cultural structure and a social structure. The cultural structure is characterized as representing culturally defined goals, those "things worth striving for," on which society places a normative value. In American society, for instance, the cultural goal for most people is material success. The social structure operates in tandem with the cultural structure in that it defines, regulates, and controls the acceptable ways of obtaining these goals. The socially prescribed manner of achieving the cultural goal of material success in American society is to complete a level of education leading to a good job and a salary that will purchase the house, automobiles, television sets, and other items that are evidence of material success. As long as individuals achieve the cultural goals according to socially prescribed modes and as long as the cultural goals satisfy the individual, an effective equilibrium in society is maintained.

Merton claims that anomie occurs when there is a breakdown in the cultural structure, particularly when there is a mismatch between the cultural goals and the socially structured capacities of people to reach those goals. Merton says this situation is most common for members of the lower class who are asked to orient their behavior toward the prospect of wealth but who at the same time are denied opportunities to do so by the social structure. A strain toward anomie subsequently results as cultural goals become incompatible with the lack of social means to achieve the goals. Although a rigid class structure could restrict opportunities to achieve such goals possibly without resulting in deviant behavior, American society emphasizes egalitarian beliefs. These beliefs maintain that Americans have the opportunity for economic affluence and social mobility, at least in theory. Of course, theory is not always reality, and many people lack the talent or financial resources to achieve the so-called good life. Therefore, the restriction of approved means for reaching approved goals is the primary factor promoting a strain toward anomie in American society if Merton's analysis is to be taken literally. Commitment to the goals is assumed; it is the means to reach the goals that are differen. ally available.

Merton identifies five basic modes of adaptation to one's prospects for achieving cultural goals. None of these adaptations is deliberately selected by the individual because all arise from strains in the social structure. First, there is *conformity*, in which an individual accepts both the goals and the means of reaching the goals. Conformity is the most common mode of adaptation and is the basis for social life, as people interact in predictable patterns according to shared norms and values. Second, there is *innovation*, in which an individual accepts the goals but rejects the means. The innovator is typically regarded as a person who breaks the law. He or she is oriented toward material success but turns to crime to achieve it because the approved means is not available. This is a normal response, says Merton, for lower-class people who lack the means to reach the goals. Third, there is *ritualism*, a situation in which the individual rejects the goals but not the means. An example of a ritualist is a person who does not strive for the goals but appears to be following the means to reach them. A low-paid clerk in a large business who has no hope of ever advancing in the job and earning a good income, yet who continues to show the appearance of doing so, would be a ritualist. Fourth, there is the mode of *retreatism*, in which an individual rejects both the goals and the means. This is a situation of hopelessness in which a person realizes he or she is unable to reach the goals because of the lack of means. But in contrast to the ritualist, the retreatist rejects the goals as well. This person most likely is an outcast such as a hobo, a bum, a skid-row alcoholic, or perhaps a mental patient. Merton's fifth mode of adaptation is *rebellion*, in which an individual rejects both the goals and the means and replaces them with new goals and new means considered more legitimate than the existing ones. Merton's typology of individual modes of adaptation is shown in Table 4–1.

Even though Merton's goals-versus-means paradigm has been highly

Table 4–1   Merton's typology of modes of individual adaptation

MODES OF ADAPTATION	CULTURAL GOALS	INSTITUTIONALIZED MEANS
I Conformity	+	+
II Innovation	+	–
III Ritualism	–	+
IV Retreatism	–	–
V Rebellion	±	±

+ = acceptance; – = rejection; ± = rejection of prevailing values and substitution of new values.

influential in deviance research, especially in studies dealing with youth and delinquency, there have been important criticisms of it. Some of those criticisms will be briefly considered here. First, it is questionable whether individuals throughout society adopt the same cultural goals to the same degree as Merton asserts. Matza (1969), for example, suggests that dominant social values are primarily "guides for action," not "categorical imperatives" requiring all to strive for their achievement regardless of the means available. With different interests, talents, and resources, different people are likely to select different goals or variations of culturally defined goals that suit their own particular purpose. Although it can be argued that many Americans are oriented toward material success, Merton's theory does not account for those who seek different standards. Moreover, some kinds of deviance (for example, homosexuality, white-collar crime) are not explained very well by Merton's typology; he also neglects the ability of the individual to choose intentionally one's own response to societal restraints and *collective* subcultural adaptations, like that of the "hippies" in the mid-1960s and "punks" in the 1980s.

Why, then, do we consider Merton's theory of anomie and social structure for our discussion of the sociological aspects of mental disorder? We do so because it adds to our insight into how large-scale societal conditions may contribute to the onset of mental illness in an individual. Merton's typology suggests that the insane belong to the retreatist form of adaptation. Although it can be argued that the insane do not merely reject society's goals and means but also are confused about what those goals are and how to reach them, the retreatist notion is not alien to such mental disorders as schizophrenia. Keeping in mind that schizophrenia is characterized by withdrawal from reality, accompanied by delusions, hallucinations, ambivalence, and bizarre activity, we can see aspects of retreatism in the very nature of the disorder. Also, the incidence of schizophrenia tends to be disproportionately large among the lower class, the segment of society that Merton identifies as having the greatest pressures and the fewest resources for adaptation.

Thus, Merton's work joins that of Durkheim to show how a functionalist orientation applies to mental disorder. This view holds that strains in the social system put pressures upon individuals, requiring them to cope with circumstances over which they have no direct control. Some people may suffer insanity as they succumb to the stress of these societal pressures. Examples of this are found in those studies linking mental disorder to social malaise and economic recession.

Anomie and Schizophrenia in Rural Ireland

Anthropologist Nancy Scheper-Hughes (1979) utilized Durkheim's concept of anomie to explain the excessive rates of schizophrenia among persons living in rural Ireland. Scheper-Hughes spent one year as a resident in a small, isolated hamlet of about four hundred persons in a remote western region of Ireland. Through participant observation, formal interviews, and a variety of projective tests, such as the Thematic Apperception Test (TAT), she studied the cultural life and social relationships of the townspeople, farmers, and patients at a nearby mental hospital and psychiatric clinic. The image of Irish rural life that emerges from this study is harsh, bleak, and especially pathogenic for the young and middle-aged bachelor farmers who form the greatest proportion of schizophrenics.

In Ballybran, the pseudonym for the village under study, the levels of stress generated by a demoralized culture had exceeded the capacity of both local institutions and individuals to cope with them. The ability of the community to sustain itself through its traditional patterns of agriculture, sheep grazing, and fishing had faltered. The farms were bolstered by government subsidies, and many people were on welfare. The government offered early retirement to the farmers through purchase of their land at the market price, supplemented by a small pension in order eventually to transfer the low-production lands to large agricultural corporations for development. The effect on the morale of the community was devastating. Scheper-Hughes reports:

> Throughout the long and discouraging winter, Ballybran farmers gathered in clusters at the pub or at each other's homes to listen to radio or public television reports decry and deride the "backwardness" and "conservatism" of the western coastal farmers, who were characterized as living like parasites off welfare handouts, grants, and subsidies, who were opposed to progress, and who hung greedily and tenaciously on to their unproductive and miserable farms. The spectre of forced and early retirement hovered over the nightly pub sessions in Ballybran, and a puritanical gloom settled like a mist into each man's pint of bitter porter. "Well, lads 'tis we're finished up now for sure," was a commonly heard refrain. The local residents read about their lives and livelihood discussed in national papers as so much debris and dead weight.[3]

---

[3]Nancy Scheper-Hughes, *Saints, Scholars, and Schizophrenics: Mental Illness in Rural Ireland* (Berkeley and Los Angeles: University of California Press, 1979), p. 43.

Only one farmer in the area retired while the study was under way, and he was subject to vicious ridicule. The retirement policy nonetheless eroded the traditional rural Irish view that there was no such status or role as "retired farmer." The elderly usually maintained some presence in the running of the farm even after they passed legal ownership to their heirs. Inactivity in this normative system was equated with immorality ("idleness is the Devil's workshop"), and retirement was associated with death. Longevity in life was ascribed to hard work in the traditional folklore of the region. "Villagers are particularly fond of repeating stories of the miraculous cures of ancient farmers," says Scheper-Hughes (1979:44), "who struggled out of their deathbeds at the last moment to check up on a favorite old cow or newborn calf, only to discover that they felt better once on their feet and involved again in the business of the farm." Thus, the older villagers clung to the familiar patterns of the past even though they were failing to sustain a viable community life and were subjected to adverse public criticism—a situation that promoted anomie.

Both economic and social conditions contributed to the flight of the young, especially women, from the area in search of greater opportunities and a less restricted lifestyle. Local girls were strongly attracted to the relative independence and higher social status of women in British and American cities and were repelled by the shyness of the village boys and the dissatisfaction of their mothers with their own lives. Many adult males tended to be cold, reserved, and awkward around women, and at most social occasions males and females would separate by sex to enjoy conversation, banter, and, for the men, drinking. Another barrier to sexual interaction, according to Scheper-Hughes, was a tradition of sexual repression, which she believed was fostered by an ascetic Irish Catholicism. This situation was evidenced in an excessive preoccupation with sexual purity and an emotional climate mistrustful of intimacy between the sexes. There were also strong family loyalties emphasizing the ties of blood over those of marriage and retarding the acceptance of "stranger" women who married into the family. Some farms were brother–sister households in which the sister's primary role was domestic care of her male siblings. One such woman was "Peggy," who, when questioned as to why she had not married despite several proposals, replied: "What! Exchange a household of four healthy, strong men—God bless them—for a household with only one?" (Scheper-Hughes 1979:114).

Few marriages, few children, and desertion by the young, plus the natural population attrition through death, have led to a rural society in western Ireland increasingly composed of bachelor farmers. It is this group that seems to have the most victims of anomie and to be the primary source of the high rates of schizophrenia. Scheper-Hughes holds responsible a guilt- and shame-oriented style of socialization that traps these men into remaining on the farms and guarantees their loyalty through scapegoating. The socialization process favors the mental health of girls and usually the first-born males, the family's so-called white-headed boy, who is treated as a pet in contrast to the leftover son, who is usually the last born. By scapegoating the leftover son as someone loved but hopelessly incompetent, the parents are often able to prevent that son from leaving home and thus to keep him to care for both them and the family farm. In this context, the child is subject to a contradictory and skewed communication system that Gregory Bateson and his colleagues (1956) call the "double-bind" hypothesis. A child may be told that he or she is loved by the mother but is put off by gestures or nonverbal behavior from showing an affectionate response. When children are confronted by such contradictory messages, they may become confused about what they should do. If they respond, they may be punished; if they do not respond, they may be punished. Hence, they are put in a double bind; they can be punished no matter how they respond. Bateson suggests that repeated exposure to this impossible situation encourages the child to respond with equally contradictory behavior, and the child may lose the ability to grasp the appropriate meanings rendered through communication with other people, which is a trait of schizophrenia. In her study, Scheper-Hughes found a similar situation for the leftover son:

> Called to his face a wretched, unfortunate, ungainly soul, a leftover, miserable remnant of flesh, the "old cow's calf" is caught in a classical double-bind in which he is damned if he does and damned if he does not. The parent can be observed belittling the runt for trying to put himself ahead and then with the same breath chiding him for not being more aggressive and achievement-oriented like his older brothers.[4]

The younger son can leave home but in doing so will be exposed to feelings of guilt for "abandoning" the parents ("Johnny, you're the *last* one we have left!"). If he stays home, he may be subjected to ridicule as being less than a man for not establishing his own independent existence (Scheper-Hughes 1979:185). The psychological defenses against this harmful situation, notes Scheper-Hughes, for children and adolescents are passive strategies of sulking and gradual withdrawal from intimate contact and for adults are feelings of self-pity and fatalism that is not their fault they are bachelors, unemployed, alcoholics, stay-at-homes, and so on.

Thus, certain individuals in the rural culture of western Ireland, specifcally the bachelor farmers living isolated and celibate lives, were most vulnerable to schizophrenia. Although many of these individuals were able to adjust to the conditions of anomie and demoralization prevalent in their community, largely through heavy drinking and socializing with peers in the local pubs, others

---

[4]Ibid., pp. 184–85.

slipped into schizophrenia. Scheper-Hughes does not deny that genetics may be responsible in·some cases of schizophrenia, but the focus of her work was to uncover the social conditions that exacerbated the tendency toward the disorder.

Mental Disorder and Economic Downturn in the United States

The relationship between economic change and abnormal behavior has been of interest to social scientists ever since Durkheim's seminal work on suicide in 1897. Yet statistical techniques capable of providing sophisticated, multivariate analysis have been employed to measure economic trends and behavioral responses only since the late 1960s. An initial study in this regard was that of Albert Pierce (1967), who correlated rates of suicide among white males with changes in the index of common-stock prices for the peacetime years from 1919 to 1940. Rates of suicide one year after changes in prices of stocks showed a significantly high level of correlation, leading Pierce to suggest that economic fluctuation, either up or down, reduced social cohesion and contributed to a higher frequency of suicide.

Studies that offer specific evidence of economic change and increased rates of mental problems are those by sociologists M. Harvey Brenner (1973) in New York State, Ralph Catalano and C. David Dooley in Kansas City (1977) and Los Angeles County (1984), and Rudy Fenwick and Mark Tausig (1994) on a nationwide data set. Brenner examined an extensive amount of data on mental hospital admissions and rates of employment in New York over a period of 127 years from 1841 to 1968. He believed that regardless of the number and combination of factors that predispose certain individuals toward becoming mentally ill, the question that needed to be answered was why mental disorder appears *when* it does. He differed from Pierce in that he felt that downward shifts in economic activity produced much greater stress than did simply economic change itself (either up or down). The data supported his hypothesis that *mental hospitalization will increase during economic downturns and decrease during upturns.* Brenner suggested that an inability to fulfill one's social role frequently results from economic downturns and that the stress produced by this experience is a causal factor in the appearance of mental illness. After finding significantly higher rates of mental hospital admissions during economic recessions and depressions, Brenner (1973:8) claimed "that a substantial fraction of *all* stress factors that precipitate mental illness in American society at present is economic in origin."

Economic downturns appeared to have a great impact upon those persons most responsible for financially maintaining their families, namely, males, the married, and the college educated. But, not unexpectedly, those persons from the higher socioeconomic groups possessed greater material and emotional resources to cope with economic adversity, thereby tending to avoid high rates of mental hospitalization. Those persons with the lowest socioeconomic status, classified as "lacking in the necessities of life" and existing largely on public welfare, had rates of mental hospital admissions twice as high as those of the other, more affluent socioeconomic groups. This finding supports the argument that a greater preponderance of mental illness is located in the lower socioeconomic class either because it faces more stressful life events or because it contains persons who have "drifted" downward from other classes. Both of these arguments will be reviewed fully in the chapter on social class and mental illness but are mentioned here to illustrate the existence of a significant relationship between poverty and mental disorder.

Brenner also suggested that economic downturns brought about increases in intolerance toward the mentally ill, which, in turn, helped to inflate the rates of mental hospitalization for those persons most marginal to a family's economic well-being. Brenner states:

> Speaking more generally, and somewhat brutally, the very young and the elderly are the most expendable members of the society at a time when emotional and financial resources are in critically short supply. One might therefore imagine that the stresses of an economic downturn, apart from those directly involved with maintaining or advancing the economic status of the family, might fall heavily upon the young and the aged in society. This might be the case particularly if, as some of the literature in this field emphasizes, a major factor possibly relating social stress to mental hospitalization is intolerance of psychiatric symptoms on the part of family and friends. It would therefore not be difficult to imagine that the psychiatric symptoms of the young and the aged would be less well tolerated than those of the higher-status age groups, and therefore that mental disturbance among these two age groups would become a particularly heavy burden on the emotional and financial resources of a family during an economic downturn. Many families, for instance, might find it easier to make excuses for the paranoia of a member who was desperately needed in order to maintain at least a marginal financial position.[5]

Brenner provided two explanations for his findings. He preferred a "provocation" hypothesis that stress resulting from being dislocated from one's usual lifestyle or prevented from improving it during a downward shift in the economy caused vulnerable people to reach the point at which they required hospitalization in a mental institution. Another explanation, also possible and described by Brenner as an "uncovering" hypothesis, suggests that economic downturns do not promote mental disorder but simply "uncover" those people already mentally ill by stripping them of their existing economic resources. These people who are mentally "borderline" may be able to support themselves during periods of economic affluence, only to become the first to lose their jobs

---

[5]M. Harvey Brenner, *Mental Illness and the Economy* (Cambridge: Harvard University Press, 1973), pp. 113–14.

when times are bad. In fact, in a declining economic cycle, mental hospitals may be attractive sources of food and shelter for these marginal individuals.

Although Brenner prefers the hypothesis that economic downturns provoke mental disorder, his data also support the finding that such downturns "uncover" mentally disordered persons. Additional research is needed to determine whether provocation or uncovering is actually at work; it may be that to a significant degree both hypotheses are relevant. The import of Brenner's work is that it shows downward trends in economic activity that may result in mental hospitalization for certain people, particularly those with the fewest financial resources. There also is strong stress for those who have some resources, yet face the threat of downward social mobility because their resources are not enough to sustain them. The stress on this latter group, essentially those in the middle class, can be very great, too. For some of these people, the stress may also influence the onset of mental disorder or remove the resources keeping them out of a mental hospital. All in all, financial adversity apparently hurts the mind as well as the pocketbook.

Another study of the effect of economic change on the psychological well-being of individuals is that by Catalano and Dooley (1977), conducted in Kansas City. This study examined the relationship between depressed moods and stressful life events as correlated with rises in inflation and rates of unemployment. Utilizing a very carefully designed approach, Catalano and Dooley found that unemployment was significantly related to depressed mood and stressful life events but that inflation was related to neither. Thus, unemployment appeared to be the strongest predictor of depression and stressful events. The study did not test Brenner's uncovering hypothesis and explored his provocation hypothesis only partially; yet the data tended to support the provocation explanation that economic change put stress on vulnerable people to the point at which they required hospitalization. In subsequent research in Los Angeles County, Dooley and Catalano (1984) produced findings that again tended to support the provocation hypothesis. Thus, the notion that economic downturns stress some people to the point of acute mental distress finds some confirmation in the research literature.

Fenwick and Tausig (1994) analyzed a nationwide data set that relates macro-level structural features of the economy to everyday job experiences of workers. They determined that when downturns occurred in the larger economy, stress was often generated that affected the routine and quality of experiences on the job. Fenwick and Tausig (1994:278) found that "whether consciously or not, firms appear to pass any increased uncertainty in the marketplace to their workers in the form of increased demands, decreased decision latitude, and increased job insecurity." Even though workers may not be laid off, the structural conditions associated with economic downturns can be stressful over a prolonged period.

Although the research of Brenner, Catalano and Dooley, and Fenwick and Tausig demonstrates how large-scale societal processes, specifically those of economic change, can be correlated with rates of mental hospitalization or with depressed moods and stressful life events, the relationship is not that simple. Among other things, it remains to be determined whether economic downturns are provocative or uncovering when it comes to mental illness, and whether it is adverse (downward) change or change per se in economic activity that has the greater impact upon the onset of mental disorders. Furthermore, it may be that the relationship between mental hospitalization and the economy is limited to those individuals who are economically active. It should also be noted that employment itself can be stressful and result in mental hospital admission (Marshall and Dowdall 1982). Therefore, the stressful effects of work, not merely its loss, need to be considered in predicting mental hospitalization. In addition, the number of people who can be admitted to mental hospitals is affected by a hospital's capacity to house new patients (Marshall and Funch 1979). Consequently, economic measures in relation to hospitalization may not indicate the full extent of the prevalence of mental disorder in a population. Another important problem with this type of research is the complexity of the causal relationship between economic change and mental hospitalization. As Brenner (1973:248) observes, it is this complexity that "probably represents the most serious barrier to the understanding and intellectual credibility of the relationship." It is very difficult to demonstrate a precise cause-and-effect relationship between a major social event like an economic depression and the mental illness of a particular individual because of the wide range of variables that may intervene in the individual's situation and modify the result.

For example, Susan Gore (1978) studied the effect of social support (that is, feelings of being loved, accepted, cared for, and needed by others) on one hundred stably employed, married blue-collar workers who had lost their jobs when two industrial plants, one in a large city and the other in a rural area, closed. These men were interviewed five times during various stages of adjustment (within six months about 90 percent had found new jobs) over a two-year period. Social support in this study was measured by an index reflecting whether the individual rated his wife, friends, and relatives as supportive or unsupportive. In comparison with the supported, Gore found that the unsupported had more severe psychological and health-related problems, felt significantly greater self-blame for being unemployed, and had a greater sense of economic deprivation. Gore suggests that the unsupported were highly dependent upon their jobs for their sense of self-worth. Once they lost their jobs, they lost their usual source of continuing self-esteem. But members of the supported group, in contrast, were able to maintain their view of themselves as valued persons because of the supportive relationships they enjoyed, even though they were unemployed for a time.

Several other studies confirm the importance of social support in lessening the impact of stress and minimizing the potential for severe depression and other forms of mental disorder in individuals (Dean et al. 1990; Gore 1981,

1989; Jacobson 1986; Lin and Ensel 1989; Lin et al. 1979, 1985; Loscocco and Spitze 1990; Matt and Dean 1993; Mitchell and Moos 1984; Norris and Murrell 1984; Pearlin et al. 1981; Thoits 1982, 1984; Turner 1981; Williams, Ware, and Donald 1981). Although the overall contribution of social support to stress reduction varied in these studies, a basic finding is that people who feel they have support from others in dealing with stress tend to have a much stronger sense of well-being than those who lack such support. This circumstance apparently lessens the degree to which psychological distress is experienced.

Macro-Level Analysis: Strength and Weakness

Social and economic circumstances beyond the direct influence or control of the average person create stressful situations that force people to respond, depending upon their individual resources. Depressions, recessions, gas shortages, labor strikes, crop failures, political turmoil, wars, and revolutions all place people in stressful circumstances requiring adjustments in their daily living. The advantage of macro-level forms of analysis is that they can show how these large-scale societal processes affect *groups* of individuals in society. Some particular groups (for example, the lower class, bachelor farmers in western Ireland, the unemployed without social support) seem more prone to mental illness than do other categories of people and can be identified as such. The greatest weakness of macro-level approaches, however, is that it is difficult to trace a direct causal relationship between a major event and the mental disorder of any one particular individual because of the possibility of a great number of intervening variables (for example, personality, social support, genetics, socialization, social class) that for certain people may modify the outcome.

MICRO-LEVEL APPROACHES TO MENTALLY DEVIANT BEHAVIOR

Micro-level approaches to deviant behavior require a shift in perspective from the macro view; here the emphasis is upon the forms and quality of interaction between individuals and within small groups of people. The concern is not so much with the effects of major societal processes upon the individual as with the style of interaction and learning experiences that people construct among themselves. The theoretical perspectives discussed in this section are those of symbolic interaction, including labeling theory, and social learning theory.

Symbolic Interaction

The symbolic interactionist perspective views society from the standpoint of the individual person, not with respect to personality but in the nature of the interaction that person has with other people (Blumer 1969; Mead 1934). It regards the individual as a creative, thinking entity able to choose his or her behavior instead of reacting more or less mechanically to the influence of large-scale social forces, as implied by functionalist theorists. Central to the symbolic interactionist's conception of human behavior is the assumption that all behavior is self-directed on the basis of symbolic meanings that are shared, communicated, and manipulated by interacting human beings in social situations (Denzin 1970a). The process of such interaction between people forms behavior in a creative fashion, rather than being merely a means by which behavior is expressed. Therefore, society is seen as a human product and people are seen as a social product, since both are formed in a continuing dialectical process in which human beings and their social environment act and react toward each other (Berger and Luckmann 1967).

Although the symbolic interactionist tradition in sociology can be traced to the ideas of William James, John Dewey, William I. Thomas, and Charles Cooley at the beginning of the twentieth century, George Herbert Mead (1863–1931) is generally regarded as the individual most responsible for its development. Mead, an American philosopher who taught social psychology at the University of Chicago between 1894 and 1931, published little; yet his book *Mind, Self, and Society* (1934), based upon student notes from his courses and unpublished manuscripts, is a sociological classic. A major interpretation of Mead's work, however, is found in the writings of Herbert Blumer, one of Mead's students, who has drawn together much of the material that is the basis of contemporary symbolic interactionist thought.

Blumer (1969), for example, explains Mead's analysis of social action by denoting its five central features: (1) the self, (2) the act, (3) social interaction, (4) objects, and (5) joint action. Mead believed that the *self* of a person is formed and develops as a result of social interaction and experience with other people; thus, the self is a social product derived from a person's relationships with others in society. In this context, the human being is able to perceive, have conceptions of, communicate with, and act toward himself or herself as a social object in relation to other people. Second is Mead's concept of the *act*. Mead insisted that human beings do not just respond more or less automatically to a given social influence but are able to interpret and define their own particular situation and organize their behavior to meet their circumstances. Blumer says:

> In order to act the individual has to identify what he wants, establish an objective or goal, map out a prospective line of behavior, note and interpret the actions of others, figure out what to do at other points, and frequently spur himself on in the face of dragging dispositions or discouraging settings.[6]

Third is the concept of *social interaction,* which consists of two forms, the nonsymbolic and the symbolic. Nonsymbolic interaction is essentially the stimulus-response paradigm in which a person makes a nonthinking response to a

---

[6]Herbert Blumer, *Symbolic Interactionism* (Englewood Cliffs, NJ: Prentice Hall, 1969), p. 64.

certain stimulus, such as stepping back from a growling dog or raising a hand to catch a baseball. Symbolic interaction, in contrast, is a situation in which human beings interpret and define actions and objects based upon symbolic meanings shared with other people. Fourth is the notion of the *object,* which maintains that objects do not possess inherent meanings but become what they are defined as by human beings interacting with each other. Thus, human beings act toward an object on the basis of the meaning that object has for them. Humans define gold as valuable and act toward it accordingly. Yet there is nothing intrinsic to gold that makes it valuable; the social meaning of gold depends upon how humans define it. Fifth is the *joint act,* which is the focal point by which symbolic interactionists judge group behavior. Each participant in a social gathering brings his or her own individual social act or line of behavior to a situation. By fitting together all of those separate acts or lines of behavior into a single collective or joint act involving each person present, it is possible to ascertain the overall direction of group behavior. The result is that group activities are socially constructed by individual people coming together and interacting with each other in respect to the overall group enterprise. Joint actions may be open to many outcomes; once started they may be interrupted, abandoned, modified, or continued as expected. What happens depends upon what those involved decide to do and how they act upon their decisions.

Joint acts contribute a sense of stability to social situations because they require a participant to identify that activity and orient himself or herself in that direction before engaging in behavior that is appropriate to the scene. Blumer (1969:71) states, "Thus, to act appropriately, the participant has to identify a marriage ceremony as a marriage ceremony, a holdup as a holdup, a debate as a debate, a war as a war, and so forth." However, as pointed out by Norman Denzin (1970b), it is necessary for the study of deviant behavior and, for that matter, all other forms of behavior to go beyond the surface of social situations and extend analysis of the joint act to the more subtle nuances of social relationships between people; for example, those verbal and nonverbal acts and gestures between two persons that signify differing interpretations of a situation in which one participant's view deviates from agreed-upon or taken-for-granted meanings.

We can see in the foregoing analysis of social action that human behavior is regarded as an ongoing process of definition, interpretation of, and calculated response to the actions of others and the conditions of the environment. *Reality is therefore socially constructed as it emanates from the perceptions and actions of those involved.* Consistent and sufficiently bizarre failure in this area is the basis for becoming defined by others as "weird," "crazy," or perhaps "insane."

Labeling Theory: Lemert and Becker

The symbolic interactionist view of deviant behavior has generally been grounded in what has become known in sociology as "labeling theory." Labeling theory is not really a theory at all; it is a view of deviance that qualifies as what Blumer calls a sensitizing concept. It is sensitizing in that it is intended to provide a *general* sense of reference and suggest directions for further inquiry; it is not intended as a definitive statement. Nevertheless, labeling theory has emerged as a major sociological approach to understanding mental disorder. The foundations for labeling theory result principally from the work of two American sociologists, Edwin Lemert and Howard Becker.

Edwin Lemert (1972) argues that studies of deviant behavior need to confront two problems: (1) how deviant behavior originates, and (2) how deviant acts become symbolically attached to certain persons and what the consequences of such attachment are for those individuals. He believes that functionalism had particularly failed to address itself to the latter. Therefore, Lemert (1951) came up with the concept of *primary deviance* and *secondary deviance*. Primary deviance is a situation in which a person who is "normal" acts differently or strangely, but the behavior is rationalized as atypical by others because it is perceived as not characteristic of the person's own true self. Secondary deviance, on the other hand, is more serious because it refers to a situation in which a person is relegated to a deviant role; that is, being deviant is thought to be a typical characteristic of that individual.

Secondary deviance occurs when a person continues over time to violate norms and is subsequently forced by the reactions of other people to assume a deviant role. Alcoholism, for example, can be regarded initially as being a case of primary deviance, but there is the possibility that a heavy drinker can be made to assume a position of secondary deviance by the reactions of others who define that person as an alcoholic. Rejected by normals, the person may be required to find a specific deviant subculture that can accommodate the deviance. Put another way, what may happen is that a person labeled by others as an "alcoholic" may find it difficult to associate with "normals" (moderate drinkers or abstainers). The result may be that the person is forced (if he or she desires companionship) to develop associations with other people who drink heavily or accept alcoholism as normative behavior. Thus, we have the stereotypical situation of the once socially acceptable person whose heavy drinking habits eventually lead to a disruption of normal relationships and downward social mobility into a world of alcoholics and "skid-row" living conditions in which heavy drinking is the norm.

Lemert also points out that the roles and relationships that are made available to the individual after labeling may be used to sustain a deviant identity. Lemert uses the example of women labeled as prostitutes who develop close "love" relationships with their pimps or perhaps with other women in lesbian relationships to resolve their conflicts about being seen by society as deviant. Although such relationships offer an emotional buffer against exclusion from the regular company of normals, they also confirm a continuing deviant status for the women. Lemert's analysis thus implicates an identity for deviants that is more or less lasting once the label has been applied.

Becker made further contributions to labeling theory through the insight in his book *Outsiders* (1973). In it he argues that social groups create deviance by making rules whose infraction constitutes deviance. *Deviance is therefore not a quality of the act a person commits but rather is a consequence of the definition applied to the act by others.* Whether an act is deviant thus depends on how other people react to it. However, the responses of other people are problematic because their interpretation of the situation is the deciding factor, and not all people see things the same way. The focus of *Outsiders* is upon marijuana smokers who view marijuana use as normative behavior in their own subculture but who are criminals in the eyes of the wider society.

Other factors may also be important to how people respond to deviance. Becker says, for instance, that responses to a particular act may vary over time; if there is a police "crackdown" on gambling, responses to gambling may be harsh, but at another time and for the same offense they could be more lenient. Responses to deviant behavior also depend upon *who* commits the act and *who* feels harmed by it. In this case, Becker observes that rules tend to be applied more to some people than to others. A lower-class delinquent male may be more likely to be arrested, convicted, and sentenced than an upper- or middle-class delinquent male committing the same offense. Also, some rules are enforced only when they result in certain consequences. Here, Becker suggests that an adolescent couple having premarital sex may suffer little social censure unless the girl becomes pregnant; then several people are likely to become upset.

Becker illustrates his view of deviant behavior as follows:[7]

Types of Deviant Behavior

	OBEDIENT BEHAVIOR	RULE-BREAKING BEHAVIOR
Perceived as deviant	Falsely accused	Pure deviant
Not perceived as deviant	Conforming	Secret deviant

In this typology, Becker notes that some behavior can be classified as obedient to rules and other behavior as rule breaking, yet whether a particular individual is defined as deviant depends upon the perceptions of others. In the category of obedient behavior we have the "conformist," who is not perceived as deviant and is not deviant in fact; then we have the "falsely accused," who is perceived as deviant but is in fact innocent. Under rule-breaking behavior, we have the "pure" deviant, who is both deviant and perceived as such and the "secret" deviant, who is deviant but not perceived as such. An example of a secret deviant would be a male who wears female

---

[7]Howard S. Becker, *Outsiders: Studies in the Sociology of Deviance* (New York: Free Press, 1973), p. 20.

undergarments in the privacy of his home or who becomes sexually aroused by leather or whips and chains but is careful to conceal that behavior from others.

Thus, the labeling approach stresses that judgments of what is deviance are relative, depending upon the perceptions of others. Therefore, the critical variable in understanding deviant behavior is the social audience that has knowledge of the act in question because the audience determines what is and what is not deviant.

But despite its merits in providing a framework to analyze the variety of perceptions people may hold about deviant acts and deviant persons, labeling theory contains some serious weaknesses. Lemert's concentration upon the transition from primary deviance to secondary deviance neglects the issue of what caused the deviance in the first place. This criticism can be applied to labeling theory as a whole because societal reaction alone does not explain why certain people commit deviant acts and why others in the same circumstances do not. A label in itself does not cause deviance. Some situations (for example, crime, homosexuality, alcoholism, drug addiction, suicide, mental disorder) are generally defined by most people as being deviant—yet people do these things regardless of how they are labeled, and their reasons for doing so may have nothing to do with the label that is attached to them. Another problem is Becker's notion of the secret deviant. If a deviant status is obtained from the reaction of the social audience, how does a secret deviant become "deviant" if no one knows about it? Becker (1973) attempts to refute this criticism by claiming that secret deviance consists of being vulnerable to discovery, that is, of being in a position in which it would be easy to make a deviant label stick. In this circumstance, the secret deviant *knows* he or she will be labeled deviant if discovered. But here again, this does not tell us how or why the deviance began in the first place. As British criminologist Ian Taylor and his colleagues (1973:153) note, the labeling approach "*avoids the question of initial deviation* and drives it towards a dubious stress on the psychological impact of social reaction" (emphasis in original). Becker adds, however, that it is not his intent to explain the cause of deviance. His intent is to enlarge the area of consideration in the study of deviant behavior by implicating the role of people other than the allegedly deviant person. Becker (1973:179) remarks that it would be foolish to propose that stick-up men stick up people simply because someone has labeled them stick-up men; hence, labeling cannot be considered the only explanation of what deviants actually do.

Another deficiency of labeling theory rests in its attempts to explain the characteristics of deviants and deviant acts. Jack Gibbs (1971) notes that if deviant acts and actors do share characteristics other than societal reaction, such characteristics are not defined or explained. Deviant behavior is often an action constructed by individuals to cope with problems brought on by a social situation over which they have little control. Other people may have similar problems and react in a similar manner. Thus, not only might there be a common "cause" for their deviant acts, but also the acts and the people committing them may share many other similarities (for example, poverty, stress, race, age, family background). Or in other cases, an individual may have control over his or her social situation but may still opt for being deviant for a variety of reasons (for example, self-punishment, thrills, personal gain). Again, there may be some sharing of characteristics concerning the deviant acts and actors, and those characteristics may be as important as, if not more important than, the reaction of the social audience. In fact, the reaction of the social audience may not be especially relevant in accounting for the type of person exhibiting deviant behavior. Gibbs thus raises the question of *what* is being explained by labeling theory—deviant behavior or *reactions* to deviant behavior? If reactions to deviant behavior is the answer, then one should ask whether deviance can be explained exclusively in terms of societal reaction. As previously noted, the best answer seems to be that it cannot.

In line with their symbolic interactionist heritage, labeling theorists also maintain that individual behavior is not automatically determined by social situations and structures; it is derived from how people define what they and others do based upon free choice. Yet once a person is labeled "deviant," labeling theorists seem to place the labeled individual in circumstances in which that person has little or no choice about what happens. That is, once labeled, the deviant person is forced to assume a deviant status in society because that is how he or she is perceived and treated by others. Although it might seem a contradiction to assert that initially people have a choice about being deviant and later they do not (when they are labeled), one strength of labeling theory lies in recognizing the transition from primary to secondary deviance. Sometimes, people do not have choices in how they are treated by others, regardless of their intentions. Ronald Akers offers the best summary of this:

> Rather, although those of this school come dangerously close to saying that the actual behavior is unimportant, their contribution to the study of deviancy comes precisely in their conception of the impact of labeling on behavior. One sometimes gets the impression from reading this literature that people go about minding their own business and then—"wham"—bad society comes along and slaps them with a stigmatized label. Forced into the role of deviant the individual has little choice but to be deviant. This is an exaggeration of course, but such an image can be gained easily from an over-emphasis on the impact of labeling. However, it is exactly this image, toned down and made reasonable, which is the central contribution of the labeling school to the sociology of deviance.[8]

Becker (1973) makes essentially the same point when he agrees that one of the most important contributions of labeling theory is that it does

---

[8]Ronald L. Akers, "Problems in the Sociology of Deviance: Social Definitions and Behavior," *Social Forces* 46 (1967), 463.

focus attention on how labeling places a person in circumstances that make it difficult to continue acting normal and to follow the routines of everyday life, thus provoking the person to act "abnormal." The example Becker uses is a former convict whose prison record makes it almost impossible to get a responsible, well-paying job and predisposes the convict to return to a life of crime.

We can see this situation clearly in David Rosenhan's (1973) study of voluntary mental hospital admissions. Rosenhan organized a group of eight supposedly normal persons—a psychiatrist, a pediatrician, a painter, a housewife, a psychology graduate student, and three psychology professors—who presented themselves for admission as schizophrenics at twelve different mental hospitals located in five states on both the East and the West coasts. All were admitted, and once in the hospital they immediately reverted to their usual normal behavior. Yet, despite their show of sanity after some initial nervousness over actually being in a mental hospital, the pseudopatients were never detected by the hospital staffs as being "fakes." Rather, it was the "real" patients who correctly identified the pseudopatients as imposters. For example, all the pseudopatients took, in an obvious fashion, extensive notes on their confinement experiences. This writing was viewed by the staffs as being just another aspect of their pathological behavior. The closest any staff member came to questioning what the note taking was all about was when one pseudopatient asked his physician about the kind of medication he was receiving. " 'You needn't write it,' he was told gently. 'If you have trouble remembering, just ask me again' " (Rosenhan 1973:252). Conversely, the real patients accused the pseudopatients of being either journalists or college professors who were "checking up" on the hospital.

Rosenhan believed that the failure of the hospital staff to discover the pseudopatients (length of hospitalization ranged from seven to fifty-two days, with an average of nineteen days) illustrates the power of labeling in psychiatric assessment. Once labeled as schizophrenics, there was nothing the pseudopatients could do to overcome an identification that profoundly affected the perceptions of other people about them and their behavior. Their release from the mental hospital was contingent upon the staff's accepting the idea that the nonexistent schizophrenia was in "remission." Rosenhan comments:

> Despite their public "show" of sanity, the pseudo-patients were never detected. Admitted, except in one case, with a diagnosis of schizophrenia, each was discharged with a diagnosis of schizophrenia "in remission." The label "in remission" should in no way be dismissed as a formality, for at no time during any hospitalization had any question been raised about any pseudo-patient's simulation.

Nor are there any indications in the hospital records that the pseudo-patient's status was suspect. Rather, the evidence is strong that, once labeled schizophrenic, the pseudo-patient was stuck with that label.[9]

Labeling Theory: Scheff and Gove

The sociologist who is best known for linking labeling theory and mental disorder is Thomas Scheff. In reviewing the labeling approach to deviance, Scheff (1984) observes that mere rule breaking is not enough in itself to cause others to respond to the rule breaker as mentally ill. Scheff, has, therefore, added the concept of *residual rule breaking* to the labeling view of mental illness. Residual rule breaking is based upon the idea that most social conventions or norms are fairly clear and understood, yet there is a residual area of social convention that is assumed to be so natural that it is part of "human nature." These residual conventions include such behaviors as looking at the person you are talking to or responding to someone who calls your name. To violate these residual conventions goes beyond just violating norms; it involves acting contrary to human nature. Such "unnatural" behavior may come to be regarded by others as mental illness.

Scheff further suggests that social stereotypes profoundly shape the symptoms of mental disorder in American society. Although he does not specify what those stereotypes are, he implies that they consist of acting bizarre or violent or some combination thereof. Scheff claims that people as young as elementary school children have grasped the literal meaning of "crazy." Such meanings are part of our culture, he says, as illustrated by the general understanding of phrases like "The boogie man will get you." Scheff goes on to point out that the cultural stereotype of insanity stays with us into adulthood and is continually reinforced through social interaction; in fact, it is often the basis for our manner of reacting to people who have already been labeled insane. Furthermore, this stereotype is available to the patient and becomes part of the patient's orientation for guiding his or her own "crazy" behavior. Thus, in brief, Scheff considers mental disorder a social role whose behavior conforms to society's expectations of people who are "crazy."

Depending upon certain contingencies, such as the identity of the rule breaker, the particular rule broken, the amount of tolerance available, any alternative explanation that might clarify or rationalize the behavior, and the social context in which the rule-breaking behavior takes place, the residual rule breaker may be publicly labeled "mentally ill." Scheff contends that when a person has been labeled "mentally ill" and people respond to that person in

---

[9]David C. Rosenhan, "On Being Sane in Insane Places," *Science* 179 (1973), 251.

accordance with that label, a deviant has been created by society. Scheff points out that at some time virtually everyone acts crazy. But if a person is labeled mentally ill and comes to the attention of a community's formal system of social control for mental illness, he argues that the person will be processed and sent to a mental hospital largely as a matter of routine. When this occurs, that person will be "launched on a career of 'chronic' mental illness" and is thus irreparably stigmatized as a mental patient (Scheff 1975a:10).

Scheff's views, however, have promoted considerable debate among scholars attempting to determine the role of labeling in cases of mental disorder. In a comparison of American (Seattle) and German (Frankfurt) high school students, mental hospital staffs, and mental patients, John Marshall Townsend (1975a, 1975b, 1978) found that stereotypes of insanity did not serve as guidelines for acting mentally ill as suggested by Scheff. The most common stereotype of mental disorder, notes Townsend, is that of wild, uncontrollable, and dangerous behavior. But that stereotype was not prevalent among students, hospital staff members, or patients. Nor were such stereotypes prevalent among Michigan high school students studied by Donald Olmsted and Dorothy Smith (1980).

In another study, of elementary school children in California, Donald Baker, John Bedell, and Lorraine Prinsky (1982) determined that young children were familiar with simple concepts like "crazy," "nuts," and "cuckoo," but not psychiatric terms like "emotionally disturbed," "insane," or "mentally ill." There was some notion of crazy behavior as residual rule breaking among the children, yet they did not appear to have learned stereotypes of mental illness from the mass media as suggested by Scheff. Rather, their concepts of mental illness appeared to have come largely from parents. The study by Baker and associates does provide partial support to Scheff's notion of residual rule breaking, but to understand mental illness, more research is needed about the manner in which people are socialized.

Walter Gove (1970a, 1970b, 1975a, 1975b) has been the leading critic of Scheff and the labeling approach to mental illness. Gove emphasizes that Scheff views mental disorder as being primarily dependent upon conditions external to the individual. Those "conditions," of course, are the responses of the social audience who base their actions toward the person in question upon the label that results from their interpretation of the situation. Consequently, Gove (1975a:67) replies: "The labeling perspective does not view the deviant as someone who is suffering from an intrapersonal disorder, but instead as someone who, through a set of circumstances, becomes publicly labeled a deviant and who is forced by societal reaction into a deviant role." Gove (1975a:48–51) suggests, in contrast, that studies providing evidence of genetics, stress from critical life events, and the expression of symptoms by mental patients indicate there is much more to mental illness than simply labeling.

Gove's argument has three central themes. First, he rejects the notion that lower-class people are more readily labeled as mentally ill than the affluent because he feels there is quicker recognition of it and less tolerance for it among members of the upper social strata. Second, being labeled mentally ill does not, in his view, result in lasting stigma for former mental patients. And third, he believes that those people who are mentally ill have an inherent mental condition quite apart from how they are labeled.

This last criticism is especially important because it recognizes that mentally ill people have something wrong with them, regardless of how they are labeled (Cockerham 1979). For example, Marvin Krohn and Ronald Akers (1977) also note that individuals are not randomly or capriciously singled out and labeled mentally ill, even though extrapsychiatric factors influence outcomes and psychiatric diagnoses, and diagnostic categories may sometimes be vague and inconsistent. Regardless of the theory involved, inferences of mental disorder are made from verbal and nonverbal behavior. These behavioral cues indicate what must be done about hospitalization or release in the first place. They indicate the ability of the person in question to affect or react to the situation. Therefore, what seems apparent is that before the onset of labeling, there may exist a troubled mind independent of the labeling process. Once the individual who possesses that troubled mind expresses his or her internal state to others, extrapsychiatric factors then intervene to influence the responses to and decisions about the individual in question.

This situation represents the most important weakness in the application of labeling theory to mental disorder. Labeling theory does not explain what actually causes mental disorder, other than societal reaction to residual rule breaking, nor does it explain why certain people become mentally ill and why others in the same social circumstances do not. Gove was clearly justified in questioning the efficacy of labeling theory. Although not all his criticisms seem warranted, particularly the issue of who in society is most likely to be committed, his criticisms pertaining to the social consequences of being labeled mentally ill and the inherent nature of mental disorders find considerable support. Yet Scheff's version of labeling theory should not be dismissed as wrong. Both Scheff and Gove note that it is not simply a case of one view being entirely false and the other being entirely correct. Both viewpoints contain important contributions. Even if Gove's position regarding the social consequences of being labeled mentally ill seems justified for the long-term situation (that the stigma gradually diminishes if the former mental patient continues to act normal over time), it does not lessen the findings from studies such as those by Rosenhan (1973) that point to the very powerful effects of labeling in temporary circumstances.

The merit of Scheff's work and of labeling theory in general is that it (1) recognizes the problematic aspects of reaction to mental disorder and (2) explains how people labeled as mentally ill may be forced into a deviant role because of how other people respond to them.

Social Learning Theory

The other micro-level theoretical perspective in sociology relevant to our discussion of mental disorder is social learning theory. Social learning theory is similar to symbolic interaction and labeling theory in that each approach focuses upon social interaction as the key to understanding human behavior. But whereas symbolic interactionists view the subjective meanings attached to behavior as a critical focus of inquiry and investigation, social learning theorists deemphasize interest in a person's subjective processes because they believe that verbal reports of internal states are suspect or unreliable. Instead, they focus on behavior that is *directly observable and measurable.*

Social learning theory is a relatively new theoretical approach in sociology and stems from learning theory in psychology, especially the work of B. F. Skinner (1971). Skinner advocates that behavior is shaped and maintained by its consequences. Briefly stated, behavior that affects the environment in such a way as to produce either positive or negative consequences is called *operant behavior.* Operant behavior is not a reflex action; it is voluntary and governed by the central nervous system. This contrasts with *respondent behavior,* which is involuntary and controlled by the autonomic nervous system. Stimuli that follow or are contingent upon an operant behavior determine the probability of that behavior occurring again because of either positive or negative reinforcement, or punishment. Besides behavior being maintained through the feedback processes of reinforcement and punishment, social learning theorists posit that it is also regulated through continuous association with a stimulus (classical or operant conditioning) or higher-level cognitive processes that specify appropriate responses according to one's tested methods of obtaining reward (Bandura 1969).

The first notable sociologist to utilize a learning perspective was George C. Homans (1961), who, following Skinner, noted that the more rewarding a social activity was, the more likely it was to be repeated. Homans's contribution was to analyze the ways in which the behavior of people in social groups influenced the actions of others who, in turn, react to influence the responses of those initiating the behavior. In regard to deviant behavior, Robert Burgess and Ronald Akers (1966) have formulated the most sophisticated statement of deviance and social learning theory to date by incorporating the principles of learning theory and Edwin Sutherland's (1939; Sutherland and Cressey 1974) theory of differential association into a single approach. Sutherland believed that people who commit criminal acts do so because they have learned from associating with others that such behavior is more advantageous than law-abiding conduct. Burgess and Akers (Akers 1977:42–43) hypothesize, accordingly, that deviant behavior is learned through the principles of operant behavior. This learning takes place in situations that can be either social or nonsocial, as long as they involve reinforcement. The core learning process occurs in those groups that are the primary source of the individual's reinforcement of behavior. Deviant behavior thus becomes a function of the effective and available reinforcers and the deviant norms, rules, and definitions that have usually accompanied the reinforcement during group interaction. Differential reinforcement of deviant over conforming behavior will increase the probability that a person will commit a deviant act. Just how strong the deviant behavior is depends upon the amount, frequency, and probability of its reinforcement.

Akers (1977; Krohn and Akers 1977) has proposed that mental disorder should be viewed sociologically as learned behavior that constitutes a form of adaptation to one's social environment. Akers explains:

> Mental illness involves one or more of the following behavior patterns: (1) autonomic, visceral, and emotional responses which have been conditioned to respond to stimuli which ordinarily do not elicit them; (2) inappropriate or unusual actions which have been learned through (a) imitation and modeling, (b) direct social attention and socialization, (c) avoiding aversive situations; (3) behavioral deficits (failures to develop adequate repertoires of social skills); (4) "delusional," symbolically constructed definitions of the situation which are directly reinforced (either positively or negatively reinforced by providing excuses for not performing roles and so on), or which are discriminative for other behavior.[10]

If a person continues to act abnormally because of one or more of the above learned behaviors, that person is likely to be labeled mentally ill and placed in the role of a mental patient. Assumption of such a role, says Akers, may be enough to cause a person to change his or her behavior so that the reinforcement sustaining the behavior is likewise changed and the behavioral problem is resolved. Or being formally labeled mentally ill may reinforce the behavior and cause that behavior to become stabilized. Akers supports his perspective by drawing upon studies that show how learning has affected the quality of symptoms among mental patients. Specifically he draws upon such situations as "token economies" in mental hospitals in which patients have been rewarded with "tokens" ("chips," "points," and the like) for normal behavior, which can be converted into privileges (abnormal behavior goes unrewarded), thus resulting in reductions of insane acts on hospital wards. He also discusses Erving Goffman's classic study *Asylums* (1961), noting the manner in which mental patients learned strategies for dealing with the conditions of their hospitalization, and a study of paranoia by Lemert (1962). According to Lemert, the paranoid was denied feedback on the consequences of his or her behavior

---

[10]Ronald L. Akers, *Deviant Behavior: A Social Learning Approach,* 2nd ed. (Belmont, CA: Wadsworth, 1977), pp. 329–30.

through exclusion brought on by acting unpleasant. Sensing rejection and exclusion, paranoid reactions are reinforced, and the paranoid person becomes more mistrusting.

Few would deny that most behavior is learned through social interaction and that people tend to repeat those behaviors they find rewarding or avoid those behaviors for which they are punished. Hence, an understanding of learning principles can provide important insight into how abnormal behavior is sustained and reinforced. Moreover, when the study of mental illness is considered, social learning theory offers the advantage of being allied with a major therapy, behavior modification, with which it shares similar conceptual principles.

Yet social learning theory has not attracted the volume of attention in sociology that it has received in psychology. Some sociologists have rejected social learning theory because it generally neglects subjective processes that determine the social meanings and attitudes that shape overt acts of behavior. Some would argue that social learning theory does not account for why certain behaviors come to be considered deviant and others do not, or how societies organize their resources to control deviance. Also, although it can be argued that symptoms of mental illness can be learned and that the probability is high that abnormal styles of behavior are shared within family clusters, social learning theory requires that the mentally ill person is able to learn or, in other words, has some ego strength that allows him or her to discriminate among conditions. In severe forms of mental disorders, especially advanced cases of schizophrenia or extreme catatonic states, clearly something is wrong with the patient beyond the mere learning and reinforcement of abnormal responses. In addition, much of the social learning perspective in psychology is based upon laboratory research on animals, which may not be translatable to the general social environment for humans. But the biggest problem with social learning theory is that it fails to determine whether mental disorders are really nothing more than learned, maladaptive behaviors acquired in the same way one acquires normal behavior (Goldenberg 1977).

Micro-Level Analysis: Strength and Weakness

Micro-level perspectives show individual people to be information-processing entities forming their responses to the social environment according to their interaction with other people. Through the cognitive processes of learning, interpreting, and defining a situation, people come to share meanings derived from common social experiences and expressed symbolically in language. Whether an individual is considered insane within this context depends upon how well that person's representation of reality compares with the conceptions held by others. Thus, the strength of micro-level theories lies in their ability to explain how people view their everyday lives, including those instances in which mental disorder becomes the focus of concern. Symbolic interaction offers a definite advantage over social learning theory in this regard because of its emphasis upon subjective processes, which form the basis for the active expression of behavior. Yet social learning theory, with its grounding in experimental psychology, has attempted to cope with concepts of personality and emotion to a much greater extent than has symbolic interaction. In essence, however, both symbolic interaction and social learning theory account for behavior patterns on an interpersonal level, which is central to understanding mental disorder. Additionally, symbolic interaction, through labeling theory, provides important insight into how people react to those labeled insane.

A major problem for both symbolic interaction and social learning theory beyond those just described is linking individual and small-group behavior to the larger social order. Just as macro-level theories have difficulty showing a direct tie to the lives of individual people, micro-level theories often do not adequately acknowledge the influence of larger social structures and organizations within which people interact with one another. However, the Scheper-Hughes (1979) study of western rural Ireland discussed earlier in this chapter is an excellent example of a work that blends macro processes (low agricultural production, migration of youth, and so on) with micro processes (the double bind of the last-born son) to explain the prevalence of schizophrenia among bachelor farmers. More research of this type is needed.

SUMMARY

This chapter has reviewed the major *macro* (conflict and functionalist) theories and *micro* (symbolic interactionism and social learning) theories employed by sociologists to study that variant of deviant behavior known as mental illness. Although no one theoretical perspective is able to provide all the answers needed to understand fully the social ramifications of mental disorder, each makes a significant contribution to the field.

5

Mental Disorder: Social Epidemiology

A major sociological contribution to the study of mental disorder has been to pinpoint and describe the most significant sociodemographic factors in determining the social characteristics of who is most likely to become mentally ill and the type of mental disorder most prevalent in a particular social group. Sociologists also estimate the prevalence of mental disorder in the general population. Accordingly, it is the purpose of this chapter to review what we currently know about the social epidemiology of mental disorder. Social epidemiology in this case pertains to the measurement and analysis of social patterns of mental disorder. This chapter will also examine some of the problems in measuring the "true" prevalence of mental disorder.

EPIDEMIOLOGICAL METHODS

Epidemiology in its most narrow sense refers to the science of epidemics. However, modern-day epidemiologists work with any health problem, whether it stems from communicable disease, chronic illnesses, mental disorder, environmental pollution, smoking, automobile accidents, suicide, or whatever. The focus of the epidemiologist is not on the individual but on the *health problems of social aggregates or large groups of people*. The role of the epidemiologist is not unlike that of a detective investigating the scene of a crime, except in this situation the criminal is a threat to the health of a group of people. Once the epidemiologists find the cause of the health problem, they can try to eliminate or control the threat. To do this, they gather information from whatever sources are relevant to the problem under investigation, including laboratory tests, clinical examinations, personal interviews, and reviews of hospitals' and physicians' records. The epidemiologists then construct a logical chain of inferences to explain the various factors and conditions in a society that cause a particular health problem.

There are several important concepts that epidemiologists use in describing the health problems of humans. One is the definition of a *case*. A *case*, in epidemiological terms, refers to an instance of disorder, illness, or injury involving a person. Another term is *risk*, defined simply as exposure to a health problem. In ascertaining the rate of admissions to state and county mental hospitals in the United States during a particular year, the epidemiologist would consider the population at risk to be the entire population at that time, and the number of cases to be the actual number of admissions to mental hospitals. To calculate the admissions rate, the number of cases (the numerator) would be divided by the number of persons in the population (the denominator), and the results would be multiplied by 1,000, 10,000, or 100,000, depending on whether the rate was being figured for the number of admissions per 1,000, per 10,000, or per 100,000 persons. The formula for computing the 1996 admissions rate for state and county mental hospitals in the United States would be as follows:

$$\frac{\text{Total state and county mental hospital admissions, 1996}}{\text{Estimated U.S. population on June 30, 1996}} \times 100{,}000 = \begin{array}{l}\text{State and county}\\\text{mental hospital}\\\text{admissions rate for}\\\text{1996 per 100,000}\end{array}$$

Computing ratios is a primary method by which epidemiologists describe the extent of health problems in a particular population. The admissions rate for state and county mental hospitals as discussed above is an example of a *crude rate*. A crude rate is the simplest ratio calculated by epidemiologists; it deals with just the number of persons (cases) who have the characteristics being measured during a specific unit of time. Birth and death rates are other examples of crude rates. Crude rates, however, may be too gross a measure to be useful in understanding significant differences within the population; therefore, other rates are used to measure specific variables such as age, sex, race, or any other characteristic of interest. *Age-specific rates* are computed in the same way as crude rates, except that the numerator and the denominator are confined to a specific age group (a similar method can be used to determine sex-specific rates, race-specific rates, and the like). To calculate an age-specific rate, the procedure is to subdivide a population by age and then compare the number of cases in that subpopulation with the total number of persons within the subpopulation. If one wanted to compute the 1996 age-specific state and county mental hospital admissions rates for all American eighteen- to twenty-four-year-olds, one would need to know how many eighteen- to twenty-four-year-olds there were in that year and the number of admissions there were in that age-specific group.

$$\frac{\text{Total state and county mental hospital admissions of 18- to 24-year-olds, 1996}}{\text{Estimated number of 18- to 24-year-olds in the U.S. population on June 30, 1996}} \times 100{,}000 = \begin{array}{l}\text{State and county mental hospital admissions rate for 18- to 24-year-olds for 1996, per 100,000 18- to 24-year-olds}\end{array}$$

Two other terms commonly used in epidemiology are *incidence* and *prevalence*. Incidence refers to the number of *new* cases of a specific health disorder occurring within a given population during a stated period of time. The incidence of schizophrenia in the United States in 1996 would be the number of people in that year first diagnosed as schizophrenic. *Prevalence*, in contrast, would be the *total* number of cases of a health disorder that exists at any given time. Prevalence would include new cases as well as all previously existing cases. Prevalence rates are sometimes expressed as *point prevalence* (the number of cases at a certain point in time, usually a particular day or week), *period prevalence* (the total number of cases during a specified period of time, usually a month or a year), or *lifetime prevalence* (the number of people who have had the disorder at least once during their lifetimes). One way to distinguish between incidence and prevalence is to regard incidence as the rate of appearance of cases, and prevalence as the rate of existence of cases. An example of the difference between incidence and prevalence would be a circumstance in which the incidence of schizophrenia in a community might be low because no new cases had developed during the period of time in question. Yet a measure of prevalence might be high because it would represent all people who are currently diagnosed as schizophrenic. Although this example pertains to schizophrenia, the same definitions and terms may apply to any epidemiological investigation.

The focus of this book, however, is not upon the general field of epidemiology or upon epidemiological research on problems of physical health. Instead, the concern here is with the social epidemiology of mental disorder and the analysis of those variables that are of particular sociological interest in such work—namely, indicators of social class, sex (in relation to sex roles), marital status, race, and so forth. The primary method of gathering data for this type of research is the survey, often supplemented by secondary sources such as health records, mental hospital admissions data, and use of key informants (other people) to verify the situations in question. The survey gathers data from relatively large selected samples of a population or perhaps from the entire population of a small community. If it is a sample of a population, that sample should be representative of the total population; that is, the background characteristics of the sample should be approximately the same as those of the larger population. The study should be designed so that every individual in the population has about the same probability of being selected as part of the sample. Strategies for accomplishing this are to use a *simple random sample* (assigning numbers to individuals or households and selecting the sample by using a table of random numbers) or an *area sample* (random selection of households within a specified geographical area, that is, certain blocks in a city). Sometimes nonprobability samples (everyone in the total population will not have the same probability of being selected) are used. These include the *stratified random sample* (only certain strata are surveyed, and a random sample is taken of that particular stratum; for example, only persons belonging to certain age groups and not to others) and the *cluster sample* (grouping individuals on the basis of common characteristics and selecting randomly within each cluster).

Interviews may be conducted by telephone, or questionnaires may be sent out through the mail, but in studies of the social patterns of mental disorder, personal, face-to-face interviews are often used. Interviewers typically gather information about the respondent's past history of mental disorder and a description of current mental health problems and also may assess the respondent's mental health. Interviewers may be trained to make such assessments; psychiatrists or other mental health professionals may be part of the interview team; or interviewers may record the respondent's reactions and possible symptoms for a psychiatrist's later determination of possible mental disorder. This presents special problems in surveys of mental health. Most epidemiological research identifies a tangible, objectively documented health threat, such as bacteria or exposure to chemical pollution of the environment. Such threats may originate in a single source and be relatively easy to find (contaminated food) or difficult to discover (Legionnaires' Disease). Or they may be derived from several sources and have a relatively complex pattern of interaction, such as that demonstrated in the Framingham, Massachusetts, heart disease research project. The Framingham study, ongoing since the 1950s, identified male sex, advancing age, high blood pressure, cigarette smoking, diabetes, and obesity as significant risk factors for developing heart disease (Sytokowski, Kannel, and D'Agostino 1990). Mental disorders, however, do not readily lend themselves to precise cause-and-effect relationships. Psychiatric disturbances, as previously discussed, may be caused by a variety of factors, such as stress, childhood experiences and developmental problems, deprivation, and genetic or biochemical defects. The exact cause or causes are not known, and the relationships between possible variables are not fully understood. Therefore, assessments of mental disorders are based largely upon subjective criteria or the opinion of the observer according to whatever evidence is available.

There are also claims that the diagnostic categories in the American Psychiatric Association's 1980 Diagnostic and Statistical Manual of Mental Disorders-III (DSM-III) are not precise enough measures of mental disorders (Mirowsky and Ross 1989a) and were not adequately tested (Kirk and Kutchins 1992). The categories for the various disorders were largely developed on the basis of clinical experience and consensus among psychiatrists and there were tests involving over six hundred patients (Klerman 1989). This was the first time an entire psychiatric diagnostic system had been empirically tested. Furthermore, some of the diagnostic categories, such as bipolar disorders, were previously supported by strong evidence of their validity (Swartz, Carroll, and Blazer 1989). And many concepts in the social sciences likewise rest on professional consensus rather than documented empirical validity (Tweed and George 1989).

Because of inconsistencies in DSM-III, revisions and corrections were made by a work group appointed by the American Psychiatric Association. That effort resulted in the publication of DSM-III-R (Revised) in 1987. Additional literature reviews, data reanalyses, and new field trials at seventy different sites involving over 6,000 subjects were subsequently incorporated into the new DSM-IV, published in 1994. DSM-IV claims that its diagnostic categories are based on empirical evidence to a greater extent than any previous classification system of mental disorders. A particular refinement is the inclusion of symptoms specific to certain cultures. However, DSM-IV also notes that it is intended as a guideline and that not all individuals having the same mental disorder will be alike. The American Psychiatric Association nevertheless maintains that DSM-IV reflects a consensus among psychiatrists at the time of its publication about the classification and diagnosis of mental disorders.

DSM-IV is not intended to be the final word on diagnosis in psychiatry, nor is it possible to have a definitive classification system at present—given the current state of knowledge about mental disorder. Yet, on balance, the DSM-IV categories are a significant improvement over past diagnostic systems; they also can be tested and modified on the basis of new research findings.

Although professionals and laypeople may agree about the mental disorder of some individuals, they may disagree about the mental health of others. Moreover, as will be discussed in the next section of this chapter, there can be a lack of consensus even among psychiatrists. Also, sufficient numbers of psychiatrists may not be available to participate in large-scale epidemiological investigations. It is then necessary to rely on trained interviewers to obtain valid and reliable information. *Validity* in scientific research pertains to an instrument's ability to measure what it is intended to measure. *Reliability* is an instrument's ability to produce consistent results over time. An instrument can be reliable (consistent) but not valid (accurate). To be considered valid, an instrument must be pretested on a representative sample of persons and refined to the point at which it accurately reflects the reality of what it is trying to measure. Response bias, which is the use of items that might be meaningful to some (for example, middle-class) and not to other (for example, lower-class) respondents, must be avoided. There are also serious questions of both validity and reliability in surveys in which psychiatrists diagnose mental disorder in people they have never seen. Nevertheless, surveys of communities are the most common method for estimating the prevalence of mental disorder in the general population (Schwab and Schwab 1978). Obviously, any survey of this nature has methodological problems, and even the most careful studies are estimates at best.

One of the most effective survey instruments yet developed is the Diagnostic Interview Schedule (DIS) used successfully in the National Institute of Mental Health's (NIMH) Epidemiologic Catchment Area (ECA) Program. This program is a continuing cooperative effort between NIMH and five universities to measure mental health in a random sample of the general population in particular cities: New Haven (Yale), Baltimore (Johns Hopkins), St. Louis (Washington), Durham, North Carolina (Duke), and Los Angeles (UCLA). DSM-III provides the diagnostic categories used in the DIS. The DIS is a survey questionnaire on which an individual's history of past mental symptoms and problems is recorded and a computer assigns a diagnosis. The interviewer does not have to be a psychiatrist, because an extensively pretested and validated computer program is used for the analysis. The ECA Program, involving the cooperation of psychiatrists, psychologists, sociologists, and other behavioral scientists, represents the most complex and sophisticated effort ever used to measure the mental health of large, noninstitutionalized populations (Eaton and Kessler 1985).

In 1990, the DIS was furthered refined into the Composite International Diagnostic Interview (CIDI) utilizing diagnostic categories in the improved DSM-III-R. The CIDI, developed and tested by the World Health Organization, is a state-of-the-art structured diagnostic interview based on the DIS and designed to be used by trained interviewers who are not clinicians (Kessler et al. 1994). The capability of survey researchers to measure mental health is consistently improving.

THE "TRUE" PREVALENCE OF MENTAL DISORDER

It is difficult (perhaps impossible) to know the "true" or actual extent of mental disorders in a large society because many disordered people escape detection. Still, estimates are needed for a variety of purposes (for example, planning, program development, estimating the need for services, and construction of facilities). Estimates of true prevalence are therefore important. Studies of admissions to psychiatric facilities on either an inpatient or an outpatient basis cannot account for the true prevalence of mental disorder because they do not include untreated cases that fail to come to the attention of mental health reporting agencies. Admissions rates may also be affected by the availability of facilities (thereby limiting the number of people who can be admitted) and by the amount of tolerance for abnormal behavior in a family or a community.

To determine the true prevalence of mental disorders, it is necessary to count both treated and untreated cases. Research conducted several years ago by Barbara and Bruce Dohrenwend (1974) identified some eighty studies published between 1900 and the early 1970s that attempted to determine true prevalence. Those studies had been carried out in several countries. Usually, they included entire populations living in a particular geographical area. Or when such studies have relied on estimates from samples of a population, those samples have generally been quite large. Not surprisingly, when information was "provided on which 'cases' were in treatment and which were not, the consistent result has been that only small minorities of the 'cases' were ever psychiatric patients" (Bruce Dohrenwend 1975:366). The great majority of mentally disordered people are untreated and at large in the community.

Although the reader might be skeptical that a mentally disordered person would be able to escape identification and treatment, consider that persons with mood, anxiety, and personality disorders might well avoid coming to the attention of mental health professionals. Instead, they might be viewed by their associates as people who were particularly depressive, or nervous, or who had some serious personality flaw. Families and communities might tolerate people whose behavior seemed "odd," "a little off," "nervous," "depressed," "strange," or "eccentric" as long as they were not exceptionally difficult, bothersome, or noticeable. This could apply also to those people with particularly severe forms of mental disorder. Consider, for example, the history of a patient suffering from paranoid schizophrenia. Obviously, that person had to be detected in order for us to know about him, but he apparently had been schizophrenic for several years.

> This patient entered a psychiatric hospital after having failed to obtain a body for his "experiments in restoring life." He had been in the army for 16 ½ months without being hospitalized, despite the fact that he had been psychotic during that entire period. The patient had a number of delusions, including one that people had been trying to kill him for about eight years. According to him, he had been changing into a woman for the last five years and would soon be able to bear children. Of interest is the fact that this patient existed in society for quite awhile before his paranoid ideas came to be known, resulting in his hospitalization.[1]

Existing studies of true prevalence have relied on both direct and indirect evidence. A few studies drew solely on the indirect evidence of records

---

[1]Kurt Salzinger, *Schizophrenia: Behavioral Aspects* (New York: Wiley, 1973), p. 4.

from hospitals, schools, social welfare agencies, the police, and other such organizations. Sometimes those records were confirmed by interviews with people working in those organizations and with people in the community. Slightly more studies interviewed people identified through records as possible psychiatric problems and others who could comment about them. Finally, a majority of studies, primarily research conducted since World War II, interviewed all people in a population or in a sample of that population. Sometimes, the interviews were supplemented by reviews of records or the corroboration of additional people in the community.

Most of these studies had psychiatrists assess whether or not the subjects of the study showed symptoms of mental disorder, and if so, what the corresponding diagnoses should be.[2] It was typically assumed that the diagnoses were valid, and usually their validity was not tested. In fact, diagnoses in psychiatry are seldom validated. But when predictive validity (the demonstration that predictions of a person's behavior derived from a diagnosis subsequently take place) has been tested, the results appear rather limited (Kendell 1975). Psychiatrists have been notoriously poor, for instance, at predicting the possibility of dangerous behavior in mental patients (Levinson and Zan York 1974; Simon and Cockerham 1977). On the other hand, tests of the effects of psychoactive drugs on behavior have relatively high rates of predictive validity. Also, for the unambiguous aspects of some mental disorders (for example, the progressive deterioration of most forms of schizophrenia), the outcome is well established, so that tests of validity (at least in the minds of psychiatrists) may not be particularly informative (Kendell 1975). When psychiatric diagnoses in epidemiological studies are the issue, however, the best that can be said is that such diagnoses represent an *approximation* of the types and extent of mental

---

[2]An example of some of the better research in this regard is Tsung-Yi Lin's (1953) community survey of schizophrenia in Taiwan. Lin gathered a random sample of twenty thousand persons from a rural village, a small town, and an urban community. Each person was interviewed by a team that included a psychiatrist. Those suspected of mental disorder were reinterviewed by Lin, who was responsible for making the final diagnosis. Forty-three cases of schizophrenia were uncovered. Rates were higher for females and lower-class persons. There was no significant difference by size of community, but all of the schizophrenics tended to live in the center, and most densely populated area, of their respective towns.

Another study, by Joseph Eaton (a sociologist) and Robert Weil (a psychiatrist), investigated the mental health of the Hutterites in the early 1950s. The Hutterites, an isolated religious sect living in the American Middle West and Canada, seemed superficially to have little mental disorder. They are a homogeneous group that supports principles of pacifism, adult baptism, communal ownership of all property, and simple living. They stay to themselves; radios and movies are forbidden. Supposedly they are free from tension and the stress of competition. Among the 8,542 Hutterites, Eaton and Weil (1955) found 199 persons (1 in 43) with active or past symptoms of mental disorders, primarily anxiety or manic-depressive reactions. The overall incidence of mental disorder, although low, was not absent, as had been claimed by some observers. Anxiety was most common among females who felt personal stress in a male-dominated society. Manic-depressive disorders were most common among those individuals who felt a strong need to live up to the social and religious expectations of their sect, yet sensed that they had somehow failed.

disorder in the population under study. Obviously, this means that the studies themselves are an approximation of reality, not a precise measure.

Measures of the prevalence of certain types of mental disorder, even if they are approximate, are more useful if they indicate specific situations and problems. It is therefore necessary to compare them with other studies and to estimate the relative importance of different variables. Although directly comparing the eighty-odd studies of true prevalence summarized by the Dohrenwends was difficult because of differences in methodology, cultures, time periods, geographic locations, and contrasting definitions of mental disorder, a particularly impressive feature of those studies is the consistent finding of significant relationships among mental disorder and three important sociodemographic variables. "These relationships seem all the more remarkable," states Bruce Dohrenwend (1975:368), "in that they hold across studies done at particular times, in different parts of the world, and using different procedures for identifying 'cases.' It is these consistent relationships that provide . . . the nearest things to truth that we have from 'true' prevalence studies." The three variables identified by Dohrenwend as the best indicators of "true" prevalence are (1) social class, (2) urban–rural location, and (3) sex.

Studies conducted since the Dohrenwends' 1974 analysis confirm their earlier summation (see, for example, Center for Mental Health Services 1992; Cockerham 1990b; Gove, Hughes, and Galle 1979; Kessler 1982; Kessler, Brown, and Broman 1981; Kessler et al. 1994; Link, Dohrenwend, and Skodol 1986; Mirowsky and Ross 1989b; Wheaton 1978). The prevalence of mental disorder in the general population is greater among lower socioeconomic groups and in cities, and there are significant differences between men and women as well.

Table 5–1 shows the results of a true prevalence study of serious mental illness of representative households in the United States conducted jointly in 1989 by the National Center for Health Statistics and the National Institute of Mental Health (Center for Mental Health Statistics 1992; National Center for Health Statistics and Centers for Disease Control 1992). A serious mental illness in this study was defined as any psychiatric disorder that seriously interfered with one or more aspects of a person's daily life. Data were collected from 113,000 people eighteen years of age or older in the noninstitutionalized general population. Table 5–1 shows that 18.2 per 1,000 persons had a serious mental illness. By age group, people seventy-five years and over had the highest rate of 25.3 per 1,000—a finding no doubt influenced by the prevalence of dementia. Females had a significantly higher rate than males (20.6 versus 15.5 per 1,000) and blacks a slightly higher rate than whites (19.7 versus 18.3 per 1,000). Of particular significance are socioeconomic differences. Table 5–1 shows that the rate for people living below the poverty line or threshold is 39.4 per 1,000, compared with 15.5 per 1,000 for people living above the poverty threshold. For education, the rates are highest for those with less than twelve years of schooling (27.2) and lowest for those with more than

Table 5–1 Number and percent distribution of the adult household population, adults with serious mental illness and rate per thousand, by selected characteristics: United States, 1989

CHARACTERISTIC	ADULT HOUSEHOLD POPULATION		ADULTS WITH SERIOUS MENTAL ILLNESS		
			TOTAL		
	NUMBER IN THOUSANDS	PERCENT DISTRIBUTION	NUMBER IN THOUSANDS	PERCENT DISTRIBUTION	RATE PER THOUSAND
Total	179,529	100.0	3,264	100.0	18.2
Age					
18–24 years	25,401	14.2	361	11.1	14.2
25–34 years	42,814	23.9	707	21.7	16.5
35–44 years	35,982	20.0	744	22.8	20.7
45–64 years	46,114	25.7	919	28.2	19.9
65–69 years	9,903	5.5	142	4.4	14.3
70–74 years	7,925	4.4	102	3.1	12.9
75 years and over	11,391	6.3	288	8.8	25.3
Sex					
Male	85,257	47.5	1,320	40.4	15.5
Female	94,272	52.5	1,944	59.6	20.6
Race					
White	153,763	85.6	2,812	86.1	18.3
Black	19,932	11.1	393	12.0	19.7
Other	5,834	3.2	59	1.8	10.1
Poverty Status					
Below poverty threshold	15,464	9.5	609	21.0	39.4
Above poverty threshold	147,070	90.5	2,284	79.0	15.5
Education					
Less than 12 years	39,809	22.4	1,083	33.8	27.2
12 years	68,563	38.6	1,120	34.9	16.3
More than 12 years	69,369	39.0	1,002	31.3	14.4

Source: Center for Mental Health Services, 1992.

twelve years (14.4). The nationwide data set displayed in Table 5–1 shows a greater prevalence of serious mental disorder among women than men and among persons in the lowest socioeconomic group.

The nationwide true prevalence study by Ronald Kessler and his associates (Kessler et al. 1994) suggests that perhaps as many as 48 percent of all Americans have experienced a mental disorder at some point in their lives. That does not mean that they are psychologically disabled; rather, it means that at some time in their lives they have experienced symptoms of a disorder. The sample consisted of 8,098 people between the ages of eighteen and fifty-four selected to be representative of the entire population of the United States. Depression was identified as the greatest mental health problem in the nation, with some 17 percent of Americans having been severely depressed at some time in their lives. Alcohol dependence was the next greatest problem, affecting some 14 percent of the population over their life course. Less than 40 percent of those with a lifetime disorder had ever received professional care. Women had significantly higher rates of mood and anxiety disorders, and men had higher rates of substance-related and antisocial personality disorders. Mental disorders were concentrated in major urban centers and among the less educated and less affluent.

Regardless of the time and place, study after study confirms this general pattern of true prevalence in populations: Important differences in mental disorder exist between social classes, men and women, and urban and rural areas. These widely accepted and confirmed findings, along with studies of the true prevalence of mental disorder according to age, marital status, and race, will be discussed in the next four chapters.

SUMMARY

This chapter has discussed studies of true prevalence. Studies of true prevalence are confronted with a variety of problems. They are difficult to design, carry out, and analyze with precision. It is necessary to seek people in the community who are not under treatment for mental disorder and yet manifest mentally abnormal symptoms. It is doubtful whether the data on such people (obtained from records, the person's past history, interviews with the person, interviews with other people who know something about the person, or all these approaches) can offer highly accurate results. The rigor required of the researcher to assess the validity of the findings is demanding and complicated by the fact that it is sometimes difficult to determine who is and who is not mentally ill. Even judgments by psychiatrists are subject to diagnostic discrepancies. Mental disorder requires a social and psychiatric judgment of the subjective condition, and exact measurement is correspondingly difficult. Therefore, epidemiological surveys of mental disorder can at best be considered only approximations of true prevalence.

What is interesting, however, is that regardless of differences in methodology, settings, time periods, and definitions of mental disorder, there have been consistent results in regard to three sociodemographic variables: social class, urban–rural location, and sex. This consistency provides the strongest indicator of true conditions in the research literature

6

Mental Disorder: Social Class

The conclusion of most studies that the highest overall rates of mental disorder are found among members of the lowest socioeconomic group has, according to Bruce Dohrenwend (1975:370), "remained remarkably persistent in the 'true' prevalence studies conducted since the turn of the century." It remains true today as well (Kessler et al. 1994). The lower social class has been observed to have the greatest prevalence of mental disorder in general and schizophrenia and personality disorders in particular. Mood disorders and anxiety disorders tend to be more common among the middle and upper classes.

THE CLASSIC STUDIES

Four of the best-known studies that helped to establish the premise that mental disorder and social class or socioeconomic status are related are those by Robert Faris and H. Warren Dunham (1939), August Hollingshead and Frederick Redlich (1958), Leo Srole and his associates (1962), and the Leightons and their associates (1963). We shall consider each of them in turn.

Faris and Dunham (Chicago)

The first systematic study of the distribution of mental disorder in a community was conducted in Chicago by Faris and Dunham in the mid-1930s. Using large maps of the city to locate the addresses of some thirty-five thousand people who had received psychiatric care from both public and private mental hospitals, Faris and Dunham found that the highest rates of schizophrenia were clustered in the slum areas of town. They hypothesized that people living in poverty were more isolated from normal social contacts and therefore were more vulnerable to developing a "seclusive" personality, which they believed was the key trait of schizophrenia. Being socially isolated, argued the authors, promoted hallucinations, delusions, and inappropriate actions, since the usual social controls that enforced normality were missing. "If the various types of unconventional behavior observed in different schizophrenic patients can be said to result from one condition," concluded Faris and Dunham (1939:173–74), "it appears that extreme seclusiveness may be that condition."

We now know that Faris and Dunham were mistaken on this point. Much more is involved in schizophrenia than simply being isolated from other people. Social isolation, moreover, is usually the *result* rather than the *cause* of schizophrenia. Dunham, commenting nearly forty years later, explains the origin of the Faris and Dunham conclusion:

> The alert reader will at this point probably have noted something that we, alas, were too young and enthusiastic to see at the time: our findings, while consistent with the notion that poor people tend to become schizophrenic, were no less consistent with the almost diametrically opposite notion that schizophrenic people tend to become poor. One should recall, however, that in 1939, at the tail end of the Great Depression, with "one third of a nation ill-clothed, ill-housed, ill-fed," many people in the social sciences (and out of them, for that matter) were intensely—and rightly—concerned about the destructive effects of poverty on families and individuals. Given the evident and easily demonstrated impact of economic deprivation on nutrition and the incidence of organic disease, they—and we—were ready to see a comparable impact on the incidence of functional psychoses.[1]

Nonetheless, the Faris and Dunham study does point to social isolation as an important factor in the experience of becoming schizophrenic. The process of isolation apparently becomes more pronounced as the disorder advances. But most important, Faris and Dunham found that the rates of schizophrenia for Chicago could be arranged into very definite patterns that closely matched the ecological structure of the city. As Figure 6–1 shows, the greatest concen-

---

[1]H. Warren Dunham, "Schizophrenia: The Impact of Sociocultural Factors," *Hospital Practice* 12 (1977), 61–68.

FIGURE 6–1   Schinzophrenia rates (all types) in Chicago, 1922–1931, per 100,000 adult population

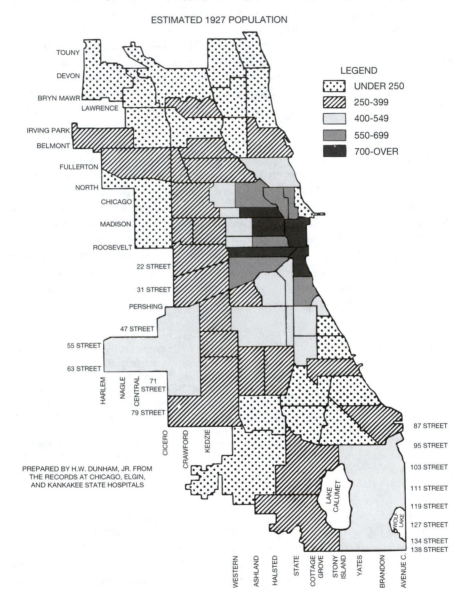

ESTIMATED 1927 POPULATION

LEGEND
UNDER 250
250-399
400-549
550-699
700-OVER

PREPARED BY H.W. DUNHAM, JR. FROM
THE RECORDS AT CHICAGO, ELGIN,
AND KANKAKEE STATE HOSPITALS

tration was in the central district of the city, where the rate for schizophrenia was 700 or more per 100,000 of the 1927 estimated adult population. The areas around the center and the south of the city had the next highest rates; the affluent districts (at that time), the lowest. For a person from the lower class, as evidenced by living in those parts of the city with the least attractive living arrangements, the more likely it was that that person or that person's neighbors were schizophrenic. The Faris and Dunham study thus established the position *that one's location in a social structure had definite implications for one's mental health* and stimulated considerable interest in the relationship between social class and mental illness.

Leo Levy and Louis Rowitz (1973) later replicated the Faris and Dunham study in Chicago with information on 10,653 city residents admitted to area mental hospitals during 1960 and 1961. Except for finding that people diagnosed as schizophrenic were not as heavily concentrated in the inner city, Levy and Rowitz essentially confirmed the results of the Faris and Dunham study with respect to the distribution of mental disorder in Chicago. Levy and Rowitz concluded that the prevalence of serious psychiatric disorders, especially schizophrenia and alcohol-related disorders, was found primarily in lower-class neighborhoods.

Hollingshead and Redlich (New Haven)

The Hollingshead and Redlich study was conducted in New Haven, Connecticut, in the 1950s and compared public and private mental patients (both inpatients and outpatients) with a sample of the general nonpatient population. No attempt was made to find untreated cases in the general population, but the comparison of patients and nonpatients was an outgrowth of the New Haven researchers' distrust of earlier studies, like those of Faris and Dunham, which were based solely on hospital admissions. The New Haven study used Hollingshead and Redlich's influential Index of Social Position, which correlated race, ethnicity, and religion with location of residence, occupation, and education to determine a person's socioeconomic status. Five principal social classes were identified: Class I (upper), Class II (upper middle), Class III (lower middle), Class IV (working class), and Class V (lower). Briefly stated, Class I (about 3 percent of the total population) consisted of wealthy families whose money was largely inherited and who dominated the social and economic life of the community. Class II (about 8 percent) was composed of families with comfortable incomes, usually from high managerial positions. Class III (22 percent) included the majority of white-collar workers, such as office and sales employees and small store proprietors. Teachers, nurses, and skilled manual laborers were also included in Class III. Class IV represented nearly one-half of New Haven's population (over 47 percent) and was composed largely of semiskilled factory workers. Class V (about 18 percent) consisted of semiskilled workers and unskilled laborers who lived in the lower-class slum areas of town. The principal characteristics of each social class in New Haven are outlined in Table 6–1.

There were also distinctions *within* Class I and Class V. In Class I, greater status was accorded to those individuals with the oldest money and from the

Table 6–1 Social class characteristics in the Hollingshead and Redlich study

SOCIAL CLASS	OCCUPATION	EDUCATION	RESIDENTIAL AREA	RACE	ETHNICITY	MAJOR RELIGION
I	Business and professional	Private university	"The Best"	White	"Old Yankee families"	Protestant (61%)
II	High managerial	State university	"Better"	Mostly white	Mixed	Protestant (45%)
III	Office and sales workers, small store owners, skilled workers	High school graduates, some attended college	"Good"	Mixed	Mixed	Catholic (47%)
IV	Semiskilled factory workers	Grade school	"Working class"	Mixed	Mixed	Catholic (63%)
V	Semiskilled and unskilled workers	Less than grade school	"Slums"	Mixed	Mixed	Catholic (73%)

Source: Adapted from August B. Hollingshead and Frederick C. Redlich, *Social Class and Mental Illness: A Community Study* (New York: Wiley, 1958), pp. 66–136.

oldest families. They were regarded as the "upper-uppers." The "lower-uppers" were people who were wealthy but who were relatively new arrivals in the upper strata of society. Sometimes this snobbery was carried to extreme lengths, as reported by Hollingshead and Redlich:

> Chronologically, wealth comes first, then one's family background is discovered, and the importance of wealth is pushed into the background. The number of generations a family has been prominent *and* resident in the community is important to the elderly arbiters of power and status. This point was well put by a distinguished matriarch while we were discussing the importance of some families in the life of the city over a number of generations. Such a family was named for illustration. The respondent closed her eyes, thought for a few moments, and resumed the discussion with, "The ——— are not really old New Haveners. They first settled in Saybrook (a pioneer settlement on the Connecticut coast) in the 1640s, but the family did not move to New Haven until 1772."[2]

Lower-class people in Class V, at the opposite end of the social scale, can be divided into "upper-lowers" and "lower-lowers," the essential difference being that the "lower-lowers" are on welfare. How long members of Class V have lived in the community is really not an issue with them. They are forced to attend to the daily demands of surviving, and their living conditions are clearly the poorest. One field worker described the typical features of a Class V home this way:

> The kitchen usually contains a refrigerator of an old vintage but still in good condition outwardly. From the ceiling hangs an old light fixture from which one bare bulb is burning. In other sockets are extension cords. One leading to a radio which is blaring and the other to the iron the housewife is using. In one corner of the kitchen is one section of a U.S. Army double-deck bed. Off the kitchen one can see into the bedroom which is crowded with sway-backed beds. Flies are buzzing around even in late fall. The breakfast set is of plastic and chrome, but the plastic is worn through and the chrome is rusted in spots.[3]

Hollingshead (a sociologist) and Redlich (a psychiatrist) found that Class I and Class II people were more aware of psychological problems and more perceptive of conflict and the nature of personal difficulties. That was in direct contrast to Class V people, who were much slower to attribute personal problems to mental disorder or to label someone as "crazy" because of the serious consequences of such a label (that is, arrest, confinement in a mental hospital). Referrals to psychiatric care for mental disorders were much more likely to come from the police or social welfare agencies for Class V patients. Private physicians or the influence of family and friends was the likely source of refer-

---

[2]August B. Hollingshead and Frederick C. Redlich, *Social Class and Mental Illness: A Community Study* (New York: Wiley, 1958), pp. 72–73.
[3]Ibid., p. 119.

Table 6–2 Percentage distribution of anxiety and schizophrenia by social class in the Hollingshead and Redlich study

	ANXIETY		SCHIZOPHRENIA	
SOCIAL CLASS	PERCENT	NUMBER	PERCENT	NUMBER
I	52.6	(10)	47.4	(9)
II	67.2	(88)	32.8	(43)
III	44.2	(115)	55.8	(145)
IV	23.1	(175)	76.9	(583)
V	8.4	(61)	91.6	(662)

Source: Adapted from August B. Hollingshead and Frederick C. Redlich, "Social Stratification and Psychiatric Disorders," *American Sociological Review* 18 (1953), 167.

rals to psychiatrists for Classes I, II, and III. Class IV was referred usually through either private or clinic physicians or the police.[4]

As for the relationship between social class and mental disorder, Hollingshead and Redlich found that for specific types of mental disorders, definite patterns emerged by social class in regard to the proportion of the mental patients with anxiety disorders and schizophrenia. This pattern is demonstrated in Table 6–2, in which 52.6 percent (10 persons) in Class I compared with 8.4 percent (61 persons) in Class V have anxiety disorders. For schizophrenia, 47.4 percent (9 persons) in Class I compared with 91.6 percent (662 persons) in Class V are afflicted. However, the proportions here are somewhat skewed because of the small number (19) of Class I mental patients. A better comparison in Table 6–2 is between Class II and the other classes. Table 6–2 shows that 67.2 percent (88 persons) in Class II have anxiety, with *decreasing* percentages for Classes III (44.2 percent), IV (23.1 percent), and V (8.4 percent). Among the schizophrenic patients, 32.8 percent (43 persons) in Class II are represented, with *increasing* percentages for Classes III (55.8 percent), IV (76.9 percent), and V (91.6 percent). The clear trend in Table 6–2 is that the lower the class, the greater the tendency is toward schizophrenia, and the higher the class, the greater the tendency is toward anxiety.

To determine the probability of schizophrenia in the general population by social class and to adjust the data to compensate for the small number of patients in Class I, Hollingshead developed a proportional index of prevalence, as shown in Table 6–3. If a social class has the same proportion of schizophrenics as there is in the general population, then the mean index score for that social class is 100. If the incidence of schizophrenia is disproportionately high for that social class, then the index is above 100. If it is dispropor-

---

[4]Interestingly enough, comparing the amount that psychiatrists and psychologists are visited shows that differences remain between high- and low-income groups, although the gap appears to be narrowing. The more affluent are still more likely to define a personal problem as needing professional help (Kulka, Veroff and Douvan 1979; Veroff, Kulka, and Douvan 1981).

Table 6–3 Comparison by social class of the distribution of schizophrenics in the general population according to the Hollingshead and Redlich study

SOCIAL CLASS	GENERAL POPULATION		SCHIZOPHRENICS		INDEX OF PREVALENCE
	PERCENT	NUMBER	PERCENT	NUMBER	
I	3.2	(358)	0.7	(6)	22
II	8.4	(926)	2.7	(23)	33
III	22.6	(2,500)	9.8	(83)	43
IV	47.4	(5,256)	41.6	(352)	88
V	18.4	(2,037)	45.2	(383)	246
TOTALS	100.0	(11,077)	100.0	(847)	

Source: Adapted from August B. Hollingshead and Frederick C. Redlich, "Social Stratification and Psychiatric Disorders," *American Sociological Review* 18 (1953), 168.

tionately low in a social class, then the index is below 100. The index of prevalence for each social class is shown in the last column of Table 6–3. The index of schizophrenia for Class I is exceedingly low at 22; for Class V it is exceedingly high at 246. Class IV comes the closest to having an index score for schizophrenia that is roughly equivalent to its proportion of the general population. Here the index of prevalence is 88 compared with the proportional score of 100. In Class I, the proportion of schizophrenia is only one-fifth of what it should be if the prevalence were proportional to the actual number of people in Class I, and in Class V the proportion is almost 2.5 times greater. In comparing Class I with Class V, we see that the prevalence of schizophrenia is over eleven times greater in the lower class than in the upper class.

Finally, it should be noted that Hollingshead and Redlich found that for treated cases of both anxiety and schizophrenia, the greatest number of patients were in Classes IV and V. Class I was relatively free of treated cases of these disorders.

The Hollingshead and Redlich study remains one of the most influential epidemiological surveys of mental health. It has received international attention and is probably the best-known study of the relationship between mental disorder and social class. As for true prevalence, however, the study is severely limited in its ability to generalize its findings to people not receiving psychiatric treatment and therefore not identified as mental patients. The Hollingshead and Redlich data are based upon cases in treatment, either as inpatients or as outpatients. Because it seems that many people are mentally ill and do not receive treatment, thus remaining at large in the general population, failure to account for those individuals prevents the Hollingshead and Redlich study from directly answering questions of true prevalence. But for those in treatment, Hollingshead and Redlich presented impressive evidence that social factors can be correlated with degrees and types of mental illness and the manner in which people received psychiatric care. Clearly, the poor were at a definite disadvantage when comparing the relative position of each social class with respect to mental health. As a result, the Hollingshead and Redlich study played a key role in the debate in the 1960s leading to the establishment of community mental health centers in the United States.

Srole and His Associates (Midtown Manhattan)

The study by Srole and associates, also conducted in the 1950s, did investigate the true prevalence of mental disorder among a cross-section of people living in the Midtown Manhattan area of New York City. Because the Hollingshead and Redlich study examined only *treated* cases of mental disorder, the Midtown Manhattan researchers felt justified in constructing a method to determine *untreated* disorders. A total of 1,660 persons between the ages of twenty and fifty-nine, constituting 87 percent of the 1,911 randomly selected households, were interviewed, and data were obtained on their personal background, past history of psychopathology and psychotherapy, and acknowledgment of current symptoms of mental disorder. The respondents were also rated by the interviewer as to their level of tension at the start and finish of the interview. All the information was given to a team of psychiatrists who assessed the respondents' psychiatric conditions. Once again it was found that mental disorders were more prevalent among the lower class than among the other socioeconomic groups. The clearest finding was that those persons aged twenty to twenty-nine and of high socioeconomic status were the most likely to be in the "well" category; those persons aged fifty to fifty-nine and of low socioeconomic origin, particularly those whose childhood was spent in poverty, were the most likely to be "impaired." In addition, it was found that those persons who were upwardly mobile in society showed fewer signs of emotional disturbances than those who had remained at the same socioeconomic level or who were downwardly mobile.

The principal hypothesis of the Midtown Manhattan study was supported:

> Sociocultural conditions, in both their normative and their deviant forms, operating in intrafamily and extrafamily settings during childhood and adulthood, have measurable consequences reflected in the mental health differences to be observed within a population.[5]

The Midtown Manhattan study was an especially large and ambitious research project. It led to the development of the Langner Scale (Langner and Michael 1963), a commonly employed measure of mental health. It also not only corroborated the findings of previous studies that more mental illness was located in the lower class, but also suggested that stress was an important com-

---

[5]Leo Srole et al., *Mental Health in the Metropolis: The Midtown Manhattan Study, Book Two,* rev. ed., ed. L. Srole and A. Fischer (New York: Harper & Row, 1975), p. 499.

ponent in mental disorder. In this instance, membership in the lower class was viewed as being a potentially stressful factor, as compared with being in the middle or upper class, in which class could be a mediating influence. In the latter, it was presumed that an individual had fewer stresses and greater resources in coping with those stresses that might arise. This suggestion helped lay the foundation for much of the current research on mental illness and life events.

Leighton and Associates (Stirling County)

One of the most thorough epidemiological investigations of mental disorder was the Stirling County study conducted in the 1950s by the Leightons and their associates (1963). Stirling County was a name given by Alexander and Dorothea Leighton and their colleagues to a rural county in the Canadian province of Nova Scotia. The population of the county numbered fewer than twenty thousand, with most of the inhabitants supported by fishing, farming, or lumber interests. The population lived in small hamlets and villages, with the only urban center having about three thousand people. The instrument measuring mental disorder was a questionnaire on the respondents' social background, concept of community, family relations, and physical and mental health, and a twenty-item inventory of psychiatric symptoms (the Health Opinion Survey). Some of the respondents were given a pretest to assess the validity and reliability of the survey instrument. The results were correlated with clinical examinations administered to the same respondents. Health records from local physicians and hospitals were also screened to determine further the validity and the reliability of the instrument.

Once the investigators were satisfied that their questionnaire measured what it was supposed to measure, 1,303 respondents, eighteen years of age or older, were selected at random to be interviewed personally in their homes. The results of the interviews were then rated by two or more psychiatrists to see if the respondent qualified as a psychiatric "case." A "case" was defined as a person having a high probability of being diagnosed as mentally ill if examined by a psychiatrist applying the standards found in the DSM-I. The results indicated an extremely high level of true prevalence of mental disorder— about 57 percent of the entire sample. However, most of those persons were only mildly impaired. Of that group, about 60 percent had psychophysiological problems (ulcers, musculoskeletal aches and pains, and the like); and only 10 percent were diagnosed with anxiety, 7 percent as depressed, and less than 1 percent as schizophrenic. The prevalence of mental disorder appeared to increase with age (until age sixty-five, when it declined) and was significantly greater for women than for men. *And, again, not surprisingly, mental disorder was most frequent among members of the lowest socioeconomic group.*

The focus of the Stirling County study was upon the degree of sociocultural integration and the extent of mental disorder in small communities of French-Canadian Catholics and English-Canadian Protestants. It was found that the French had much lower rates of mental disorder, especially among the women. The Leightons and their associates hypothesized that these families were somewhat more stable and that there was less confusion about the role of women (the women were expected to occupy traditional roles, that is, mother, housekeeper). The English families had a more worldly view; that is, they had more interest in events outside the county, and they were more equivocal about the role of women in the culture.

Although the methodological approach of this study was more comprehensive than those of the preceding studies, the results were still dependent upon the psychiatrists' assessments of what constitutes a "case." As previously discussed, psychiatric diagnoses are known to often have relatively low levels of validity and reliability. Furthermore, a particular problem with the Stirling County findings is their attempts to equate social disintegration with mental disorder. The difficulty here, which the study failed to resolve, is that social disintegration may be as much a result of mental disorder as it is a cause. Nevertheless, the Stirling County study is a relatively sophisticated endeavor to deal with the methodological problems inherent in studies of true prevalence.

EXPLANATIONS OF THE RELATIONSHIP

The Faris and Dunham study in Chicago and the Hollingshead and Redlich study in New Haven can, of course, be criticized for investigating only treated cases of mental disorder. The Midtown Manhattan study by Srole and his associates and the Stirling County study by the Leightons and their colleagues can be faulted for relying upon psychiatrists' subjective and somewhat incomplete judgments. Nor did Faris and Dunham, Hollingshead and Redlich, and Srole and his associates attempt to measure all forms of mental disorder. There is some evidence, for example, that social class is related to some mental disorders (especially schizophrenia) but possibly not to others (Rushing and Ortega 1979). Yet the central results of these studies have been confirmed by several other investigators to the extent that the trend is marked: Although there are some differences between the classes, in general there is *more* mental disorder among the lower class (see, for example, Carr and Krause 1978; Cockerham 1985, 1990b; Dohrenwend and Dohrenwend 1974; Dohrenwend 1975; Eaton 1974b, 1980b; Gallagher 1987; Kessler 1979, 1982; Kessler and Cleary 1980; Kessler et al. 1994; Kohn 1972, 1974, 1976; Liem and Liem 1978; Link et al. 1986; Link, Lennon, and Dohrenwend 1993; Turner and Gartrell 1978; Warheit, Holzer, and Schwab 1973; Wheaton 1978; Wilkinson 1975).

The research cited above represents findings for studies whose focus is the United States or Canada. Yet when studies from other nations are considered, the results are the same. For example, research in both the Netherlands (Wiersma et al. 1983) and Taiwan (Lin 1953) found a significantly greater prevalence of schizophrenia among the lower class. Other research involving respondents from Great Britain (Cooper 1961; Eaton 1980a; Goldberg and Morrisson 1963) and Mexico (Mirowsky and Ross 1983; Ross, Mirowsky and Cockerham 1983) likewise found a higher level of psychological distress among lower-class people. In Germany, studies of the true prevalence of mental disorder in the states of Bavaria (Dilling and Weyerer 1984) and Northrhine-Westphalia (Cockerham, Kunz, and Lueschen 1988) and the city of Mannheim (Schepank et al. 1984) identified more psychiatric problems among the lower class. Other research in Mannheim involving the elderly (Häfner 1984) and mentally retarded children (Cooper and Lackus 1984) had similar findings.

For those nations of the world in which behavioral research is well established and not constrained by politics or ideology, the existing data clearly show that those people who inhabit the lower rungs of society are more susceptible to mental disorder in comparison with other social classes.

Three rationales have been advanced to explain the relationship between social class and mental disorder. First is the *genetic* explanation, which holds that as a result of genetic inheritance, there is a greater predisposition toward mental disorder among the lower classes. But studies of monozygotic (identical) twins have shown that genetics alone is not sufficient to account for schizophrenia and other mental disorders (Shields, Heston and Gottesman 1975; Snyder 1980). Genetic studies have established that some people have a specific vulnerability toward a particular mental disorder, but this vulnerability is essentially a predisposition. Psychological, social, or other factors apparently are needed to trigger the onset of symptoms. Only about 50 percent of monozygotic twins in families with histories of schizophrenia, for example, develop the disorder, and for dizygotic (fraternal) twins the average is about 10 to 15 percent (Snyder 1980). Therefore, although genetic mechanisms are significant, psychological and social factors are also important (Bruce Dohrenwend 1975; Dunham 1977; Eaton 1980a; Kohn 1972, 1974, 1976; Rainer 1985; Snyder 1980; Weiner 1985).

Second is the *social stress* explanation. The social stress explanation is a type of social causation explanation. It suggests that members of the lower class are subjected to greater stress as a result of living in a deprived life situation and having to cope with this deprivation with fewer resources. Thus, stress affects the emotional ability of the poor more severely than it does the upper classes (Kessler 1979; Kessler and Cleary 1980; Mirowsky and Ross 1989b). Examples of this are found in several studies of the poor and their emotional problems. For instance, of the twenty lower-class schizophrenic Puerto Rican families studied by Rogler and Hollingshead (1965), all had succumbed to the stresses of their environment. One of those families was the Padillas, of whom Mrs. Padilla became schizophrenic:

A complicated pregnancy was followed by the death of a baby under provocative circumstances; unemployment decimated the family's meager store of economic resources, and Mrs. Padilla's children suffered; when Mr. Padilla did find work he shared his earnings with a concubine; the interpersonal relations of the Padillas underwent a series of stress-provoking incidents; as Mrs. Padilla became more disturbed over her husband's behavior she began to quarrel with the neighbors. Her dream of a legal marriage to him has never been realized—she goads him; he retaliates with infidelity.

The breaking point was reached when Mrs. Padilla returned from the hospital and found her "lazy sister" sitting in the middle of the floor reading with the house "torn to pieces," the 17-day-old twin of the sick infant screaming in the basket, and food and dishes scattered over the floor by the older children. The last link connecting Mrs. Padilla with reality broke when the baby died.[6]

The experiences of Mrs. Padilla show how a person living in poverty can finally reach the point at which he or she can no longer cope with the pressures of daily living. Research by Leonard Pearlin and Carmi Schooler (1978) on coping as a protective process to keep from being psychologically harmed suggests that individuals cope most effectively when dealing with problems within the close interpersonal areas of marriage and child rearing. People are least effective when dealing with the more impersonal problems found in work situations, although males, the well educated, and the affluent usually have the most effective modes of coping in this context. But if individuals cope best in circumstances like marriage and family in which they are committed to and engaged with others most relevant to their lives, presumably failure in this area would produce the greatest amount of psychological harm. At least, this is what we see in the case of Mrs. Padilla as her family situation became intolerable, regardless of the effects on her of the impersonal wider society.

Yet the social stress explanation as illustrated by Mrs. Padilla does not account for those persons living in poverty and having the same life experiences who do not become schizophrenic. The difference between the lower-class schizophrenic and nonschizophrenic families in the Rogler and Hollingshead study was that those who became schizophrenic, like Mrs. Padilla, were *overwhelmed* by a series of related problems they could not solve. So stress by itself, particularly in a circumstance where many are stressed, does not appear to be an exclusive answer. Consequently, other factors, such as genetics, must also be considered. Whether the schizophrenics in the Rogler and Hollingshead study had a genetic predisposition toward the disorder and stress acted to trigger that condition is not known, but a combined genetics-stress theory may be the most likely overall explanation of the lower-class–schizophrenia relationship. In the meantime, more extensive research is needed to verify the role of stress in mental disorder.

Third is the *social selection* explanation, which maintains that there is more mental disorder in the lower class because mentally ill persons tend to

---

[6]Lloyd H. Rogler and August B. Hollingshead, *Trapped: Families and Schizophrenia* (New York: Wiley, 1965), pp. 196–97.

"drift" downward in the social structure (the "drift" hypothesis), or conversely, mentally healthy individuals in the lower class tend to be upwardly mobile, thus leaving behind a "residue" of mentally ill persons (the "residue" hypothesis). The best support for the social selection explanation suggests that the primary effect of abnormal behavior is to retard upward social mobility rather than to contribute to downward mobility (Harkey, Miles, and Rushing 1976; Wiersma et al. 1983). Thus, the "residue" hypothesis seems to be a somewhat better explanation than the "drift" hypothesis.

However, despite some evidence supporting a relationship between social mobility and mental disorder (Bruce Dohrenwend 1975; Eaton 1980a; Kohn 1972, 1974; Srole et al. 1975; Srole et al. 1962; Turner and Gartrell 1978), social selection in itself does not seem to be a fully adequate explanation. John Fox (1990), for example, has determined in a new analysis of the Midtown Manhattan study that mentally ill people are not especially mobile, either up or down, in the class structure. Neither the social selection nor the drift hypotheses were supported. As Melvin Kohn explains in the case of schizophrenia, the weight of the evidence

> clearly indicates either that schizophrenic individuals have been no more downwardly mobile (in fact, no less upwardly mobile) than other people from the same social backgrounds, or at a minimum, that the degree of downward mobility is insufficient to explain the high concentration of schizophrenia in the lowest socioeconomic strata.[7]

When the question is whether social class position helps to promote mental disorder (social causation) or whether mental disorder causes social class position (social selection), most likely the former (social causation) is correct. That is, social class position contributes to the onset of mental disorder to a more significant degree than mental disorder causes social class position (Fox 1990; Link et al. 1986; Wheaton 1978).

Nonetheless, social selection and genetic and social stress factors all may be involved in some fashion in the concentration of mental disorder among the lower classes. Considered separately, none of the explanations is at present sufficient, but all warrant serious consideration in future research.

One line of inquiry in regard to the social class–schizophrenia relationship is Melvin Kohn's (1974) approach. He suggests that the constricted conditions of life experienced by people in the lower socioeconomic classes encourage the formation of limited and rigid conceptions of social reality that inhibit such persons' ability to deal effectively with problems and stress. His earlier research (Kohn 1969) notes that the lower a person's social class

---

[7]Melvin L. Kohn, "Social Class and Schizophrenia: A Critical Review and a Reformulation," in *Explorations in Psychiatric Sociology*, ed. P. Roman and H. Trice (Philadelphia: Davis, 1974), p. 118.

position is, the more likely that person is to value conformity to external authority and to believe that such conformity is all his or her own capacities and resources will allow. The social psychological orientation of the lower-class person therefore includes a rigidly conservative view of life marked by fear, distrust, and "a fatalistic belief that one is at the mercy of forces and people beyond one's control, often, beyond one's understanding" (Kohn 1974:129).

Kohn does not argue that his orientation applies to all members of the lower class or that it is a philosophy to which lower-class people subscribe exclusively, but simply that the perception of social reality he has described is more common to the lower class. Kohn suggests that the family is particularly important in this scheme because of its role in transmitting its unique conception of social reality to the young. By transmitting a learned conception of reality that is too limited and too rigid to deal effectively with complex and changing stress-inducing situations, lower-class families may well contribute to the onset of schizophrenia among those genetically susceptible persons who experience great stress.

For instance, Thomas Langner and Stanley Michael (1963) believe that social class membership affects behavior through the internalization of values, beliefs, and norms that originate early in a person's socialization experience and continue to influence the person throughout his or her life. They suggest that greater impairment is found among the lower classes because they tend to respond to stress as a result of socialization more often with coping behaviors that resemble psychotic symptoms (for example, withdrawal from reality) than upper-class persons do. Upper-class persons, on the other hand, may respond more often with neurotic (anxiety) responses. Richard Sennet and Jonathan Cobb reinforce this theme in their book *The Hidden Injuries of Class* (1972) by arguing that lower-class manual workers tend to withdraw psychologically from their work situation by separating their "real" selves from their "performing" selves. By acting as if his or her work or acceptance by superiors has nothing to do with the "real self," the worker supposedly is better able to handle the tension of being in a dependent state.[8] The more a person is emotionally depen-

---

[8]Some jobs leave little possibility of viewing oneself as a "good" person, thus reinforcing the tendency to withdraw. In *Worlds of Pain: Life in Working Class Families* (New York: Basic Books, 1976), p. 158, Lillian Breslow Rubin reports:

> The men who hold these jobs often get through each day by doing their work and numbing themselves to the painful feelings of discontent—trying hard to avoid the question, "Is this what life is all about?" Unsuccessful in that struggle, one twenty-nine-year-old warehouseman burst out bitterly: "A lot of times I hate to go down there. I'm cooped up and hemmed in. I feel like I'm enclosed in a building forty hours a week, sometimes more. It seems that all there is to life is to go down there and work, collect your paycheck, pay your bills, and get further in debt. It doesn't seem like the circle ever ends. Every day it's the same thing; every week it's the same thing; every month it's the same thing."

dent on rewards from a higher authority, the more that person is dependent for self-respect on someone else or something else that is impersonal, uncontrollable, and potentially threatening.[9]

Sennett and Cobb state:

> The loss of "I" defends a person from two threats. First of all, it wards off social isolation. If I act as though my "real" self is someone divorced from the person who does well in situations when higher authority asks it, if my competence or power to cope is held at arm's length, as though it were a power external to me as a human being, then when I achieve a new position or other reward from a higher power, I can pass it off as something *I* didn't do.
>
> Advancement through approval, promotion, even such mundane cues as having a superior ask one's opinion or advice, now do not have to get in the way of fraternity with those around me who have not changed. I can still be accepted as a friend, as someone who is not deserting them or putting them in a bad light, because "I" really have not done anything to make this change occur. Passivity has a real place in the life of men who want friends, because the institutions in which men pass their days make it so.
>
> This language of self also deals with the threat of being accepted as an individual—in the sense of a special person, passivity shields the person from a wound contained in a seemingly flattering state.[10]

The division of the lower-class person's notion of "self" into "real" and "performing" aspects can have the effect of diminishing involvement and reducing vulnerability to stress. But the divided self-defense, as Sennett and Cobb explain, may be short-term because it does not change the situation that required the defense in the first place. If it fails, it is because the reorientation of one's feelings was unable to provide an escape from an intolerable social circumstance. If the defense succeeds, it may suggest that lower-class people can readily accommodate themselves to stress. Consequently, it might be argued that lower-class people are more flexible and less rigid than upper-class people in dealing with comparable stresses. Ronald Kessler (1979) claims that this is the case and that the poor are less likely to be extremely distressed when exposed to common stresses than the affluent are, although the poor still report more extreme distress because they are

---

[9]Sennett and Cobb (1972:197) describe a middle-aged asbestos worker who was once a hero in the navy, having saved his ship from exploding because of a malfunctioning heating system. He was decorated for that act and promoted several times during his four years in the navy—all in all, an outstanding record. Yet he treats his record in an offhand manner, most likely because at the time he wanted to keep his friends and not become too dependent on the navy for his ego strength. When asked about how he felt about the navy, the man replied that he had got through it all right. "I kept my nose clean, I didn't get involved, I didn't let nothing go to my head," he said. "You 'go Navy' like in the ads, . . . there's nothing left of you!"

[10]Richard Sennett and Jonathan Cobb, *The Hidden Injuries of Class* (New York: Random House, 1972), p. 196.

exposed to greater amounts of stress. This, of course, goes against Kohn's (1974) thesis that the lower class has a more rigid outlook. Kessler's argument is that the poor are more flexible but go under because they are hit much harder with more stress. "The much greater exposure of the poor to stressful experiences," says Kessler (1979:265), "cancels out their relative advantage in effectively buffering stress impacts."

Whether lower-class people have more rigid or more flexible patterns of coping with stress is unresolved. The crucial variable appears to be the amount of personal resources, social or economic, available to contend with stressful conditions—a situation that clearly goes against the poor. Socialization is still important because it is the means by which the young are taught to perceive social reality and use whatever resources they have to reduce threats to their well-being.

The relevance of having limited personal resources and poor coping abilities to a person's mental health is that this condition tends to promote feelings of fatalism. Fatalism is a term used to describe the belief that outcomes of situations are determined by such external forces as fate, luck, chance, or other, more powerful people (Rotter 1966). Several studies have found that people in the lower social classes are more fatalistic than those in the middle and upper classes and that this sense of fatalism is associated with higher levels of psychological distress (Kessler and Cleary 1980; Mirowsky and Ross 1983, 1984, 1989b; Ross, Mirowsky and Cockerham 1983; Turner and Noh 1983; Wheaton 1980, 1983). This research shows that many persons in the lower social classes learn through recurrent experiences that they have limited opportunities, that no matter how hard they try they cannot get ahead, and that more powerful people and unpredictable forces control their lives. These beliefs can be realistic perceptions of their position and are most likely reinforced in day-to-day living. People not in control of their lives tend to show higher levels of depression (Mirowsky and Ross 1990), which is clearly seen in a study of the homeless in Birmingham, Alabama (La Gory, Ritchey, and Mullis 1990).

By continually experiencing failure, people in low-status situations learn that their actions are not generally associated with successful outcomes. This situation not only is depressing and demoralizing but also can degrade the will and ability to cope with life's problems (Pearlin and Schooler 1978; Wheaton 1980). Goals seem unattainable regardless of effort. The result is greater susceptibility to psychological distress as one's ability and motivation to cope are diminished.

Therefore, it is apparent that future investigations of the relationship between social class and mental disorder need to consider the social psychology that underlies class-based conceptions of social reality. This suggestion appears to be especially appropriate for schizophrenia because (1) most schizophrenia occurs in the lower class, (2) the lower class contends with the harshest and most discomforting forms of social reality, and (3) schizophrenia is a mental disorder characterized by *withdrawal from reality,* accompanied by delusions, hallucinations, ambivalence, and bizarre activity.

SUMMARY

The discussion in this chapter focused on social class. It is clear that greater amounts of mental disorder are found in the lower class in general, with schizophrenia and personality disorders being exceedingly more prevalent among the lower rungs of society than in the upper echelons of social strata. The common explanations for this are (1) genetic, (2) social stress, and (3) social selection (the "drift" and "residue" hypotheses). Most likely, all three are necessary to some degree to explain the relationship of mental disorder to social class, but none of the three is totally satisfactory. The best explanation is probably some combination of genetics and stress. Another argument was that different types of socialization also influence the handling of stressful circumstances and that lower-class techniques may be more rigid, thereby contributing to higher rates of schizophrenia. Future research on class differences should take into account class-oriented perceptions of reality.

7

Mental Disorder: Age, Gender, and Marital Status

This chapter discusses current findings in sociology exploring the relationship between mental disorder and age, gender, and marital status. Age is important because future trends in longevity point toward greater numbers of mentally distressed elderly people. Although men and women seem to share equally in certain types of disorders, there are significant differences between the sexes in regard to other mental problems. This chapter will also examine the extensive literature on male–female differences in psychological distress, as well as the effects of marital status, which has been identified in recent studies as an increasingly important variable for mental health.

AGE

The relationship between age and mental health is becoming increasingly important because of the growth of the aged population. The worldwide trend in aging is toward larger and larger numbers of elderly people. In the United States, for example, some 12.6 percent of all Americans were age sixty-five and over in 1991—a percentage that is expected to rise to 13.1 by the year 2000. Extremely rapid growth occurs in the early twenty-first century as the percentage of Americans age sixty-five and over reaches 21.8, or one-fifth of the entire population, by 2050. This is a significant trend because increased numbers of elderly people signal increased demand for mental health services by the aged in the future.

Another reason for analyzing age and mental health is that certain mental disorders are more prevalent in particular age groups than in others. The nationwide study by Kessler et al. (1994) found the highest prevalences of mental disorder generally among people aged 25 to 34, followed by declining prevalences thereafter. This overall pattern is seen in Table 7–1, which shows resident patients by age and primary diagnosis in state and county mental hospitals for 1992. Table 7–1 shows that age groups 18–24 and 25–44 have the highest percentages of resident patients in most of the diagnostic categories of mental disorders. Schizophrenia, the largest primary diagnosis in state and county mental hospitals, peaks in the 25–44-year-old age group. Exceptions include mood disorders and preadult disorders, which are more prevalent in the under-18 resident-patient age group, and alcohol-related disorders and dementia, which are highest in the 65-and-over group.

As noted in DSM-IV, infancy, childhood, and adolescence constitute the period of life when mental retardation and disorders involving learning, motor skills, communication, attention-deficit, disruptive behavior, and eating problems first become apparent. Negative childhood experiences, especially family violence and physical and sexual abuse, can produce traumatic emotional effects lasting into adulthood (Kessler and Magee 1994; Pilgrim and Rogers 1993). Substance-related, mood, and anxiety disorders, along with schizophrenia, become more prevalent in late adolescence and early adulthood and are significant in middle age as well. Old age is characterized by an increase in dementia of the Alzheimer's type, which often requires institutional care in a nursing home or a mental hospital. Table 7–1 shows, for instance, that 27.5 percent of all state and county mental hospital resident patients have dementia as a primary diagnosis. As people move through the life course, certain mental disorders tend to be more prevalent at some ages than at others.

Aging and Mental Health

People age sixty-five and over accounted for 16 percent of all residents in inpatient psychiatric facilities in the United States in 1992. The majority (52 percent) were in state and county mental hospitals, followed by general hospital psychiatric units (23 percent), veterans' hospitals (13 percent), private mental hospitals (11 percent), and multiservice mental health organizations (1 percent). As discussed in Chapter 5, patients in psychiatric facilities do not identify the true prevalence of mental disorder in a population because they do not include untreated cases or outpatients. When it comes to the true prevalence of mental disorder among the elderly, 15 percent of all aged persons are estimated to be in need of mental health services. Mood disorders, especially depression, are the most common form of mental disorder among

Table 7-1 Resident patients in state and county mental hospitals, by mental disorder and age, United States, 1992

MAJOR DIAGNOSIS	NUMBER	UNDER 18	18-24	25-44	45-64	65 & OVER	ALL AGES
Mental retardation	2,575	2.0	6.0	3.5	2.9	1.2	3.1
Alcohol-related	2,077	0.9	2.8	2.3	3.0	3.2	2.5
Substance-related	1,491	2.1	4.1	2.5	0.6	0.3	1.8
Dementia	7,418	2.4	5.1	4.6	9.0	27.5	8.9
Mood disorders	9,892	20.2	12.3	10.0	13.3	11.1	11.9
Schizophrenia	40,417	9.7	36.2	56.7	54.2	38.1	48.5
Other psychotic	3,612	4.5	7.2	4.6	3.7	3.2	4.3
Anxiety/Somato./Dissoc.	292	1.2	0.6	0.3	0.3	0.3	0.4
Personality disorders	1,227	2.3	4.3	1.6	0.8	0.3	1.5
Preadult disorders	2,121	27.1	1.8	0.6	0.5	0.3	2.5
Other nonpsychotic	3,063	19.8	6.8	2.6	1.5	1.0	3.7
Social	246	0.7	0.7	0.3	0.2	0.1	0.3
No mental disorder	440	1.0	0.7	0.5	0.4	0.3	0.5
Deferred/undiagnosed	8,449	6.1	11.4	9.9	9.6	13.1	10.1
TOTALS:	83,320	100.0	100.0	100.0	100.0	100.0	100.0

Source: Center for Mental Health Services, 1994b.

the elderly (Cockerham 1991; Mirowsky and Ross 1992). Also significant are dementia, alcohol and substance-related disorders, and suicide.

The high prevalence of mood disorders among the aged is related to the fact that a sense of loss is particularly common for older people (Matt and Dean 1993). The elderly frequently are confronted with multiple and simultaneous losses, such as the death of a spouse, relatives, or friends, declines in physical health, changes in status, or difficulty in dealing with retirement. Many elderly may cope satisfactorily with feelings of loss, but it is natural that feelings of depression would be generated in such circumstances, and, for some, their emotions may produce extreme sadness and grief. Losses in late life can cause older people to expend large amounts of emotional and physical energy in grieving and resolving grief; therefore, it is not surprising that mood disorders are the primary mental health affliction of the old.

Suicide, which is often associated with depression, is also an important problem. Between 1981 and 1986, suicide rates among aged Americans increased from 17.1 per 100,000 to 21.3 per 100,000—an increase of 25 percent. This was a surprising development, since no other Western country was experiencing such a trend. It suggested that the quality of life available to aged Americans was not especially appealing, but the reasons for the rise in suicides was not known. Since 1986, however, the suicide rates have been declining somewhat and stood at 20.2 suicides per 100,000 persons in the age category of sixty-five and older in 1991. Despite the slight decrease, the elderly, especially aged males, are more likely to take their own lives than any other age group.

The mental problem most often associated with aging is the onset of senility or dementia, one example of which is Alzheimer's disease. According to DSM-IV (1994), the essential features of dementia include memory impairment and a disturbance in mental functioning. Memory impairment is, in fact, required to make a diagnosis of dementia; individuals with dementia may also become spatially disoriented, show poor insight and judgment, fail to recognize people and objects, and exhibit changes in personality—perhaps becoming more violent or suicidal.

Although dementia is a particularly terrible affliction of old age, it is not a normal feature of the aging experience. According to DSM-IV, only about 3 percent of the aged population have severe cognitive impairment caused by dementia. An additional 5–10 percent may be mildly or moderately impaired.

GENDER

Most studies of the true prevalence of mental disorder by sex clearly indicate (Aneshensel, Rutter, and Lachenbruch 1991; Dohrenwend and Dohrenwend 1974; Dohrenwend 1975; Dohrenwend and Dohrenwend 1976; Kessler et al.

1994; Rosenfield 1989) that (1) there are no consistent differences by sex in regard to rates of schizophrenia, (2) rates of mood and anxiety disorders are consistently higher for women, and (3) rates of personality disorders are consistently higher for men. Also, it should be noted that substance-related disorders are more common among men and that dementia is slightly more common among women. Sarah Rosenfield (1989:77) summarizes the mental health differences between men and women by concluding that these differences exist "across cultures, over time, in different age groups, in rural as well as urban areas, and in treated as well as untreated populations."

Whereas there are distinct differences between men and women in the prevalence of particular mental disorders, past studies have usually not supported the claim that the sexes are significantly different when it comes to overall rates of mental disorder (Dohrenwend and Dohrenwend 1974, 1976; Dohrenwend 1975). More-recent research disputes that and holds that women have greater tendencies toward mental disorder than men. A review of relevant studies conducted nationwide and in the National Institute of Mental Health Epidemiologic Catchment Area (ECA) Program suggests that females are generally more vulnerable to mental disorder than males (Center for Mental Health Services 1992; Kessler et al. 1994; National Center for Health Statistics and Centers for Disease Control 1992; Reiger et al. 1988; Stroup and Manderscheid 1988).

For example, a true prevalence survey of representative households throughout the United States conducted jointly by the National Center for Health Statistics and the National Institute of Mental Health identified 1.32 million males and 1.94 million females with a serious mental illness (Center for Mental Health Services, 1992; National Center for Health Statistics and Centers for Disease Control 1992). Overall rates of mental disorder were 15.5 per 1,000 for males and 20.6 for females. The ECA study of 18,571 persons at each of their five sites (Baltimore, Durham, Los Angeles, New Haven, and St. Louis) found rates of 14.0 per 1,000 for males and 16.6 per 1,000 for females (Reiger et al. 1988). Rates for females were higher than those for males in each age group. The nationwide Kessler et al. (1994) study likewise found that women had higher prevalences of more mental disorders on both a lifetime and a twelve-month basis than men. An impressive body of evidence is now developing that holds that the number of females in the general population with mental disorders exceeds the number of males at any given period (Center for Mental Health Services 1994c; National Center for Health Statistics and Centers for Disease Control 1992; Reiger et al. 1988; Stroup and Manderscheid 1988).

Of course, it might be thought that women tend to report more mental disorder because they are more expressive. A man, more than a woman, might feel that admitting to psychiatric symptoms of mental disorder is a sign of personal weakness. In that case, differences in rates of mental disorders could be due to underreporting by men rather than to real differences. However, as Myrna Weissman (1979) observes, research on both treated and untreated cases of mental disorder typically finds real differences between the sexes in regard to certain mental disorders. This is particularly true of studies of depression (Aneshensel, Frerichs, and Clark 1981; Avison and McAlpine 1992; Bart 1974; Gore, Aseltine, and Colton 1992; Newmann 1984; Roberts and O'Keefe 1981; Warheit et al. 1973; Weissman and Klerman 1977; Weissman and Paykel 1974). Other research by Kevin Clancy and Walter Gove (1974) has found that differences between men and women in the reporting of psychiatric symptoms are real, and not an artifact of response bias. Ronald Kessler and his associates (1981) found in a national sample that women did indeed have a greater tendency to seek psychiatric help, but they also had more emotional distress than men. Furthermore, when it comes to the use of outpatient psychiatric clinics and visits to the offices of psychiatrists and clinical psychologists, women are represented in far greater numbers than men (Center for Mental Health Services 1994a; Kessler, Reuter, and Greenley 1979; Veroff et al. 1981).

Despite the identification of higher overall rates of mental disorder among females, males are more likely to be admitted to state and county mental hospitals (Center for Mental Health Services 1994c). Table 7–2 shows admissions (which includes readmissions) to state mental hospitals (or county facilities if they are functionally equivalent) for the period 1881 to 1990. For each year shown, male admissions exceeds those of females; moreover, since the mid-1960s, the gap between male and female admissions has increased. Table 7–2 shows that the male–female ratio (the number of male admissions divided by female admissions multiplied by 100) for 1960 was 121 and the corrected male–female ratio (the ratio of males per 100,000 of the general population divided by the female rate multiplied by 100) was 124. The number of males admitted per 100,000 persons in the total population in 1960 was 135.4, as compared with 116.2 females. Table 7–2 shows that by 1990, the male–female ratio had risen to 172 and the corrected ratio to 183 in favor of males. Some 146.6 males per 100,000 of the general population had been admitted to state mental hospitals, compared with 80.3 per 100,000 for females.

The exact reason for significantly more male than female admissions to state mental hospitals, including the current upturn, is not known. The explanation given, however, is that males are perceived by society as being more dangerous and more likely to commit antisocial acts; therefore, males are more likely to be placed in public mental hospitals (Stroup and Manderscheid 1988). Several studies report that males are more likely to be hospitalized in public facilities because mental disorder in males is seen as more serious, threatening, or disabling (Clausen 1983; Gove 1972; Gove and Tudor 1973; Rushing 1979a). Another possible reason is that females are more prone to anxiety and mood disorders (primarily depression) and that those conditions can be more readily controlled with drugs and are less threat-

Table 7–2 Admissions and male–female ratios per 100,000 population, state mental hospitals, United States, 1881 to 1990

YEAR	MALES	FEMALES	MALE–FEMALE RATIO (× 100)	MALES PER 100,000	FEMALES PER 100,000	CORRECTED MALE–FEMALE RATIO (× 100)
1881	8,874	7,743	115	34.6	31.3	111
1885	12,153	9,455	129	42.2	34.3	123
1890	14,389	11,255	128	44.9	36.8	122
1895	17,268	13,514	128	48.7	39.9	122
1900	21,408	19,435	110	55.1	52.2	106
1904	23,131	18,260	127	54.9	45.6	120
1910	30,008	23,444	128	63.1	52.3	121
1915	37,965	28,967	131	73.6	59.1	125
1922	42,570	30,493	140	76.2	56.3	135
1930	40,743	32,709	140	73.4	53.8	136
1935	51,422	38,542	133	80.2	61.0	131
1940	62,307	47,812	130	93.9	72.7	129
1945	59,694	55,693	107	85.2	79.7	107
1950	79,992	66,646	120	105.9	87.5	121
1955	95,282	78,841	121	116.2	94.7	123
1960	120,961	99,655	126	135.4	109.1	124
1965	145,707	115,609	126	152.4	117.1	130
1970	274,761	184,762	149	274.0	176.6	155
1975	248,937	136,300	183	239.9	124.6	193
1980	239,400	129,649	185	217.6	111.3	196
1985	212,085	113,855	186	185.0	93.0	199
1990	175,647	102,166	172	146.6	80.3	183

Source: Center for Mental Health Services, 1994c.

ening to society, thereby allowing patients with those disorders to have a higher probability of being treated on an outpatient basis.

Biological Factors

Differences between males and females in relation to specific types of mental disorder may be due to biological and sociocultural factors. States of depression and anxiety in women may be influenced by hormonal changes in the body, such as those occurring during menstruation and menopause. However, the evidence in this regard is insufficient at present. Many women become irritable and depressed during menstruation, but there is no strong evidence that the onset of depressive disorders can be correlated with the menstrual cycle (Weissman 1979; Weissman and Klerman 1977; Weissman and Paykel 1974). Conversely, it may be that psychological distress has an important effect on menstrual problems (Fuller et al. 1993). There is some evidence that some women with a prior history of psychiatric disorder may develop depressive symptoms when taking oral contraceptives, but again it is unlikely that this would result in a full-blown depressive episode. Furthermore, women have had high rates of depression both before and after the introduction of oral contraceptives, and the rates have remained unchanged in those countries where birth control pills are not in widespread use (Weissman 1979). Another possible source of depression related to hormonal change is the period following pregnancy. Yet the so-called new-baby blues, or mild postpartum depression, is so common as to be considered normal. Usually, it disappears without treatment in about six weeks or less.

As for menopause, Weissman (1979) points out that several careful studies have shown that women are no more likely to become depressed at that time than at any other. Mary Lennon (1982) found in a national sample of American women that when menopause occurs on time, that is, during midlife, it is not associated with psychological distress. Menopause, however, can be stressful if it occurs either early or late in life, but generally there is no peak period when it causes depression. Furthermore, although women tend to show higher rates of depression than men, these rates gradually increase with age for both sexes until leveling out at around age fifty-five. This gradual increase, indicates Weissman (1979), is most likely related to an awareness of the aging process itself, as the individual copes with the loss of youth and what it signifies about lessened sexual attractiveness and physical energy.

For males, research on animals has suggested that the male hormone androgen stimulates aggression, and this may be a factor in the greater prevalence of personality disorders for men. Yet a biological basis for enhanced aggression in animals does not guarantee that a similar process is operative in human beings, and so we are left without any conclusive evidence (Mazur and Robinson 1972). Also, there is a highly speculative theory that the *Y* (male) sex chromosome is an "aggression" gene. Data supporting such a premise are derived from studies of *XYY* genotypes (males with an extra male chromosome in contrast to the normal male *XY* genotype). The *XYY* genotype tends to be overrepresented in penal and mental institutions. A 1965 study in Scotland, for instance, found no *XYY* genotypes in a sample of adult males in the general Scottish population and only 0.14 percent *XYY* genotypes among a sample of male infants; in mental hospitals and prisons 3.6 percent of the inmates were classified as *XYY* genotypes (Hook 1973). A particular shortcoming of *XYY* genotype studies is that the number of such individuals is extremely small in relation to the total population, and the evidence is dubious at best. When a comparison was made between the first-order relatives of hospitalized *XYY* males and a control group of normal males hospitalized for the same reason, there were six times more family histories of criminal convictions in the control group (Hirsch 1970). As for women and the possibility of a sex-linked pattern of inheritance for depression related to the *X* chromosome (the normal female has an *XX* genotype), there are few data to support such a conclusion.

There is evidence that the sexes may differ in the way they think, perceive, aspire, daydream, experience anxiety, and play competitive games (Hochschild 1973). A study by Janet Lever (1978) of the complexity of children's play and games found significant differences between the sexes. Using school-playground observations, interviews, written questionnaires, and diary records maintained by the children, Lever studied some 180 predominantly white and middle-class ten- and eleven-year-olds at three schools—two urban and one suburban. Boys' play was found to be more complex than girls' play, as illustrated by greater role differentiation, interdependence between players, size of play group, explicitness of goals, number of rules, and team formation. Lever suggests that the boys' games are a valuable learning experience. Boys, more than girls, learn to deal with diversity in group membership in which each person is required to perform a specialized task, to coordinate actions and maintain cohesiveness among group members, to cope with impersonal rules, and to work for collective as well as personal goals. Lever states:

> Team sports furnish the most frequent opportunity to sharpen these social skills. One could elaborate on the lessons learned. The rule structure encourages strategic thinking. Team sports also imply experience with clear-cut leadership positions, usually based on universalistic criteria. The group rewards the individual who has improved value skills, a practice which further enhances a sense of confidence based on achievement. Furthermore, through team sports as well as individual matches, boys learn to deal with interpersonal competition in a forthright manner. Boys experience face-to-face confrontations—often opposing a close friend—and must learn to depersonalize the attack. They must practice self-control and sportsmanship; in fact, some of the boys in this study described the greatest lesson in team sports as learning to "keep your cool."
>
> Girls' play and games are very different. They are mostly spontaneous, imaginative, and free of structure or rules. Turntaking activities like jump rope may be played without setting explicit goals. Girls have far less experience with interpersonal competition. The style of their competition is indirect, rather than face-

to-face, individual rather than team affiliated. Leadership roles are either missing or randomly filled.

Perhaps most important, girls' play occurs in small groups. These girls report preferring the company of a single best friend to a group of four or more. Often girls mimic primary human relationships instead of playing formal games, or they engage in conversation rather than play anything at all.[1]

The differences in the complexity of the children's play as reported by Lever are most likely due to socialization as much as or more than to biological factors. Lever notes that male children are quick to learn that displays of athletic skills earn the praise of adults, especially fathers. Girls, in contrast, may be discouraged from participation in sports to avoid the "tomboy" label. Whether the sexes develop different social skills through play in childhood that carries over and influences adult behavior is primarily speculation, as Lever mentions. Nevertheless, the differences in play are striking and are similar to adult behavior patterns for each sex.

In the classroom, girls seem to start out ahead of boys in nearly all subjects, and then fall behind boys in some subjects, beginning in the late high school years. Studies comparing sex differences in intelligence, for example, show that despite a more or less equal distribution of boys and girls in superior performance, there are substantial differences between the sexes in specific abilities (Boocock 1972). Males tend to outperform females on mathematical reasoning, judgment, manipulation of spatial relations, and mechanical aptitudes. Females tend to outperform males on vocabulary, verbal fluency, and memorization tasks. Eleanor Maccoby (1966) has found that sex differences in scholastic performance may be attributed to boys' more aggressive and active behavior, whereas girls exhibit greater dependency, anxiety, and passivity. These tendencies could be significantly related to more depression and anxiety disorders among women and to more personality disorders, which are characterized by active and antisocial behavior, among men. Again, whether these behavioral differences between males and females are mostly the result of innate biological qualities or of sociocultural influences is not known.

Sex-Role Socialization

As for sociocultural factors, sex-based differences in behavior appear to be the result of socialization into the socially prescribed roles for men and women. Sex-specific behavior in human society is strongly influenced through the process of sex typing, in which boys are taught to be men and girls to be women, with all that those roles imply about masculine and feminine attributes. The sex role for men clearly offers an advantage in self-direction and professional opportunities, yet may lend itself to increased susceptibility to per-

---

[1]Janet Lever, "Sex Differences in the Complexity of Children's Play and Games," *American Sociological Review* 43 (1978), 480–81.

sonality disorders. Conversely, the sex role for women may lend itself to increased depression and anxiety.

In a review of the sociological and psychological literature on stress and mental disorder in the young, Walter Gove and Terry Herb (1974) explain how this might happen. Gove and Herb suggest that life initially tends to be more stressful for young boys than for young girls because their intellectual and physical development is slower, yet they are expected to perform as well as girls. For instance, girls not only learn to say their first words sooner than boys but also progress much more rapidly having once reached that stage. There are similar differences in perception, emotion, and cognition. A second problem for young boys is their aggressiveness. "Virtually all the evidence," say Gove and Herb (1974:257), "indicates that boys have a lower frustration threshold, that they are more impulsive and more aggressive and that they get into fights more often than girls." This tendency most likely gets boys into more trouble with their parents and teachers, thereby increasing the amount of stress they experience.

Finally, a third factor that raises the stress levels for young boys is that the character of their sex role is more stringent. Little girls are allowed and perhaps encouraged to participate in traditionally masculine activities (for example, being a "tomboy"), but little boys are expected to act like "men" and to earn their masculine identity. Little boys are actively discouraged from and often punished for acting in feminine roles, but the taking on of more masculine roles by little girls is not considered serious until adolescence. Moreover, little boys usually spend most of their time in environments such as nurseries, preschools, schools, or home, where the most constant presence is that of an adult woman. In a predominantly feminine world, they may run into obstacles in expressing and adopting a masculine identity and thus perhaps are unsure and frustrated as to how they should behave. This situation is compounded by the fact that young boys are more limited by their sex role in the range of behaviors they can employ in overcoming their problems.

In midadolescence, there is a change in the relative stress experienced by the two sexes. Boys begin performing better in school as their physical and cognitive development begins to match that of girls. In addition, school subjects supposedly become more masculine, for example, mathematics and science. Boys begin to see their education as more relevant to their interests and presumably to their careers; girls begin to show signs of being less adept and less interested in the "masculine" subjects. Girls also may tend to see a disparity between school activities and their long-range goals, for it is at this time that girls are subject to more pressure to adopt the traditional feminine role (that is, deference to men, motherhood, family aspirations, dependency on males) and to abandon attempts to compete in a masculine world, despite being told they are the equals of men and have an equal opportunity to achieve career goals outside the home. Thus, girls become confused over whether they should act as "women" and defer to men, or be less feminine and compete with men.

And as part of this process, girls find that their roles require them to develop and maintain interpersonal ties with boys, as girlfriend or spouse, which often depends on the actions of *boys*. All in all, the adolescent girl experiences greater stress than her male counterpart does as she adjusts to a set of expectations that may oppose her predispositions. A particular source of stress is the state of dependency that evolves for the female. Gove and Herb state:

> Just as young boys have a personality trait, aggressiveness, that tends to get them into trouble, girls have a trait, dependency, that would appear to create problems for them in adolescence. Research uniformly indicates that boys are much more independent and autonomous than girls and that by adolescence they have become fairly self-sufficient. Girls, in contrast, are generally quite dependent on others and tend not to establish an independent identity and self-esteem. Furthermore, they tend to lack confidence in their ability to meet goals and are relatively unwilling to attempt new or difficult tasks.[2]

Gove and Herb therefore hypothesize that young boys have higher rates of mental disorder than young girls because of the greater amounts of stress they experience, but in adolescence this is reversed, with girls showing the higher rates because of greater stress. This hypothesis is supported by data Gove and Herb obtained from the National Institute of Mental Health on cases of mental disorder for persons nineteen years old or younger treated in public and private mental hospitals, general hospitals, and outpatient clinics. Before five years of age, the rates are exceedingly low for both sexes, but between the ages of five and nine, males had higher rates of disorders than females in all treatment settings. With increasing age, rates for both sexes likewise increased; yet by ages fifteen to nineteen, females were found to have caught up with males and overall showed rates as high if not higher. An exception was personality disorders, which remained predominantly male. For females, the trend upward was particularly marked for those disorders that involved anxiety.

More-recent data, collected as part of the Epidemiologic Catchment Area (ECA) Program in Los Angeles, support the Gove and Herb results by showing stress to be significantly related to anxiety and mood disorders in women and substance-related disorders in men (Aneshensel et al. 1991). Stress therefore appears to push many men and women toward different mental health outcomes.

Sex Roles and Work

Other indicators of how women's sex roles lead more readily to depression and anxiety are suggested by Walter Gove and Jeannette Tudor (1973) in regard to adult women. They summarized this as follows: (1) For women who are restricted to a single occupational and social role—that of being a house-

---

[2]Walter R. Gove and Terry R. Herb, "Stress and Mental Illness among the Young: A Comparison of the Sexes," *Social Forces* 53 (1974), 259.

wife—sources of gratification are severely limited; (2) being a housewife is frustrating because it requires limited skill and has low prestige; (3) the role of the housewife is relatively unstructured and invisible; (4) when a woman is employed outside the home, she is typically in a less satisfactory position than a married male; (5) the expectations for women are unclear. Thus, we see that to be a housewife is to have limited involvement with people outside the home. The activities themselves also may be boring and lonely for many women.

Many married women who work outside the home are viewed as working primarily to supplement the family income rather than as working toward specific career goals. Employed women may also be discriminated against in salaries and promotions when competing with married men in the same company. And working wives usually have to maintain the house as well as perform satisfactorily on the job, which, in essence, is tantamount to having two full-time jobs. What happens when the wife is more financially successful than the husband? Does the husband then assume greater responsibility for housework? Julie Brines (1994) finds that the more a husband relies on his wife for economic support, the less housework he does. This situation was found to be particularly true in low-income households. There is research showing that men have diminished feelings of psychological well-being when their wives earn more money than they do (Glass and Fujimoto 1994; Rosenfield 1992a). It may be that one way men, especially working and lower-class men, compensate for feelings about not being the primary breadwinner is to resist housework (Brines 1994). Regardless of a woman's income, it appears that housework generally remains "woman's work." This situation led Catherine Ross, John Mirowsky, and Patricia Ulbrich (1983:681) to conclude that "if a married woman gets a job to bolster the family income or find self-expression through occupational achievement, or both, she finds that the wife is now more like a husband but the husband is not more like a wife." There is research that shows the strain of working and doing the majority of work associated with raising children increases psychological distress among some married women—particularly those from low-income families (Cleary and Mechanic 1983; Gore and Mangione 1983; Parry 1986; Ross and Huber 1985; Shehan, Burg, and Rexroat 1986; Thoits 1986; Turner and Noh 1983). Therefore, it may be that working wives are under greater strain than their husbands. All in all, whether in the home or on the job, the lives of women are often dependent on what others (usually men) do; hence, they cannot control the possibilities for satisfaction as much as men can.

Not only are social roles generally more limited for women than for men, but also those women who choose motherhood as their primary role are particularly vulnerable to depression when their children leave home to pursue adult lives. Several studies indicate that the loss of the maternal role is a significant factor in the depression of many middle-aged women. For example, Pauline Bart (1974) studied 533 women in Los Angeles between the ages of forty and fifty-nine who had no prior history of hospitalization for mental disorder and yet were being treated at the time of the study in one of five local mental hospitals. In comparing the women with diagnoses of depression with those with other diagnoses, it was found that the depressed women were more likely to have had role loss or to sense an impending role loss—primarily loss of the maternal role. This was common among housewives who were overprotective or overinvolved with their children. Jewish women were more likely to be affected in this regard than either Anglo-Saxon or black women. Bart noted that the Jewish mother tended to be very overprotective toward her children and often felt like a "martyr" when the children did not react with what the mother thought was appropriate attention. Bart reports:

> Although she was a patient and I was an interviewer and a stranger, one Jewish woman forced me to eat candy, saying, "Don't say no to me." Another gave me unsolicited advice on whether I should marry and to whom, and a third said she would make a party for me when she left the hospital. Another example of the extreme nurturant patterns was shown by a fourth who insisted on caring for another patient who had just returned from a shock treatment while I was interviewing her. She also attempted to find other women for me to interview. The vocabulary of motives invoked by the Jewish women generally attributed their illnesses to their children. They complained about not seeing their children often enough. The non-Jewish women were more restrained and said they wanted their children to be independent. Two of the Jewish women had lived with their children, wanted to live with them again, and their illness was precipitated when their children forced them to live alone. However, living with their children was not a satisfactory arrangement for the women in the sample, since the few women having this arrangement were all depressed.[3]

This situation indicates that the *quality* of social relationships is also significant to female depression, particularly for those women who require involvement, like the Jewish women in the Bart study. The George Brown and Tirril Harris (1978) study of depression in London, England, found that although all of the female sample had experienced stressful life events, not all had suffered a major depressive episode. The essential difference between those who became seriously depressed and those who did not was the lack of an intimate, confiding, and supportive relationship. In this study, it was the relationship with the husband rather than with the children that was at issue. As housewives, these women had limited opportunities for developing friendships outside the home because of their responsibilities for caring for the children and the house. Without close involvement with their husbands, they tended to be both socially and psychologically isolated. Women working outside the home were less likely to suffer from depression, but the most important factor for all remained the quality of the personal relationship with a man.

Men apparently can tolerate an unsatisfactory relationship better than

---

[3]Pauline B. Bart, "The Sociology of Depression," in *Explorations in Psychiatric Sociology*, ed. P. Roman and H. Trice (Philadelphia: Davis, 1974), pp. 151–52.

women because they are more likely to have other outlets. A man has greater freedom in locating sources of personal satisfaction outside the home through work, career, social activities, and recreation. If a man finds one role unsatisfactory, he can focus on another. A woman is more likely to be tied to the home as the focal point of her life, particularly if she has small children. Women also appear more dependent than men on the support of other people for psychological well-being (Flaherty and Richman 1989). Thus, it seems highly probable that the disparity between men and women in depression is due at least partially to the different social roles and sociocultural expectations for each sex. Research conducted by René Levy (1976) in Switzerland on a nationwide sample of married couples found, for instance, significantly more indicators of psychophysiological problems among women who both played the traditional sex role of the woman in the family setting and were most accepting of that role. The greater the integration into the "normal" (traditional) role arrangement, the more likely it was that psychophysiological symptoms (for example, nightmares, trouble falling asleep, becoming easily exhausted, dizziness/nausea, hand trembling, heart palpitations) would occur. Levy (1976:131) concluded that "coincident structural and normative integration provokes symptoms if the situation in which one is integrated is pathogenic in itself."

Difficulties stemming from the traditional sex role of the woman, however, are not confined to those women who are locked into the housewife role. Professional women, including physicians, were found in a St. Louis study to have significantly higher rates of psychiatric problems than women in the general population (Welner et al. 1979). One hundred eleven women with M.D. degrees and 103 with Ph.D. degrees were interviewed. Among the physicians, 51 percent were found to have significant psychological distress. That compared with 32 percent of those with Ph.D.s. The most commonly reported disorder was depression, and it was particularly frequent and severe among the female physicians. Depression was greatest among those women reporting prejudice and discrimination in their employment and was even higher among those with children. In this case, for women who are in a position to reject the traditional sex-role stereotype rather than to accept that role, depression seems to be related more to role strain and the conflict between professional aspirations and family responsibilities. Perhaps they feel guilty about not completely fulfilling the maternal role and placing their career on a level that limits their family involvement. If the Switzerland and St. Louis studies can be generalized to most women, it would appear that they are in a "double bind" in that they may experience frustration in the traditional woman's role in the family and also if they leave that role for a career.

However, some studies have found that employment outside the home has enhanced the overall psychological well-being of women (Kessler and McRae 1981, 1982; McLanahan and Glass 1985). Other research suggests that women occupying nontraditional (typically male) roles are especially better off psychologically than women in traditional roles (Rosenfield 1980). But findings in this regard are controversial because there is evidence that women manifest more depression than men in both traditional and nontraditional roles (Roberts and O'Keefe 1981). Furthermore, many jobs that women perform have low levels of complexity, which reduces the possibilities for satisfaction (Lennon 1987). Consequently, the degree to which employment outside the home has resulted in improved mental health for women is generally not clear. What is clear is that increased employment for women has not had a negative impact on the psychological well-being of the great majority of women working outside the home.

Some women are no doubt content to be wives and mothers; other women may find more satisfaction in establishing a career outside the home or combining a job with being a housewife. But others appear to be torn between being a homemaker and being a career person and thus experience emotional conflicts regardless of their choice. Married women do have less control over their lives because of the demands of marriage and family and dependence upon the careers of their husbands. This lack of control has been found to make women particularly vulnerable to psychological distress (Kessler and McLeod 1984; Mirowsky 1985; Rosenfield 1989; Thoits 1987). Conversely, studies of employed wives show that having some degree of control at work moderates the psychological effects of demands put on the woman by her family (Lennon 1994; Lennon and Rosenfield 1992). Therefore, in comparison with men, women are more prone to psychological distress and mental disorder in general and to anxiety and mood disorders in particular. The social role of the woman appears highly significant in this process.

The "Double Standard" in Mental Health

If women seem to be caught in a double bind in regard to their role aspirations, they face a similar situation in standards for mental health. Research by Irene Broverman and her associates (1970) suggests that women are also subject to a "double standard" in mental health evaluations. Broverman and her associates studied the responses of a sample of male and female psychologists who were asked to describe character traits of men and women. The psychologists were divided into three groups. The first was asked to select the degree to which certain traits were indicative of the mature, healthy, socially competent male. The second group was requested to do the same for the mature, healthy, and socially competent female, and the third group was to do likewise in regard to the mature, healthy, and socially competent adult. The psychologists generally agreed on the traits considered most representative of the healthy male, female, and adult of either sex. Yet, although the descriptions of the male and the adult were not significantly different, the descriptions of the female were quite different. The female was seen as being more submissive, less independent, more easily influenced, less aggressive, less competitive, more excitable in minor crises, more emotional, more conceited, and less objective. The male and the adult traits were the reverse of the female traits. The ideal personality for the adult was that of the male, leaving the "normal" female model as less than positive.

Other studies also show the existence of a double standard in mental health evaluations. For example, Derek Phillips (1964) presented hypothetical case descriptions to a group of subjects without telling them that the descriptions pertained to mentally disturbed people. Half of the descriptions were of males and half of females. The rejection of males exhibiting abnormal behavior was much greater than for females. Phillips concluded that standards of normal behavior for females comes closest to including behavior that is symptomatic of mental disorder. In another study, Sandra Bem (1974) had a sample of college students rate characteristics thought to be desirable for males and females in American society. The students thought that males should be assertive, athletic, individualistic, and self-reliant, among other things. The ideal female characteristics included loyalty, affection, understanding, and compassion. Although the female traits were not seen as negative, the male traits were viewed as more valuable because they were thought to serve the needs of society better than those of the female.

Kay Deaux summarizes this situation as follows:

> Men, for example, are viewed as independent, objective, active, competitive, adventurous, self-confident, and ambitious. Women are seen as possessing the opposite of each of these traits. They are characterized as dependent, subjective, passive, not competitive, not adventurous, not self-confident, and not ambitious. In each instance, people have indicated that the trait the male possesses is the more desirable trait for someone in our Western culture. Women are not seen as all bad, however. There is a cluster of positively valued traits that people see as more typical of women than men; these traits generally reflect warmth and expressiveness. Women are described as tactful, gentle, aware of the feelings of others, and able to express tender feelings easily. Men in contrast are viewed as blunt, rough, unaware of the feelings of others, and unable to express their own feelings. Yet while women are credited with a number of positive traits, the numbers are still less. Furthermore, some good things may be better than others, and, in a competitive society such as ours, competence seems to be a more highly valued trait than warmth.[4]

The double standard for mental health places the female in a double bind. If feminine traits are followed, the woman has less desirable characteristics; if masculine traits are followed, the woman is deviant. Hence, here again there is a "damned if you do and damned if you don't" situation.

If normal female traits are more similar to mentally disordered behavior than normal male traits are, it would suggest that males are more likely to undergo psychiatric treatment when they act abnormal. As previously mentioned, there is research indicating that this is what happens (Doherty 1978;

---

[4]Kay Deaux, *The Behavior of Women and Men* (Monterey, CA: Brooks/Cole, 1976), pp. 13–14.

Gove 1972; Gove and Tudor 1973; Rosenfield 1982; Rushing 1979a). When both men and women perform acts indicative of mental disorder, men are more likely to be perceived as mentally ill because symptoms of distress and disorganization are considered to be more usual among females. William Tudor, Jeannette Tudor, and Walter Gove (1977, 1979) investigated this situation in regard to anxiety, psychotic symptoms, and mental retardation. They hypothesized that role expectations for women are such that females are generally expected to be less competent than males; therefore, societal reaction to disturbed males is more prompt and severe. In other words, people are more tolerant of bizarre behavior among females. Their hypothesis was supported. The data showed that males with psychotic symptoms were hospitalized more readily and tended to have longer hospital stays than psychotic females. For anxiety, usually self-limiting, more common to females, and often not requiring hospitalization for treatment, it was found that if hospitalization was necessary, there was no difference in the frequency with which males and females entered the hospital. But males tended to remain hospitalized longer. As for mental retardation, Tudor and his associates (1979) found that mentally retarded males tended to be institutionalized more often than mentally retarded females and that for males institutionalization took place, on the whole, at earlier ages and for milder conditions.

Conclusion

Even though males may be more likely to be admitted to mental hospitals, females have a particular disadvantage in regard to the stress associated with their gender role and the double standard that influences how their mental health is perceived. From a social standpoint, gender can be depicted as an enduring ascribed characteristic that cuts across all social classes and racial/ethnic groups to affect the evaluations of people in all areas of life and to form the basis for persisting sexual divisions of labor and gender-based inequalities. This situation, combined with biological differences, undoubtedly contributes to the varying incidence between men and women of certain mental disorders. The task currently before sociologists is to help isolate the relative contributions of male–female differences in those disorders in which gender is known to be an important variable. These differences apparently not only cause differences in particular forms of mental disorder but also contribute to the greater overall prevalence of such disorders among females.

MARITAL STATUS

Another major variable that is commonly employed in epidemiological surveys of mental disorder is marital status. A consistent finding is that married people have better mental health than unmarried people. The rationale behind this finding is that the married have greater social and emotional support and therefore are better able to cope with psychological trauma and stress. To a limited extent, that probably is correct. As we saw earlier in the discussion of the social stress model of mental disorder, sources of social support like families and spouses can help mitigate the effects of stress and assist in deflecting tendencies toward psychological difficulties (Kandel, Davies, and Raveis 1985; Kessler and Essex 1982; Turner and Marino 1994). Conversely, families and spouses can also be the sources of stress, and impaired relationships in this context can be precipitating factors in the onset of abnormal behavior. Situations leading up to divorce and their aftermath, for example, are known to cause increased depression—especially for women (Aseltine and Kessler 1993). The association of psychological distress with poor marriages is common among both African Americans and whites (Williams, Takeuchi, and Adair 1992a). Therefore, it seems safe to assume that if marital relationships are stable, affectionate, and supportive, tendencies toward mental disorder are likely to be somewhat reduced or at least are not aggravated by what occurs in the home.

A study of this situation was conducted by Leonard Pearlin and Joyce Johnson (1977) in the Chicago area, where they interviewed twenty-three hundred persons in regard to their conflicts and problems of daily living, the manner in which those conflicts were handled, and their symptoms of emotional stress and disturbance. The focus of the study was on the relationship between marital status and noninstitutionalized cases of depression. It was found that the lowest scores for depression were recorded by the married and the highest scores by the formerly married (widowed, divorced, or separated). The never-married scored somewhat lower on depression than the formerly married. Perhaps the formerly married were pressured by the transition from marriage to being single so that their self-concepts may have suffered, their social networks became disrupted, and their usual patterns of life changed. Pearlin and Johnson conclude that marriage functions as a protective barrier against threats (for example, social, economic) outside the marital relationship. Married persons had the advantage, in comparison with the unmarried, of being able to draw emotional support and other help from spouses. "Marriage does not prevent economic and social problems from invading life," report Pearlin and Johnson (1977:714), "but it apparently can help people fend off the psychological assaults that such problems otherwise create."

Other research suggests that women are more likely to show signs of distress than men whether they are married or not (Fox 1980). But among persons who are married (women as well as men), the quality of the relationship with the spouse appears especially important in maintaining a positive level of mental health (Gove, Hughes, and Style 1983; Vanfossen 1981). Ross, Mirowsky, and Huber (1983) have found that both spouses are less depressed when the wife's employment outside the home is consistent with their preference. And both spouses are less depressed if neither dominates the marriage (Mirowsky 1985).

The possible supportive nature of the marital relationship, however, accounts only partially for the interplay between marital status and mental disorder because it leaves two other issues unresolved. The first issue is whether there is a difference between men and women by marital status in rates of mental disorder. The second issue pertains to whether marital status is a truly relevant variable. If insane people are less likely to be married, marital status may not be particularly important to understanding madness.

Data for 1980 from the National Institute of Mental Health (1986) on admissions to state and county mental hospitals by marital status remain the most recent report on this topic. These data show that 25.7 percent of all admissions were married females as contrasted with 18.2 percent for married males. Half (51.5 percent) of the male patients admitted had never been married, compared with 34.2 percent of the females. The percentages of separated/divorced patients were about equal by sex (27.9 percent of males and 29.7 percent of females), whereas more women (10.4 percent) than men (2.3 percent) were widowed. If marriage conferred any special benefits on women in avoiding mental hospitalization, these data do not support that conclusion. But they also do not support the conclusion that marriage promotes mental disorder for women. Public mental hospital admissions data alone cannot prove this point, and the disparity between married male–female admissions in the existing data is not great. Higher rates of mental disorder among women cannot be attributed to their being married (Warheit et al. 1976).

The other issue that demands our attention is whether marital status is in fact a highly significant variable in relation to mental disorder. It has been suggested that people with mental problems are more likely not to be married in the first place (Martin 1976; Rushing 1979b; Turner and Gartrell 1978). A certain amount of social competence seems necessary if a person is going to be able to attract a spouse. So although it may seem that marriage is an important protection for some in regard to mental disorder, that may be somewhat deceiving. Possibly, social selection is operative (the mentally ill are selected out of marriage) in that the married are more likely to be socially competent and therefore less susceptible to mental disorder. R. Jay Turner and John Gartrell (1978) argue for the social selection hypothesis. They suggest that marital status is pertinent because it does reflect important differences in social competence. They insist there is no reason to believe there is anything about marriage per se that significantly affects the amount of time a person spends in a mental hospital. "The more symptomatic and/or ineffective an individual," state Turner and Gartrell (1978:378), "the less likely he will find a marital partner, achieve higher class levels and work consistently and the more likely he will spend extended periods in the hospital."

The social selection approach clearly places the locus of the problem in the individual and not in the marriage. The assertion is accurate that the mentally ill are more likely to be unmarried, either through failure to court a spouse successfully or through divorce. Nevertheless, although being married may not affect the length of time one is hospitalized, marital status most likely plays a limited role in helping a person to avoid hospitalization. Overall, marital status does not seem to be as strong a predictor of mental disorder as social class and gender.

SUMMARY

This chapter has examined the relationship between age, gender, marital status, and mental disorder. The highest prevalences of mental disorders generally are found among people in the 25–34-year-old group. Dementia, especially of the Alzheimer's type, is the mental disorder most often associated with aging. About 3 percent of the aged population have severe cognitive disorders resulting from dementia, and an additional 5–10 percent may be moderately or mildly impaired. Mood disorders are the most common disorder among the elderly. It was found that gender is also a highly significant and consistent predictor of certain mental disorders. New findings suggest that women in general are more likely to become mentally disordered even though females are not represented in public mental hospitals in significantly greater numbers than males. Women are more prone to anxiety and depression than males; males are more prone to personality disorders and substance-related disorders. Reasons for these differences between men and women may be traced to both biological and social factors (especially sex roles), but the relative contribution of each has not been determined, and there is as yet no specific information that allows a definitive conclusion.

Marriage can be a protective factor in psychological distress if the quality of the relationship is good. The marital status variable, however, is questioned because social selection indicates that the married are less likely to be mentally ill in the first place because of their demonstrated social competence in obtaining a spouse.

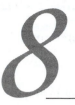

Mental Disorder: Urban versus Rural Living and Migration

This chapter reviews what is known about the psychological well-being of people who live in urban areas as compared with those who reside in rural settings. The chapter will also examine patterns of mental health among migrants who leave their home country and typically move to a more affluent nation, especially the United States or one of the Western European countries, to flee persecution or to obtain jobs and greater economic opportunities.

URBAN VERSUS RURAL LIVING

The widely held assumption that the stress of urban living is responsible for high rates of mental disorder and that rural areas are relatively free of such problems is not entirely accurate. Past studies suggest that schizophrenia, anxiety, and personality disorders are more common in urban areas, and mood disorders (especially depression) are higher in rural environments (Dohrenwend 1975). However, recent research finds that mental disorders in general, including problems in mood, are more prevalent in major metropolitan centers than anywhere else (Kessler et al. 1994). Disagreement therefore exists over whether higher rates of mood disorders prevail in rural areas than in urban locales. What seems certain is that when specific types of mental disorders in rural areas are considered, mood disorders stand out as a particular problem—whether or not there may be more of it in cities.

Mental Disorder and Rural Living

According to the Bureau of the Census, 24.8 percent of the American population could be classified in 1990 as rural in that they live in places with fewer than twenty-five hundred people. Such people would be those that live in sparsely settled areas, wide-open spaces, relatively isolated communities, and small towns and small suburban areas in or near larger metropolitan areas. At first glance, the rural population of the United States would appear to be exceedingly heterogeneous and very difficult to characterize in any general manner. The values and culture of a Maine fishing village, for example, differ from those of farmers and ranchers in the Midwest or in the intermountain West (Flax et al. 1979). Even if one attempts to focus on a particular region like the rural South, one can come up with differences in values and traditions between such areas as the Tidewater, Piedmont, or Delta South. Nevertheless, some broad generalizations are possible. Rural values emphasize the following themes: humankind's subjugation to nature, fatalism, an orientation to concrete places and things, distrust of outsiders, and human relationships as grounded in personal and friendship ties (Flax et al. 1979).

Other research suggests that rural people, as compared with urban residents, *tend* to be more conservative, religious, puritanical, work oriented, ascetic, ethnocentric, isolationist, intolerant of heterodox ideas and values, prejudicial, uninformed, authoritarian, and family centered (Hassinger 1976). The emphasis is on *tend* because in contrasting rural–urban values, it is not that all or most rural people are one way and most urban people are another. Instead, the differences are a matter of degree. No doubt, there are also variations within overall patterns.

Differences in urban–rural values, although informative, are not held up as the cause of significant differences in mental disorders. They do point toward possible differences in psychological orientation among people in rural areas subject to more isolation from mainstream society than urban residents. Two studies that explore this situation are those by Claude Fischer (1973) and Stephen Webb and John Collette (1977). Fischer reviewed several American and foreign surveys of urban and rural residents to determine whether the size of one's community promoted personal unhappiness. What was evident was not that urban dwellers were particularly unhappy but that feelings of malaise (defined as a psychological state of dissatisfaction, unhappiness, despair, and melancholy) in rural areas might be worldwide. In fact, people in cities across the world seemed more content generally, especially because of economic opportunities, than those in the countryside. Although there was evidence of some urban malaise in the largest cities, the effect was small and was usually restricted to the center of the city. Fischer concludes that city life per se does not generate malaise, although very large cities may be too large and contribute modestly to unhappiness.

The Webb and Collette study investigated the use of stress-alleviating drugs (tranquilizers) in urban and rural areas of New Zealand as an indicator of stressful living conditions. Data were obtained from pharmacists throughout New Zealand and consisted of the name of the drug prescribed, sex of the client, and daily dosage for every tranquilizer prescription filled on an average day. The data showed that the larger the locality was, the lower the mean monthly rate of prescriptions filled. Particularly noteworthy was the finding that the number of prescriptions filled in rural areas (under twenty-five hundred population) was almost double that of the largest cities (one hundred thousand or more persons). Females used a far larger proportion of tranquilizers than males. Webb and Collette suggest that

> lack of stimulation and the routinization of an isolated life-style may account for the greater prevalence in rural communities of the symptoms of stress. Through the predominantly urban mass media, ruralists may be exposed to life-style aspirations beyond their reach; and their relative deprivation may engender feelings of frustration, alienation, and isolation. We might also speculate that rural residents are more likely to be exposed to a larger number of situational and continuous stresses. The crowding of rural housing, an inability to escape easily to distracting amusements, and the stifling social pressure of small towns may combine with other factors to produce a highly stressful environment.[1]

This quotation may be the most accurate description of why mood disorders—as compared with other mental disorders—are a particular problem in rural areas. Although rural areas may be more peaceful, they are also more isolated and perhaps even boring for some people because social and cultural stimulation is lacking.

Mental Disorder and Urban Living

Most people in the United States live in what is known as a Standard Metropolitan Statistical Area (SMSA), a classification scheme devised by the Bureau of the Budget. An SMSA is a county or a group of contiguous counties that contains at least one city of fifty thousand or more persons, except for New England, where SMSAs consist of towns or cities only. The surroundings of urban life vary from so-called concrete jungles of the inner city to urban or suburban areas where the countryside is nearby. A common notion of city living, at least in very large cities like New York, Philadelphia, Chicago, and Los Angeles, is that of human beings packed into overcrowded areas and caught up in the "rat race" in which the pursuit of success is everything. The casualties of this environment are those people who finish up in the slums, in prison, or

---

[1]Stephen D. Webb and John Collette, "Rural–Urban Differences in the Use of Stress-Alleviative Drugs," *American Journal of Sociology* 83 (1977), 706.

in mental hospitals. Those who adapt may seem distrustful, selfish, cynical, aloof, superficial, and perhaps mercenary. Of course, that, like most stereotypes, is inaccurate—many people in big cities do not have those traits, but the image remains nonetheless. Cities offer much of both the best and the worst that is available in society; the best cultural, intellectual, and economic opportunities are found in cities, but so is the most crime, environmental pollution, and overcrowded housing.

Overcrowded housing A particular aspect of urban living and mental health that has caught the attention of social scientists is the possible effects of a highly dense population and overcrowded housing. Some studies maintain that high levels of density present serious psychological problems for human beings (Baldassare 1978; Freeman 1984). These studies attempted to test the theory that people living in large communities find themselves in a locale that is relatively confining in relation to the number of people present and the amount of space available. The greater the density, the more "crowded" people feel. It is therefore thought that perhaps the tension brought on by this situation will become so stressful that physical or mental problems will result. "Relief must somehow be found, for example, by aggression or withdrawal," says Fischer (1976:155) as an illustration of this approach, "or the stress will result in mental or physical illness."

But is this actually the case? Does overcrowding cause mental disorder? Some research suggests that it may not have a particularly strong effect. In Detroit, Stanislav Kasl and Ernst Harburg (1975) surveyed a cross-section of married residents living in four carefully selected census tracts. Two tracts were predominantly black, and two were almost exclusively white; each was either a high-stress or a low-stress neighborhood as determined by social class, crime rates, divorce, and residential stability. It was found that residents of high-stress neighborhoods had more negative evaluations of their neighborhood, but there was little evidence of poor mental health and psychological well-being. What few differences existed were slight and pertained mostly to women. Yet when the effects of overcrowding are considered, *the variable of major importance seems to be overcrowding in the home rather than in the neighborhood* (Booth and Cowell 1976; Carnahan, Gove, and Galle 1974; Galle and Gove 1978; Gove et al. 1979). That is so because relationships in the home are more important and contribute more to shaping the behavior of the individual. As Walter Gove and his associates (1979:59) observe, "Disruption of these relationships due to overcrowding is thus apt to have serious consequences." Such studies of overcrowding in the home are more analogous to the numerous studies of overcrowding done with animals, especially rat studies in which rats have been found to act in pathological ways simply because there are too many of them.

Studies of the overcrowding of humans in their homes, however, have produced inconclusive results. In a comprehensive review of the literature and a secondary analysis of survey data derived from various studies, Mark Baldassare (1978) found that overcrowding in the home was related to poor interpersonal relationships but not to poor mental health. Other research carried out in Toronto and published in a series of papers by Alan Booth and his associates (Booth 1976; Booth and Cowell 1976; Booth and Edwards 1976) likewise discovered modest effects at best on mental health because of overcrowding. In general, Booth stated that crowding has little or no effect on family relations, although in a later paper he noted that the lack of space and the availability of privacy was modestly associated with psychiatric impairment among women (Duvall and Booth 1978). It is noteworthy that differences between men and women keep recurring in regard to the effects of overcrowding. Some research suggests that men are more affected overall by crowding in the home (Booth and Cowell 1976) and the constraints of apartment living (Edwards, Booth, and Edwards 1982), but other research indicates that women are more affected by building density and height. For example, in a study of high-rise housing and psychological strain, A. R. Gillis (1977) found in a sample of public housing residents in the Canadian province of Alberta that the higher the building, the greater the psychological strain on women. In addition, women with young children are particularly stressed in overcrowded homes (Baldassare 1981).

Although there may be differences between the sexes in how they are affected by overcrowding in housing, the question still remains as to whether overcrowding can be linked to mental disorder. In a well-designed study of census tracts in Chicago, Gove and associates (1979) found that both objective crowding (persons per room) and subjective crowding (excessive social demands and lack of privacy) were strongly related to poor mental health, poor social relationships in the home, and poor child care. Less strong, but still significant, was the discovery of a relationship between poor physical health and poor social relations outside the home. Gove and his associates suggest that crowding results in physical withdrawal, a lack of effective planning behavior, and a general feeling of being "washed out." They argue that crowding does have substantial effects and that it is time to end the debate over whether overcrowding is pathological and to study factors important in magnifying or minimizing that pathology.

In fact, in subsequent research, Hughes and Gove (1981) studied the psychological effects of living alone among unmarried persons and found them to be in no worse, and in some ways in better, mental health than unmarried persons who live with others. Persons living together who are not part of a nuclear family (parents and their children) experience a greater lack of privacy and have to make more adjustment to the presence, habits, and personalities of those sharing the living space. This includes not only grandparents, aunts, uncles, and other relatives but also friends and roommates. Therefore, Hughes and Gove conclude:

In contrast to what one would anticipate on the basis of the literature on social integration, living alone does not appear to be particularly problematic. Indeed, there is some evidence that it may be a somewhat better living arrangement for those who are not married than is living with others. This makes a great deal of sense if we assume that the benefit of families to members is particularly a benefit to spouses and minor children and not necessarily to other persons in the household.[2]

Overcrowding in the home is a negative situation. Whether it leads to mental disorder is still not clear, but it seems likely that overcrowding at least exacerbates the social conditions that foster mentally abnormal episodes of behavior. Thus, we can see that overcrowding may well promote schizophrenia as a flight from reality and anxiety disorders as a form of tension. Moreover, overcrowding may contribute to the strained social relationships that are common in personality disorders. Consequently, the three disorders most prevalent in urban areas— schizophrenia, anxiety disorders, and personality disorders—may be associated with crowding. Unfortunately, it is not entirely clear whether the association is direct or indirect. Fischer (1976) explains, for example, that the people who lack space in their lives (that is, the poor, the minorities, and persons who are socially, physically, and psychologically handicapped) are generally those who also lack the other good things in life. "It is more nearly the case," states Fischer (1976:162) "that suffering people come to live densely than that density causes suffering." Nevertheless, the relationship between mental strain and overcrowding appears real, regardless of whether overcrowding causes strain or strain causes overcrowding or both.

Another factor relevant to our discussion of mental disorder in urban areas is the well-established finding that schizophrenia tends to be more prevalent in the inner city (Eaton 1974b; Faris and Dunham 1939). Studies tracing the ecological distribution of schizophrenia consistently find higher rates of it in the central areas of large cities, and the rates drop significantly as the pattern of schizophrenic residencies is followed to the suburbs and rural areas. This finding is presumably tied to that of social class, with the lower class most likely to be both schizophrenic and residents of the inner city.

MIGRATION

A variable related to location of residence that has attracted the attention of some researchers is migration. Migration studies usually examine patterns of either internal or international migration. As for internal migration in the United States, one rationale previously discussed in this section, which sometimes is used to account for the greater prevalence of certain mental disorders

[2]Michael Hughes and Walter R. Gove, "Living Alone, Social Integration, and Mental Health," *American Journal of Sociology* 87 (1981), 69.

(for example, schizophrenia, anxiety disorders) in urban areas, is that rural people with those problems tend to move to the cities. Consequently, urban rates may be falsely inflated by the presence of mentally disturbed migrants whose mental disorders had their origin in rural living conditions.

A similar argument is found in the research literature pertaining to international migration, especially those studies done in the 1930s (for example, Faris and Dunham 1939), which suggest that foreign-born persons in the United States show higher rates of mental disorder than native-born persons do. For instance, a 1932 comparison of Norwegian-born immigrants in Minnesota with native-born Minnesotans and Norwegians in Norway found that mental hospital first-admissions rates were highest for the immigrant group (Ödegaard 1932). Yet other research has found that Swedes and Danes moving into rural areas of Norway had lower first-admissions hospital rates than did native-born Norwegians (Astrup and Ödegaard 1960) and that immigrants to Canada between 1958 and 1961 had lower admissions rates than did native-born Canadians (Murphy 1969). Also, research on Jewish immigrants to Israel after World War II found Jews of European descent to have about the same rates of mental hospitalization as those for native Israelis, but Jews of Asian and African descent had somewhat higher rates (Murphy 1969). And Mexican immigrants to the United States have been found to have better mental health than native-born Mexican Americans (Burnam et al. 1987).

A problem with migration in relationship to mental disorder is that although some mentally disturbed people may be predisposed by their disorder to move, it also may be true that perfectly stable individuals move to improve their chances for upward mobility through enhanced economic, social, and cultural opportunities elsewhere (about 20 percent of the American population change their residence each year, and the majority do so for reasons that are not indicative of mental disorder). Or people move simply to survive, like the flood of refugees from Southeast Asia following the end of the Vietnam War in 1975 and the Vietnamese invasion of Cambodia in 1978.

Also, in the 1980s large numbers of people fled to the United States because of poverty in Haiti, communism in Cuba and Poland, guerrilla warfare in Central America, and serious economic downturns in Mexico and the Philippines. This situation has caused some experts (Oxford Analytica 1986) to conclude that the United States' biggest import is people, with about 450,000 arriving legally every year and an additional 1.5 million entering the country illegally. The United States, with about 5 percent of the world's population, takes in about 50 percent of the world's immigrants. This situation is expected to continue through the 1990s as the population of Mexico and the Caribbean continues to grow faster than the number of available jobs. Because of immigration and a high domestic birthrate, Hispanic Americans will become the nation's largest minority group in the twenty-first century.

Consequently, the mental health of immigrants and the difficulty of adjusting to their new society are topics that are likely to continue to be of interest to sociologists. One study is that of Alejandro Portes, David Kyle, and William Eaton (1992) on Cuban and Haitian refugees in south Florida. Significant differences were found in the utilization of mental health services by the two immigrant groups. Haitians experienced significant barriers in obtaining care because of a general lack of familiarity with mental health services and bureaucratic requirements; also ethnic tensions with African Americans who received care at the same facility discouraged utilization by Haitians. Cubans, in contrast, had prior experience in their homeland with mental health services, and they were treated in a mental health center in Miami's "Little Havana" that was oriented toward helping Cubans. This facility had Cuban-American staff members, Spanish was spoken, and Cuban culture was not denigrated. The Cuban refugees had greater need for care and received better services than the Haitians because of the more supportive environment in which care was rendered. The Cubans therefore found it easier to adapt to their new circumstances.

Another study of mental health and migration is that of Wen Kuo and Yung-Mei Tsai (1986) who investigated psychological problems among newly arrived Asian immigrants in Seattle. Kuo and Tsai noted that existing studies usually treat emigration as a process of uprooting to emphasize the social stress that is involved in leaving one's native land and resettling elsewhere. That stress can include feelings of isolation, cultural conflict, poor social integration and assimilation, role change and identity crisis, low socioeconomic status, and racial discrimination. Yet Kuo and Tsai remind us that the change associated with resettlement is not always bad; gains in one's quality of life can be achieved.

Among the Chinese, Filipinos, Japanese, and Koreans in the Kuo and Tsai study, about 35 percent reported adjustment difficulties with finances, the English language, homesickness, American food and lifestyle, climate, and isolation from their ethnic group. The remaining 65 percent were able to adjust relatively well. Kuo and Tsai came to two conclusions. First, immigrants can live apart from the larger society and not suffer from severe social isolation, especially if they are able to become part of a social network of others of the same ethnic background. And second, personality seems to be a migratory selection factor. Those migrants with the hardiest personalities were able to avoid the stress of migration the best. Persons who were rugged, active, and willing to risk change had the best mental health.

What is suggested by findings such as those of Kuo and Tsai is that many migrants are able to escape the mental stress associated with being uprooted from their native environment. Some migrants, however, do suffer considerable hardship, particularly those forced to leave their homes because of tyranny, injustice, poverty, or racial, ethnic, political, or religious persecution. These people most likely experience considerable psychological distress associated with their situation. But to claim that migration per se causes mental disorder for most migrants is incorrect. Research linking mental disorder with migration patterns has produced inconsistent findings, and to date no clear association can be proved (Gallagher 1987; Schwab and Schwab 1978).

SUMMARY

This chapter discussed the relationship between mental disorder and whether a person lives in a city or in the country. Rural life was found to be a state of living that was not completely free from mental problems. Mood disorders are more common among rural populations than urban, and some of the reasons for that might be the greater social isolation and lesser cultural stimulation of the countryside, but no one knows for sure. As for urban conditions, schizophrenia and the anxiety and personality disorders are more prevalent among city residents. Much of the investigation in urban areas is of the effects of overcrowding, although the stress and competition of the city may also be pertinent. Overcrowding in the home seems much more significant than overcrowding in the neighborhood in regard to emotional disturbances. The evidence from crowding studies is not conclusive, yet enough data have been gathered to suggest that overcrowding is indeed stressful and most likely has some influence on mental disorder, even if it does nothing more than simply aggravate the problem. As for location of residence in the city, higher rates of schizophrenia are usually found in the inner city. This is likely related to being also from the lower class. Migration studies are inconclusive.

9

Mental Disorder: Race

Claims that members of racial minority groups in the United States have higher rates of mental disorder than whites are not borne out by the research literature—although controversy and debate on this topic continue. Admittedly, many studies involved in this argument have had imprecise methodologies and theoretical formulations, but most of the better studies provide little or no support for the claim that there is a significant relationship between mental disorder and race (Dohrenwend and Dohrenwend 1969, 1974; Frerichs, Aneshensel, and Clark 1981; Kessler 1979; Kessler et al. 1994; Roberts 1980; Warheit et al. 1973; Warheit, Holzer, and Avery 1975). Therefore, as William Grier and Price Cobbs, two African-American psychiatrists, conclude about the mental health of African Americans:

> There is nothing reported in the literature or in the experience of any clinician known to the authors that suggests that black people *function* differently psychologically from anyone else. Black men's mental functioning is governed by the same *rules* as that of any other group of men. Psychological principles understood first in the study of white men are true no matter what the man's color.[1]

---

[1]William H. Grier and Price M. Cobbs, *Black Rage* (New York: Basic Books, 1992), p. 154.

Yet other research maintains that racial differences in mental health between blacks and whites exist. Ronald Kessler and Harold Neighbors (1986) analyzed data from several prior surveys of mental health in the United States and found that among the lower class, blacks showed more psychological distress than whites. The authors suggest that perhaps the combined effects of poverty and racial discrimination produce greater distress for poor blacks in comparison with poor whites. Additional research in Tennessee (Neff 1984; Neff and Husaini 1987) found greater depression among blacks than among whites, but this finding was primarily due to the responses of rural blacks. Rural blacks showed significantly more depression than either urban blacks or rural and urban whites. And, in north central Florida, Patricia Ulbrich, George Warheit, and Rick Zimmerman (1989) found greater psychological distress among blacks with low incomes and occupational status than among whites with similar low-status characteristics or among affluent blacks. Other research has found that although lower-class blacks may have higher levels of psychological distress than lower-class whites, they do not have higher rates of mental disorder (Williams, Takeuchi, and Adair 1992b). However, in Illinois, the author (Cockerham 1990b) found a lack of significant difference in psychological distress between low-income blacks and whites; in fact, the higher the income for blacks, the lower their distress in comparison with whites. So although there is some evidence of greater psychological distress among lower-class blacks, that evidence is not yet conclusive.

Furthermore, studies showing differences between people within special population groups, namely, between the poor or rural dwellers, do not change the general position in the literature that there is no difference *overall* between blacks and whites with respect to mental health. But they do point toward some possible exceptions to the general situation and are likely to cause renewed interest in the study of race and mental health. The research that helps put this debate into perspective is the recent nationwide study by Kessler and his associates (1994). This study provides strong evidence that there are no mental disorders for which either lifetime or active prevalence is significantly higher among blacks than among whites.

The primary reason that race is associated with mental disorder is that many racial minority people are found in the lower class, and class position is a much stronger predictor of mental disorder than is race. For example, in a well-known study by George Warheit and his colleagues (1973), blacks showed more depression than whites, but the difference was due primarily to the fact that the blacks were also lower class. Even though this study is more than twenty years old, it is still considered an important work and illustrates that class is of greater importance than race as a predictor of mental disorder.

When treatment as an inpatient in a mental health facility is considered, the data shown in Table 9–1 reinforce the importance of social class position over that of race. Since nonwhites are more likely to be poor, historically they have been placed in public facilities rather than in private institutions (Warheit

TABLE 9–1 Distribution of resident mental patients in selected psychiatric treatment settings by race, 1990

TREATMENT SETTING	WHITES		BLACKS		NATIVE AMERICANS		ASIAN/PACIFIC ISLANDER	
	PERCENT	NUMBER	PERCENT	NUMBER	PERCENT	NUMBER	PERCENT	NUMBER
State and county mental hospitals	46.4	64,181	64.6	24,377	54.3	614	50.5	712
Private mental hospitals	18.9	26,064	8.3	3,146	20.9	237	14.6	206
Nonfederal general hospitals	23.7	32,657	14.0	5,284	10.0	113	21.1	298
Veterans hospitals	8.7	12,045	11.8	4,446	10.7	121	8.9	124
Multiservice mental organizations	2.3	3,249	1.3	493	4.1	46	4.9	69
TOTALS:	100.0	138,196	100.0	37,746	100.0	1,131	100.0	1,409

Source: Adapted from Center for Mental Health Services data.

et al. 1975). This is seen in Table 9–1, which shows the number and percentage of resident mental patients in selected psychiatric treatment settings for whites, blacks, Native Americans, and Asian/Pacific islanders in 1990. The data show that 46.4 percent of all white patients received care in state and county mental hospitals—a lower percentage than that of Asian/Pacific islanders (50.5 percent) and Native Americans (54.3) and especially lower than that of blacks (64.6 percent). For private mental hospitals, Table 9–1 shows that the reverse is true, with 18.9 percent of all white patients in private hospitals, compared with only 8.3 percent of all black patients. Native Americans actually had the highest percentage (20.9) of private patients, and Asian/Pacific islanders show a percentage of 14.6 for private hospitals. Given the small number of Asian/Pacific islanders and Native American patients, the best comparison is between whites and blacks. Table 9–1 shows that, in comparison with whites, the highest percentage of blacks are in public hospitals and a much lower percentage is in private hospitals.

Further support for the argument that social class is more significant than race in predicting mental disorder is found in the few carefully designed studies of true prevalence dealing with this issue. One of those studies is by Warheit and his associates (1975), who interviewed a randomly selected sample of 1,645 persons living in a county in the southeastern United States. Their sample included 1,267 whites and 366 blacks, all of whom were tested on five scales measuring psychiatric impairment. When the data were not controlled for other variables, blacks scored significantly higher than whites on each of the scales. However, when the data were controlled for variables like age, sex, and social class, the statistical significance of race generally disappeared, and the authors noted that race as an independent variable was not an important predictor of mental disorder. Warheit and his colleagues (1975:255) state that, for the present, "we can conclude that race, along with the other sociodemographic variables included, tends to be symptom specific and relegated to a subordinate position in the equation when socioeconomic factors are included."

Consequently, almost all of the data and research that currently record differences in mental disorder between races show there is no significant difference in general between whites and members of racial minority groups. And those differences that do exist are caused more by social class than by race. We will consider this situation further in the next two sections by examining differences in mental health between racial minority groups and levels of self-esteem in such groups.

DIFFERENCES BETWEEN RACIAL MINORITY GROUPS

African Americans

As previously discussed, the research literature on African Americans shows that, in general, there are no significant differences between blacks and whites with respect to overall rates of mental disorder (Cockerham 1990b;

Dohrenwend and Dohrenwend 1969, 1974; Frerichs et al. 1981; Grier and Cobbs 1992; Kessler 1979; Mirowsky and Ross 1980; Neff and Husaini 1980; Roberts 1980; Warheit et al. 1975; Warheit et al. 1973). The Kessler et al. study (1994) suggests that blacks have a lower prevalence of mood and substance use disorders than whites but finds no disorders in which the prevalence for blacks is higher.

Other research shows that blacks do tend to utilize the services of psychiatrists and other sources of professional help for mental problems when needed. Blacks may use these services, on the average, somewhat less than whites, but the differences appear to be more the result of socioeconomic factors (for example, poverty and less education) than of race (Veroff et al. 1981). Blacks may also seek help from mental health specialists for economic reasons and for problems of physical health more than whites (Broman 1987), whereas black women are more likely than black men—just as white women are more likely than white men—to use mental health services (Neighbors and Howard 1987). Research on the social support available to psychologically distressed blacks through extended family networks suggests that such support is often minimal in the face of persistent economic difficulties for the family as a whole (Brown, Gary, Greene, and Milburn 1992). Although some family members may be able to provide assistance, they may not be able to sustain it over time—especially when the circumstances of family members may not be substantially different from those they are trying to help. Consequently, close family ties have been found to not be particularly responsive to offsetting the effects of chronic economic strain on levels of depression among blacks (Brown et al. 1992).

In considering the mental health of blacks in American society, it is also important to discuss the psychological implications of current trends in the increase of the black underclass. The term "underclass" describes that segment of society that has fallen out of the class structure to a point on the fringe of or perhaps even beyond the lower class because of a total lack of prospects for employment and social advancement. In essence, the underclass consists of people who have dropped out of society and, because of their lack of education, job skills, and social attributes, find it impossible to improve their situation.

According to William Julius Wilson (1987), the social conditions facing poor urban blacks since the mid-1960s have deteriorated to the extent that rates of unemployment, out-of-wedlock births, households headed by females, dependency on welfare, and violent crime have increased to their highest levels ever. Wilson blames the situation not so much on racism as the fact that both middle-class black professionals and working-class blacks have moved out of ghetto neighborhoods in the inner city, leaving behind a high concentration of the most disadvantaged segments of the black urban population. At the same time, the American economy has been changing from one based on manufacturing to one based on service and information. This situation has produced extraordinary rates of joblessness for those persons lacking the education and skills to adapt to the broader economic changes in society. One result is that blacks still have more poverty and unemployment, more substandard housing, and higher mortality rates than do whites.

Therefore, it is not surprising that studies of psychological well-being and quality of life in the United States show blacks scoring consistently lower than whites on these measures, even when social class, age, and marital status are controlled (Thomas and Hughes 1986). Of course, lower scores on feelings or self-assessments of psychological well-being do not necessarily translate into higher rates of mental disorder. They may mean little more than unhappiness, mild depression or anxiety, or simply greater dissatisfaction with life. In an extensive review of the research literature, Melvin Thomas and Michael Hughes (1986) determined that the relationship between race and psychological well-being does not apply to mental disorder. That was because social class was seen as a better explanation of mental illness among racial minorities than race itself. Thomas and Hughes claim that indicators of psychiatric symptoms and quality-of-life variables measure different, not similar, dimensions of life experience. "Based on this interpretation," state Thomas and Hughes (1986:839), "we conclude that while being black does not lead to psychopathology it is associated with a less positive life experience than being white."

Therefore, life may be harder, more stressful, and less satisfying for some blacks—especially low-income blacks. Although researchers generally agree that this situation has not provoked higher overall rates of mental illness among blacks in comparison with whites, there is, as discussed in the introduction to this chapter, some recent disagreement about whether this situation has caused more psychological distress among low-income blacks. According to John Mirowsky and Catherine Ross (1989b), psychological distress is conceptually distinct from mental illness in that the term *psychological distress* does not include problems like personality disorders, dementia, extreme mood swings (bipolar disorders), alcoholism, or schizophrenia. Rather, psychological distress refers to a highly adverse mental state involving marked depression and/or anxiety. Psychologically distressed persons may not be mentally ill in a full-blown clinical sense, but they are clearly mentally disturbed.

On the basis of that definition, the studies by Kessler and Neighbors (1986) and Ulbrich and associates (1989) measure psychological distress to a greater degree than more advanced forms of mental illness. Thus, it may be that when the lower class as a whole is considered, more psychological distress is found among blacks than whites, even though there is evidence to the contrary (Cockerham 1990b). It may be, however, that if lower-class blacks (and perhaps rural blacks, who are also likely to be poor) show more psychological distress than lower-class whites, it is because the socioeconomic situation in the lower class is much worse currently for blacks than for whites. Thus, any differences may still be due to socioeconomic factors rather than race. As previously discussed, when differences in rates of mental disorder between blacks and whites have been observed, the results have usually been attributed to socioeconomic causes. Blacks are more likely than whites to be poor, and poor people have higher overall rates of mental disorder. Therefore, researchers have generally concluded that social class is more important than race in determining differences in the prevalence of mental disorder between blacks and whites in America. As Grier and Cobbs (1992:30–31) point out in their discussion of the mental health of black males, the black man most likely has no special psychological or genetic determinants toward enhanced mental disorder, but "if he undergoes emotional conflict, he will respond as neurotically as his white brother."

Hispanic Americans

Hispanic Americans, consisting largely of Mexican and Cuban Americans and Puerto Ricans, are replacing blacks as America's largest racial/ethnic minority. If current demographic trends continue, Hispanics will surpass blacks as the the nation's largest minority group by 2020. One review of the mental health of Spanish-speaking people in the United States *rejects* the idea that Latinos have fewer mental health problems than Anglos (arguing that they are subject to more stress) and the role of folk healers (although recognizing that it is difficult to know just how effective they are) as the principal reasons why Spanish-speaking people are underrepresented in rates of admissions to mental health facilities (Padilla and Ruiz 1973). Instead, the argument is that the underrepresentation of Spanish-speaking people is mostly because of problems in the delivery of professional psychiatric services, that is, accessibility, language and cultural differences between the health care providers and their patients, diagnostic decisions based on middle-class values, problems with therapists concerning prejudice, and the neglect of potentially significant ethnographic factors in their disorders. Other research (Kessler et al. 1994; Roberts 1980) likewise suggests that levels of psychological difficulties for Mexican Americans are equal to if not greater than similar problems among Anglos. However, the bulk of the current literature on the mental health of Hispanic Americans, including studies of the true prevalence of mental disorder in the general population, does not show a high prevalence of mental disorder.

Most studies of the mental health of Hispanics in the United States are primarily studies of Mexican Americans, who constitute the largest Hispanic group in the United States. The most recent studies on the mental health of Mexican Americans do not find that mental disorder is a widespread problem. Quite the contrary, studies comparing Mexican Americans with non-Hispanics have typically shown either no difference between the two groups or even that Mexican Americans tend to have even less psychological distress generally than non-Hispanics (Aneshensel et al. 1991; Antunes et al. 1974; Burnam, Timbers, and Hough 1984; Mirowsky and Ross 1980, 1984; Ross,

Mirowsky, and Cockerham 1983; Ross, Mirowsky, and Ulbrich 1983). Moreover, immigrants from Mexico to the United States tend to show more relatively positive levels of mental health (Burnam et al. 1987). And employment outside the home does not appear to be particularly stressful for Mexican-American women (Krause and Markides 1985), nor is the Mexican-American housewife as likely to suffer from stress associated with family roles (Ross, Mirowsky, and Ulbrich 1983).

Findings documenting low rates of psychological distress among Mexican Americans differ from what would be expected because Mexican Americans typically show lower socioeconomic status and higher levels of fatalism than non-Hispanics (Mirowsky and Ross 1980; Ross, Mirowsky, and Cockerham 1983). This result (low psychological distress) appears typical even though Mexican Americans for generations have been subjected to low incomes, unemployment, underemployment, poor housing, limited educational opportunities, prejudice, discrimination, and linguistic barriers. Therefore, Mexican Americans appear to be an important exception to the general finding that lower-class people show more psychological distress. It may be that Mexican culture includes some protective feature that is missing from Anglo and black cultures. John Mirowsky and Catherine Ross (1984) investigated this situation, and they suggest that Mexican culture emphasizes exceptionally strong personal relationships with family and friends. Anglos, in contrast, tend to be more on their own when it comes to dealing with psychological problems. Mirowsky and Ross concluded that the overall effect of Mexican culture was contradictory; that is, Mexican culture fostered greater depression because of its association with fatalism and low socioeconomic status but decreased anxiety because of the association with strong family and friendship ties.

Mexican Americans and other Hispanics in the United States may not necessarily be free of psychological problems. Yet current research suggests Hispanic Americans do not have especially high rates of mental disorder, even though many have low socioeconomic status.

Native Americans

There is a lack of data about the prevalence of mental disorder among Native Americans. It is known that their children from five to eight years of age show approximately that same prevalence of severe emotional problems as do children in the majority culture; but from the age of ten until twenty, emotional difficulties, drug and alcohol use, and delinquency escalate perhaps beyond that of white teenagers (Yates 1987). Psychological distress is also seen in the high rates of alcoholism among Native Americans, which is two to three times the national average; the high rate of alcohol-related problems (75 percent of all accidents and 80 percent of all homicides by Native Americans are alcohol related); and suicide as the second major cause of death (accidents are the leading cause of death).

The death rate for suicides for Native Americans age 15–24 years in 1989–91 was 26.3 per 100,000, which is twice as high as that of whites the same age. Within some tribes, the rate is even higher. Native American victims of suicide tend to be younger than most other suicide victims. The problem of Native American suicides is concentrated largely among young males, which is a highly negative indication of the quality of life available to them.

More research, however, is needed on other forms of psychological distress, such as schizophrenia and the mood and anxiety disorders, before we can fully assess the rate of mental disorder among Native Americans. But the information on hand strongly implies that Native Americans have significant mental health problems.

Asian Americans

Compared with other racial/ethnic minority groups, Asian Americans are a distinct contrast when it comes to mental health. Asian Americans have the highest levels of income, education, and employment of any minority group in American society, often exceeding levels achieved by the white population. Furthermore, when it comes to mental health, the prevalence of mental disorders for Japanese Americans is exceedingly low. Japanese Americans, in particular, have strikingly low rates of mental hospital admissions, perhaps because of an extremely stable family structure that exercises considerable control over the behavior of its members and the strong social solidarity the Japanese-American communities seem to exhibit (Gallagher 1987; Kitano 1969, 1985).

However, mental hospital admissions rates for Chinese Americans have been found to be increasing in recent years, perhaps because of a reduction in the cohesion of Chinese-American families and communities (Kitano 1969, 1985). Estimates of mental disorder in the People's Republic of China show not only relatively low rates of such disorders but also extremely strong social networks of family, friends, and fellow workers that place considerable pressure on individuals to control their behavior (Cockerham 1984; Livingston and Lowinger 1983). Such intense control is lacking among Chinese in the United States, which may partially account for differences from residents of mainland China. Yet estimates of mental disorder in China remain only estimates because reliable data are not available (Cockerham 1984). Some research has suggested that mental disorder among the Chinese in China should be considered on a par with studies of Chinese living in Hong Kong, Taiwan, Singapore, and the United States, which would suggest that the Chinese have about the same proportion of schizophrenia as Western populations but considerably less alcoholism and sexual deviance (Kleinman and Mechanic 1979).

Nevertheless, the overall prevalence of mental disorder among Asian Americans appears low in relation to other racial/ethnic minority groups in

American society and to whites as well. This statement appears to be especially true of Japanese Americans. When the racial minorities are considered separately, it appears that African Americans and Native Americans have the highest prevalence of mental disorder, followed by Hispanic Americans and Asian Americans. But in general, there appears to be little or no significant difference between the pattern of mental disorder for members of American racial/ethnic minority groups and those of the white population.

MINORITY STATUS AND SELF-ESTEEM

Theoretical efforts to link adverse mental health to members of racial minorities have often focused on the issue of self-esteem. The rationale behind this approach is that minorities tend to feel less self-esteem because of their subordinate position in society. According to Mary and Robert Jackman (1983), who conducted a nationwide study of class awareness in the United States, people are more likely to give emotional priority to those group memberships that lie at the subordinate rather than dominant end of a relationship of inequality. So instead of being equally sensitive to all their group affiliations, people tend to care more about those that place them in a disadvantaged position. Jackman and Jackman found, for instance, that middle-class blacks identified more with being black than with being middle class. They used this finding to support their contention that subordinate status is experienced more sharply than is dominant status.

When minority status is used as the basis for understanding mental disorder, it is argued that minorities tend to have mental problems because of self-hate, a sense of inferiority, and a negative view of self brought on by the norms, values, and definitions of the wider white society. A common theoretical explanation for negative self-images among minority youth is Erik Erikson's (1968) concept of "identity diffusion." Erikson, revealing his Freudian orientation, believed that during the developmental stage of puberty and adolescence, minority youth sense they are trapped in a cultural conflict between their own world and the dominant white culture. Erikson hypothesized that every person's concept of self contains a hierarchy of both positive and negative elements, resulting from the fact that as the child becomes older, he or she is presented with both socially disapproved and ideal role models. The individual belonging to an oppressed and exploited minority, who is aware of the dominant cultural ideas but is prevented from emulating them, is likely, according to Erikson, to merge inferior role models with his or her own identity. Consequently, the person is supposed to experience self-hate and to define one's self negatively.

The relevance of Erikson's theory lies in its description of the possible implications for the self-esteem of racial/ethnic minority members when confronted with a majority racial/ethnic group designation of social inferiority.

The implication is that such contact promotes negative feelings of self. Erving Goffman (1963) presents a similar argument in his discussion of the moral career of stigmatized persons. Goffman suggests that persons who have a particular type of stigma, like race, tend to have similar learning experiences regarding their stigma and similar changes in their self-concepts. Through socialization they learn and incorporate the viewpoint of the "normal," thereby acquiring the beliefs of the wider society and obtaining knowledge of the consequences of not measuring up. At some point they learn that they, too, are deficient according to society's standards and that their social identity is "spoiled." The result is that they supposedly develop feelings of devaluation and diminished self-worth.

A problem with this approach is that it is not at all conclusive that members of racial minorities accept majority definitions of "self" as correct or that they internalize a sense of negativeness in the manner described above. For instance, the National Study of American Indian Education, conducted by Estelle Fuchs and Robert Havighurst (1973), firmly rejected the claim that Native American youth generally have a negative view of self. According to their test, Fuchs and Havighurst found that the great majority of Native American youth in their national sample viewed themselves as fairly competent persons within their own social world. An exception was observed among urban Native Americans, who expressed more alienation from white culture than did the more geographically isolated rural Native Americans. Fuchs and Havighurst suggest that only when Native American youth came into close contact with white culture and the urban-industrial environment did they begin to feel some doubts about their competence and self-esteem. Their self-doubt was largely based upon a realistic view of their disadvantages in competing for jobs and income. "They are not," report Fuchs and Havighurst (1973:156), "depressed, anxious, paranoid, or alienated as a group." In essence, they had the same problems as any other low-income group, and these problems were complicated somewhat by their also being Native American.

As Anselm Strauss (1969) explains, the self is not simply a mirror image of the evaluations and definitions of other people. Instead, the self is a multifaceted social object arising from interaction and interpersonal relationships with others. The responses of others may not be compatible with one's own expectations, thereby causing reevaluation, acceptance, or rejection of the identity they offer. Factors such as time, place, degree of involvement, and type of social situation are also important. Thus, for Native Americans and other racial minority groups in the United States, the generalization that whites define them as inferior does not mean that all whites agree (thus failing to provide reinforcement) or that all (or most) minorities accept that definition as correct and incorporate a sense of inferiority into their own idea of self. Furthermore, it may be that an individual's attitude toward self, either positive or negative, is influenced less by the larger society and more by significant others in the immediate environment. For racial minorities, these significant others are more likely to be of their own race and socioeconomic status. Roberta Simmons describes the situation for many black children:

> The black, particularly the black child, tends to be surrounded by other blacks. Thus, those persons who matter most to him—parents, teachers and peers—tend to be black and to evaluate him as highly as white parents, teachers and peers evaluate the white child. In addition, although his race, family structure and socioeconomic status may be devalued in the larger society, in his immediate context most others share these characteristics. Comparing himself to other economically disprivileged blacks, the black child does not feel less worthy as a person on account of race or economic background.
>
> In fact, encapsulated in a segregated environment as are most urban black children, they may be less aware of societal prejudice than is assumed. Even if aware, they may attribute blame to the oppressor rather than to themselves. Militant black ideology is aimed at just this end, at encouraging the disprivileged to internalize blame for their low societal rank and thereby protect their self-esteem. Whether the ideology has accomplished this end and actually led to higher self-esteem or whether other factors are responsible for current research findings, the problems of minority status and the self-picture remains an intriguing one.[2]

The research findings that Simmons refers to in this quotation are the growing number of studies that suggest that the self-esteem of black children is as high as if not higher than that of comparable whites (Baughman 1971; Rosenberg and Simmons 1972; St. John 1975; Simmons 1978). Other research points to similar findings for Native American school children (Cockerham 1978; Cockerham and Blevins 1976; Fuchs and Havighurst 1973; Trimble 1987). It is not known, as Simmons indicates, whether this is due to new ideology (for example, "black power" and "red power" movements) or other conditions, but the argument that minority youth generally feel depressed and alienated and are more subject as adults to mental disorder is not strong. Although there is some suggestion that blacks are more likely than whites to exaggerate their responses of self-esteem tests, scores for blacks on such tests when extreme response styles are excluded still do not show blacks scoring significantly lower than whites (Bachman and O'Malley 1984). Overall, tests of the self-esteem of minorities do not indicate that they view themselves negatively.

The case has been presented thus far that although some members of racial minorities, such as lower-class blacks and perhaps adolescent Native American males, may tend to manifest somewhat higher signs of mental distress in contemporary American society, no particular race appears to have a greater abundance of overall psychological impairment than any other. In fact, a possible advantage that lower-class racial minority group members may have in relation to poor whites is the availability of lay practitioners such as folk heal-

---

[2]Roberta G. Simmons, "Blacks and High Self-Esteem: A Puzzle," *Social Psychology* 41 (1978), 56.

ers and *curanderos*. These practitioners may serve as alternative sources of treatment for emotional problems for which many other Americans would probably seek out a psychiatrist. In this context, there is no separation between the psychological and the total well-being of the individual, and treatment is rendered in accordance with the normative values of the racial/ethnic community. Studies of black folk healers in Chicago and Mexican-American *curanderos* in the American Southwest describe this process.

URBAN BLACK FOLK HEALERS

According to Loudell Snow (1978), there are many low-income black Americans who believe that sorcery can cause illness. These people are characterized by Snow as subscribing to a belief system that, unlike modern medicine, does not differentiate between science and religion. All events, including illness, are viewed in relation to the total environment as either natural or unnatural, good or evil. Being healthy is an instance of good fortune, like having a good job, a faithful spouse, and so forth. Being sick is an example of misfortune, like unemployment and marital strife. Thus, life is *generally* good or bad, and the cure for *one* problem, says Snow, might cure *all* problems.

Additionally, Snow notes that the folk diagnosis of a health problem emphasizes the *cause* of the problem, not the symptoms. Having a body rash might be seen initially as stemming from a lack of cleanliness but might come to be defined as the result of black magic. In this belief system, what is important is not the rash, but what or who brought on the rash. Snow offers the following example:

> Even when a direct cause-and-effect relationship is known which is equivalent to the professional view this may be supported by religious or magical overtones. The sister of one of my informants died of bacterial meningitis, an etiology clearly understood by the family. But why did the organism invade her system at all? In their view to punish the father for "drinking and running around with women."[3]

Also significant is the idea that all illnesses can be cured, if not by medicine then by magic. This belief is supported by the aforementioned notion that illnesses are either natural or unnatural. Natural illnesses are those maladies caused by abusing the natural environment (for example, staying out too late, eating too much, failing to wear warm clothing) or brought on as a punishment by God for sin or for not living up to the Lord's expectations.

---

[3]Loudell F. Snow, "Sorcerers, Saints, and Charlatans: Black Folk Healers in Urban America," *Culture, Medicine, and Psychiatry* 2 (1978), 71.

Thus, in the case of divine punishment, the afflicted person must make contact with God either directly or indirectly through an intermediary such as a faith healer. "Prayer and repentence," reports Snow (1978:73), "not penicillin, cure sin."

Unnatural illnesses are outside "God's plan" and beyond self-treatment or the treatment prescribed by friends and relatives. And if the mind is affected, unnatural illnesses are thought to be beyond the capabilities of physicians, who are usually associated just with natural illnesses that have obvious physical symptoms. The cause of an unnatural illness can be worry or stress, but often the etiology is ascribed to evil influences or acts of sorcery. When black magic is suspected, it is necessary to find a healer with unusual magic or religious powers who can successfully intervene for the victim.

In the black community, however, Snow observed that the term "healer" included a bewildering array of persons performing different healing rituals. The variety of healers is reflected in the number of descriptive terms given them, such as healer, herb doctor, root doctor or root worker, reader, adviser, spiritualist, or conjure man or woman. If voodoo is practiced, a male healer may be called *houngan* or *papaloi,* and a female healer would be a *mambo* or *maraloi.* Few of them refer to themselves as "doctor" because healing is only part of their services. Instead, their given name is likely to be prefaced by a kinship, religious, or political title, for example, Sister, Brother, Mother, Reverend, Bishop, Prophet, Evangelist, Madam. These healers will depend on word of mouth for patient referrals, or they may advertise by newspaper or leaflet. They will claim to have received their ability to heal as a result of (1) learning (which confers little status because most anyone can be expected to learn); (2) an altered state of consciousness, such as a profound religious experience or a divine "call" to healing; or (3) conferral at birth. According to Snow (1978:79), "they will probably have in common only the assertion that the abilities are a gift from God."

Many healers do not require direct personal contact with the recipient of services but will conduct business over the telephone or by mail. If the individual's complaint includes sorcery, then the use of some substance, such as oils, potions, or perfumes, will be required; if witchcraft is at work, a thought, prayer, or verbal spell is necessary. For witchcraft, it might be necessary to purchase candles to assist the healer in effecting a solution. For example, when Snow complained in a letter to "Sister Marina" that she had problems sleeping and eating, was losing weight, and did not seem to enjoy life anymore, Sister Marina replied:

> I am so sorry I took so long to write but I had to take your letter into my church to see if what I suspected about your case was true. I had suspected an unnatural problem and I was right. But writing everything to you that I have learned would have to fill 10 pages of paper and maybe you still would not fully understand so I

am asking you to phone me so that I can explain to you better the history of your case and let you know what will be needed to help you. I have lit a special candle for you and my spirits have told me since you have written to me you have felt slightly better. But if you want to be helped call me.[4]

Snow wrote back asking if Sister Marina could help her by mail, and she received a warning by return mail that if she did not hurry it might be too late to save her. Sister Marina wrote:

> In order for me to take your case I must burn 9 candles for you to find out just what it is I must do to get rid of this UNNATURAL PROBLEM and remove this EVIL! And each candle cost $10.00 each it would come up to $90.00 to help and if you do not either bring it to Chicago or send it within a week and 1/2 which would be about 11 days I cannot except your case because you might get too bad off and then no one will be able to help if you decide to come to see me please call me a day ahead of time and let me know.[5]

How effective black folk healers like Sister Marina are in treating their clients is not known. Some of these healers are likely to be frauds; but the advantage they offer to their clients is that they are readily available, the results are usually quick and sometimes guaranteed, and they claim to be able to solve any problem. Their abilities are supposed to be derived from divine authority, and if they fail, they can attribute the failure to the will of God. However, what is particularly significant in their practices, as Snow comments, is the recognition that health problems are an integral part of other problems of daily life, like lack of money, a straying spouse, loss of a job, or envious relatives or neighbors. Thus, black folk healers treat the "whole" person, not just a single symptom as is often the case with a physician. In essence, what black folk healers appear to accomplish, as described by Snow, is the lessening of their clients' anxieties in a fashion not unlike those of witch doctors.

> "Get what you want," reads a flyer from a South Chicago store dealing in occult items, "New Car—Better Job—Big Apartment Building—The One You Love—We Deliver." The store sells candles, oils, incense, soaps and lotions, and aerosol sprays as aids in specific purposes; to keep evil spirits at bay, attract a mate, keep a spouse at home, bring luck at bingo or the races.[6]

There are two distinct types of black healers in the United States: (1) traditional and (2) Caribbean. The traditional form has been discussed above. The Caribbean form consists of several variations, such as voodoo (Haiti), Santeria (Cuba), and Obeah (West Indies). What these Caribbean approaches to folk healing have in common is that they are based on native African beliefs

---

[4]Ibid., p. 99.
[5]Ibid., p. 99.
[6]Ibid., p. 75.

and are part of the Caribbean's past slave culture. Each uses rituals, charms, herbs, concoctions, and prayer to prevent or cure illness by healing the mind and spirit, along with the body (Laguerre 1987). These healing practices are all part of a larger system of religious and spirit beliefs that are largely restricted in the United States to small numbers of black Americans with ties to the Caribbean. Cities like Miami, New Orleans, Chicago, Philadelphia, and New York show the largest concentrations of these practitioners.

THE CURANDEROS

There are also healers, known as *curanderos,* practicing folk medicine among Mexican Americans in the United States. Both males *(curandero)* and females *(curandera)* can become curanderos, and their healing powers are supposed to be gifts from God. Like black folk healers, curanderos blend religion and folk medicine into a singular therapeutic approach. They, likewise, classify illnesses primarily by *what* causes the disorder rather than by the symptoms, and they do not separate the natural from the supernatural in diagnosis and treatment. Most of their patients are from the lower class. Unlike black folk healers, the curanderos normally do not charge for their services, although they may ask for a small donation (perhaps a dollar) for expenses such as candles, or they may accept a small gift such as food (vegetables or a chicken).

Curanderos also appear to use religion to a much greater extent than do black folk healers. Ari Kiev (1968) points out that religion of the curanderos, based upon a Spanish Catholic tradition, is central to their belief that life is ordained by the divinity and that good health and happiness can be achieved only by those who keep God's commandments. A patient who suffers, therefore, is seen as helping God's plan for the universe because it is believed that God allows people to suffer so that they may learn. The example of Christ suffering on the cross is often used to illustrate that suffering and illness can be a worthwhile experience. Thus, the curandero views helping the patient accept suffering as a major task. In this context, suffering is explained as being part of the patient's burden for the world's sin and ignorance and a necessary role in God's plan for the universe. The more religious the curandero appears to be and the more convincing he or she is in influencing others to accept the will of God, the more highly regarded the curandero is as a healer. One effect the curandero uses to help accomplish this is to establish a work setting that supports his or her image. Kiev describes it thus:

> Each curandero works in his own unique setting, depending usually upon his degree of affluence. The basic atmosphere created is invariably the same. In general, the curandero sees patients in part of his home set aside for treatment. These rooms, even in poor slums, are distinctive because of the great number of religious objects contained in them. The presence of numerous pictures and stat-

ues of the Virgin Mary and Jesus, of various sized crosses and religious candles, which are often arranged around an altar in a corner of the room, creates an atmosphere of religious solemnity which makes one forget the poverty of the slum or the humble shack of the curandero. Indeed, in such treatment rooms one feels as if in a church, and cannot help but view the curandero with awe and respect.

The therapeutic effect of this "temple in the home" cannot be minimized. The quiet calm can invoke a feeling of security and protectiveness in the frightened and anxious. . . . [P]erhaps most important is the authority the curandero derives through his relationship to the setting. It makes him the object of respect and awe and puts him in command of much of the power that derives from the patient's response to the setting and the symbolism. By relying upon religious symbols and objects that have great meaning for the patients, he can immediately establish himself as a man of wisdom and authority, which undoubtedly increases the patient's willingness to cooperate and his expectations of relief.[7]

Besides prayer and religious counseling, the curandero employs a variety of folk drugs and herbs to produce a cure (for example, rattlesnake oil, mineral water, garlic, sweet basil, wild pitplant, licorice, camphor). To a very large extent, this approach is based upon sixteenth-century Spanish medicine, derived largely from Greek and Arabic sources, and influenced by Mayan and Aztec beliefs. Dominant in this view is the Hippocratic notion of bodily equilibrium. As mentioned in Chapter 1, Hippocrates, a famous physician of ancient Greece, believed that good health resulted from the equilibrium in the body of the four humors of blood, phlegm, black bile, and yellow bile. Important, too, was the harmony of the body with living habits and the environment. As long as the four humors were in balance, the body was healthy. If there was an imbalance, more of one type of humor than another, a person was sick. Because the body is perceived as being a mix of cold and hot conditions, curanderos use "hot" foods and medicines to treat "cold" conditions (for example, drowsiness, chills) and "cold" foods and medicines to treat "hot" conditions (for example, fever, hypersexuality).

Curanderos also believe that intense emotions like anger, hostility, and grief can bring on sickness, especially mental disorders. Likewise significant are excessive feelings of guilt. Other causes of mental disorder are preoccupation with sex or, conversely, inadequate sexual gratification and overexposure to the sun (causing a fire in the head). Dreams, in contrast, offer a path of discharge from emotions and are considered necessary for good mental health. The cessation of dreams is viewed as a loss of intellect. Curanderos believe, too, that they themselves can become insane through misuse of their powers as a form of punishment from God.

The most dreaded form of disorder, either physical or mental, is that caused by witchcraft. Witches, or *brujas*, are evil persons who have supposedly

---

[7]Ari Kiev, *Curanderismo: Mexican-American Folk Psychiatry* (New York: Free Press, 1968), pp. 129–30.

made pacts with the Devil and use supernatural powers in the forms of curses, magic, herbs, or ghosts to harm other people. According to William Madsen (1973), who studied Mexican Americans living in southern Texas, even though belief in witchcraft is more strongly denounced by the churches and in newspapers and schools than other folk theories of disease, conservative lower-class Mexican Americans almost universally accept the existence of witchcraft. Hence, curanderos are needed to provide "good" power to offset "evil" influences.

Kiev (1968) comments that *curanderismo* persists in the American Southwest because it works in many cases. Kiev states that the curandero is at a distinct disadvantage in treating mental disorders requiring precise biochemical intervention, such as that needed for organic psychoses and certain other psychotic moods and thoughts in the schizophrenic and mood disorders. But he adds that the curandero is probably just as effective as many modern psychiatrists in treating anxiety disorders, mild paranoid reactions, and schizotypal personality disorders. The advantage the curandero brings to therapy, like that of the witch doctor, is that he or she works in a subculture that supports beliefs in the effectiveness of the curandero's methods. Especially important is the anxiety-reducing approach of the curandero carried out within the context of family and friends that defines the treatment as therapeutic and positive according to the norms and values of the Mexican-American community. Although Anglos may view illness as impersonal and unemotional in origin, lower-class Mexican Americans may see illness as related to one's interpersonal relationships, community life, and religion. Community norms are, therefore, central to recovery. Consider the following example, described by Madsen, of "Catalina," a twenty-year-old Mexican-American girl committed for paranoia to a state mental hospital. After two years of treatment with no improvement, Catalina's parents had her released to their custody. She was returned home and placed under the care of a curandera. Madsen states:

> The treatment that Catalina received under the curer's care would be regarded as barbaric by most psychiatrists but it was successful. When she had won the confidence of her patient, the *curandera* learned that Catalina believed the world hated her because she had committed a sexual perversion with an Anglo during her teens. She was laden with guilt and self-recrimination. On hearing Catalina's confession, the *curandera* registered emotions of horror and disgust. "No wonder everybody hates you!" she exclaimed, "God hates you too." . . . The *curandera* did not conceal her own contempt for Catalina but announced that she would help the girl because it was her duty to God who had given her the power to cure.
>
> The treatment consisted of a painful program of penance and self-debasement accompanied by prayer. Catalina was allowed to wear only the dark color of mourning and she was required to spend hours on her knees praying for forgiveness. When the *curandera* discovered Catalina's fondness for the rabbits her father raised, the patient was ordered to cut open the head of a rabbit every morning and eat the raw brains from the skull. This act caused Catalina extreme anguish and considerable nausea. Aside from the rabbit brains, the patient was

kept on a rigid and tasteless diet. She was denied permission to indulge in any frivolous or pleasurable activity. To complete her miserable existence, the patient was ordered to report for regular floggings at the home of the *curandera.*

The *curandera* never revealed the nature of Catalina's sin to anyone else for had it been known the girl would have been an outcast forever from respectable society. Instead, the *curandera* leaked out the information that Catalina was being punished for failure to demonstrate the proper respect for her parents. As the story spread, many listeners felt that the penance imposed on Catalina was too severe. Women who knew her went out of their way to demonstrate their friendliness and respect to Catalina for the suffering she had endured to repair the injury to her parents. Catalina came to believe that she was no longer hated by everybody. The *curandera* became more and more affective in her relations with the patient and held forth the hope of divine forgiveness.

The treatment ended six months after it began. When Catalina came one day for her appointed flogging, the *curandera* instead asked the patient to join her in prayer. Whey they rose after the prayer, the *curandera* laid her hands on Catalina's shoulders and solemnly announced that God had forgiven her. With tears of joy in her eyes, the *curandera* embraced her patient and whispered that God loved Catalina for so faithfully repaying the world for her sin. . . . A week later, Catalina's parents gave a party to thank God for his blessing. Society welcomed Catalina home again.[8]

The continued ability to attract clients is testimony to the effectiveness of black and Mexican-American folk healers in meeting the needs of low-income minority groups. Traditionally, the poor have been unable to afford the services of trained psychiatrists, who are typically white and male and practice according to the norms of the majority culture. Use of folk healers is a means by which racial minorities have coped with psychological distress and is an example of how some disadvantaged groups have established their own approach to mental health. The use of folk healers may have historically been one way minorities have narrowed the gap between themselves and more affluent groups in society in relation to mental health. Thus, folk healers exist because they serve a purpose for socially and economically disadvantaged persons.

SUMMARY

One should not conclude that racial minorities are relatively free of mental health problems associated with prejudice and discrimination. The extent of the mentally disordered among minorities may be greater than is known at present, and discrimination may be a particularly important favor in the insanity of some. But to date, race alone does not appear to produce higher rates of mental disorder for particular groups. Therefore, it does not seem that race

---

[8]William Madsen, *The Mexican-Americans of South Texas,* 2nd ed. (Holt, Rinehart & Winston, 1973), pp. 80–81.

per se is a significant variable in determining whether a person is or will be mentally disordered. Theoretical approaches that argue that less self-esteem among minorities, children in particular, leads to mental disorder are questionable as well. Mental disorders among members of racial minorities seem to be largely due to also being poor, a condition that racial prejudice and discrimination have fostered.

10

Help-Seeking Behavior and the Prepatient Experience

The initial decision that a particular person is mentally disordered usually takes place within the context of social groups, such as family or friends, in which that person participates. But the difficulty in deciding what is or is not mental disorder often creates indecision and contributes to the uncertainty that sometimes characterizes attempts to label someone "mentally ill." Generally, a person is started on the route to becoming so labeled when his or her inability to respond "normally" in a given situation becomes a consistent pattern of behavior and is recognized as such by other people. At other times, individuals may come to view themselves as mentally ill by comparing their own behavior with that of others or with how they themselves performed in past circumstances. In this chapter, we shall examine the reasons often given for why individuals decide to seek treatment for mental problems and shall explore some of the experiences people may have in becoming mentally disordered.

THE DECISION TO SEEK TREATMENT

The decision to seek treatment for a psychiatric condition is a process that is not fully understood. Some mentally disturbed people make the decision on their own, but often a person is defined as abnormal by others in the community and on that basis is directed to mental health services. The help-seeking process, however, is complicated not only by the problem of not knowing *what* actually constitutes mental disorder but also by the vast differences among people, both individually and as a group, in their capacity to tolerate difficult behavior. The tendency of others, particularly relatives, to "normalize" difficult behavior patterns through rationalization until those patterns can no longer be tolerated is a major reason there often is a delay in seeking psychiatric treatment.

The Uncoerced Situation

After they recognize that they need it, some people will seek help for mental problems completely on their own and without coercion from others. Others have to be coerced into obtaining care, either through threats or deception on the part of significant others or through force (for example, arrest, involuntary commitment). This section will examine what we know about the uncoerced decision to seek psychiatric care.

Although some individuals will recognize the symptoms of a health problem and seek out a health care provider for treatment, others with similar symptoms will not do so. This is true for problems of mental as well as physical health. Although the exact factors that motivate a person to turn to a psychiatrist or another mental health professional for treatment have not been completely identified at present, there are enough data on the subject to allow some generalizations. As James Greenley and David Mechanic (1976a) explain, persons seeking help on their own for psychological problems have different sociocultural and attitudinal profiles from other persons in the community not seeking comparable assistance. In a review of several epidemiological surveys, Greenley and Mechanic found that women, Jews, people with low religiosity, residents of urban and suburban areas, and people with more education and income were more likely than anyone else to seek out psychiatrists for mental and emotional problems.

Greenley and Mechanic (1976b) also conducted their own study of help seeking for psychological problems among a group of 1,502 randomly selected university students. Two hundred seventy-four of those students were located two years later and retested to search out any possible changes over time. All students were asked about their utilization of a variety of services—psychiatric, counseling, religious, medical, and other formal agencies—for personal problems. It was found that sociocultural characteristics, attitudes, knowledge, reference-group orientations, and degree of psychological problems all had independent effects on the use of such services. The strongest variables were being female, having an attitudinal propensity to seek help for psychological problems, and being oriented toward people who tended to be introspective as a reference group. Students most attracted to seeing psychiatrists were women, Jewish or of no religious affiliation, and of relatively higher social status.

A major nationwide survey of help seeking for psychological problems was undertaken by Joseph Veroff and his associates (1981). Veroff and his colleagues investigated patterns of help seeking in 1976 and compared the results to earlier data collected in 1957. They found that Americans in 1976 were more likely to seek both formal and informal help for mental distress than they had been twenty years earlier. Sources of help were diverse—from spouses, family, and friends to psychologists and psychiatrists as well as other physicians. But the greatest change was in the increased use of mental health specialists. Most people in 1976 who sensed they were having a nervous breakdown were still more likely to consult a medical doctor who was not a psychiatrist, but utilization of the services of psychiatrists and psychologists had significantly improved since 1957. Veroff and his associates (1981:73) concluded that "people are now more willing to accept the view that emotional problems should be referred to more specialized professional resources (mental health specialists) for treatment rather than to more general professional help resources, such as doctors or clergy."

Acceptance of psychiatric help, however, was not universal. Men tended to be more isolated in times of personal crisis because of a reluctance to share their problems with other people or even to acknowledge that they needed help. The poor also tended to be isolated in that, compared with the affluent, they prayed more and talked less to others about their mental state. Veroff and his coworkers suggest that perhaps people living in low-income neighborhoods are less comfortable with their neighbors and less likely to talk over their problems with them. As for education, less educated people were more likely than better-educated people to be passive about psychological distress. This suggested that denial was a more common method of dealing with problems for those Americans who are not well educated.

Overall, Veroff and his associates found that when people suffer from psychological difficulties, they initially seek advice from family and friends. When the decision is made to seek professional help, they turn most often to physicians, but use of psychiatrists and other mental health specialists is on the rise. Women, the well educated, and the more affluent were most likely to seek help from specialists, with men, less well educated persons, and the poor least likely.

What is indicated from studies such as those by Greenley and Mechanic and Veroff and colleagues is that social and cultural factors seem to be most important in deciding *where* to seek help, rather than in deciding *whether* to seek help. What is likely to be the most important factor in the decision to seek help is the degree of psychological distress the person suffers. It has been found, for instance, that psychological distress negatively affects a person's overall perception of his or her physical well-being (Tessler and Mechanic 1978). Mechanic (1975) reminds us that a highly consistent finding in studies of help-seeking behavior for physical illnesses is that people are most likely to be distressed and seek professional treatment for symptoms that most disrupt usual functioning. The more bizarre and disturbing the symptoms of mental disorder are, the more probable it is that a person experiencing those symptoms will seek psychiatric services or be required by others to seek those services.

Unfortunately, as Mechanic notes, the study of how people conceptualize experiential change has been neglected. This becomes particularly apparent when considering the literature on how people attribute mental disorder to themselves. One of the few studies that attempts to explain the attribution process of individuals in relation to their own possible mental disorders is Charles Kadushin's *Why People Go to Psychiatrists* (1969). Kadushin suggests that an individual's decision to seek psychiatric therapy has five stages: (1) The person decides whether he or she has a problem and whether that problem is emotional; (2) the person decides whether and to what extent to discuss the problem with relatives and friends; (3) the person decides that personal efforts to deal with the problem are inadequate and that professional help is required to relieve the symptoms; (4) the person next decides what type of facility or practitioner would most be helpful; and (5) the person decides what particular practitioner should be consulted. Kadushin focuses on the idea that people in particular social circles will have a high probability of seeking psychotherapy if others in that circle have either sought or known others who have sought similar treatment. Moreover, he found that people of high socioeconomic status and low religiosity tended to be drawn to psychoanalytic therapists. Lower-status and more religious people favored religious counseling services. In essence, Kadushin believes that people tend to seek help from therapists who are similar to themselves.

Other research on help seeking and mental disorder shows that people seek help because of troublesome feelings and interpersonal difficulties that they recognize as abnormal (Thoits 1985). This is especially the case when the problems associated with these feelings and difficulties begin to increase and the reality of the symptoms intensifies (Whitt and Meile 1985). The social networks or family and friendship groups in which the person participates will try to make sense of the situation when the abnormal mental state becomes apparent, and those persons emotionally closest to the individual will be most likely to insist on some type of medical help (Perrucci and Targ 1982). Therefore, it is clear that people do label themselves mentally disordered (Thoits 1985). Some of them turn directly to professionals for help, but the majority appear to initially cope with their symptoms within their social network before seeking treatment from a specialist (Grusky and Pollner 1981; Perrucci and Targ 1982; Veroff et al. 1981).

Other people, however, do not willingly seek treatment. This includes those who deny they are mentally ill (a common occurrence) or whose state of mind is so severely disturbed that choice is not possible. For these people, treatment is initiated when others bring them to a mental health practitioner or facility.

The Coerced Situation

It is probable that the great majority of mental patients are coerced in some way to obtain treatment for a psychiatric condition. That coercion may be loving and gentle, such as a spouse delicately pressuring a person to seek help, or it may be brutal. A person may be threatened with divorce, unemployment, loss of friends, or arrest, or may in fact be divorced, fired, friendless, or arrested because of abnormal behavior.

One study that helps to describe the role of others in seeking care for psychological problems is Allan Horwitz's (1977) interviews with 120 outpatients and short-term inpatients and some of their friends and relatives at a community mental health center in New Haven, Connecticut. Horwitz compared lower-middle- and working-class male and female patients in the differing pathways each followed to the treatment setting. He found that women were more likely (1) to have recognized the existence of a mental problem in themselves; (2) to have discussed their problems with and sought help from family, intimate friends, and professionals; and (3) to have entered treatment voluntarily. Women followed primarily two paths into treatment. Either they defined their own problem as psychiatric in nature and sought professional treatment, or they discussed their problem with others and accepted when offered a psychiatric definition of their difficulties. Men, on the other hand, rarely placed themselves in treatment or even discussed their problems with others. At some time, their mental state became visible, and the disruption they caused in their families or on their jobs forced others to take action to control the problem.

The Horwitz study dealt with relatively mild cases of mental disorder in an outpatient treatment setting. When hospitalization is involved, as Erving Goffman (1961) explains, few people come into the mental hospital willingly because of their own idea that it will be good for them or because they are in wholehearted agreement with their families that this is what should be done. This situation presents special problems for the family and often rips at the very social and emotional ties that keep the family together. Consequently, there is often considerable tolerance in the family for bizarre behavior.

Family disruption   The reluctance to label a family member as having a mental problem is aptly illustrated in studies of the wives and husbands of mental patients. Marian Yarrow and her associates (1955) studied the process by which wives attempted to cope with their husbands' mental illness and found that it usually had five major stages: (1) The wife first recognized that the husband's behavior was not understandable or was unacceptable; (2) the wife adjusted her own expectations of her husband to account for his deviant responses; (3) the wife's interpretation of the husband varied; sometimes the husband was seen as normal and other times as abnormal; (4) the wife tried to adapt to the husband's behavior and became defensive about it with other people; (5) finally the wife was no longer able to sustain a definition of normality and to cope with the husband's behavior. The fifth stage would generally be the prelude to intervention by outside authorities.

Yarrow and her associates illustrated this with the case of Mr. F. Mr. F was a thirty-five-year-old unemployed cab driver at the time of the study. He had contracted malaria during World War II and did not work regularly, supposedly because of recurring malaria attacks. Mrs. F noticed very early that he appeared to be prone to nervousness but rationalized that she was perhaps too happy-go-lucky. Over a period of three years, he seemed to become more nervous and resisted his wife's attempts to get him to see a doctor. He increasingly complained of severe headaches and nightmares and went on a trip to talk to a famous person (Albert Einstein) about his ideas.

Three days before his admission to a mental hospital, Mr. F stopped taking baths and changing his clothes; two days before admission, he awakened his wife to tell her that a book he was writing had nothing to do with science but was about himself and what he had been worrying about for ten years. Not overly impressed, she suggested that he burn his book, and it was on the following morning that she noticed his behavior was particularly "rather strange." The day before his admission, he went shopping with her (something he never did) and worried that he might lose her; that night he thought that a television program was about him and that the television set was "after him." She clearly recognized the bizarre nature of his behavior. But also that night

> Mr. F kept talking. He reproached himself for not working enough to give his wife surprises. Suddenly he exclaimed he did have a surprise for her—he was going to kill her. "I was petrified" and said to him, "What do you mean?" Then he began to cry and told me not to let him hurt me and to do for him what I would want him to do for me. I asked him what was wrong. He said he had cancer. . . . He began talking about his grandfather's mustache and said there was a worm growing out of it. She remembered his watching little worms in the fish bowl and thought his idea came from that. Mr. F said he had killed his grandfather. He asked Mrs. F to forgive him and wondered if she were his mother or God. She denied this. He vowed he was being punished for killing people during the war. "I thought maybe . . . worrying about the war so much . . . had gotten the best of him. . . ."[1]

Here Mrs. F was trying to understand his behavior as somehow normal (that is, as a reaction to the war). She had to extend her range of definitions for normality to do this. She saw him as abnormal after this discussion, but

---

[1]M. Yarrow et al., "The Psychological Meaning of Mental Illness in the Family," *Journal of Social Issues* 11 (1955), 13.

later that night he seemed to "straighten out," and the next morning he drove her to work. At this point, she returned to seeing him as normal and used this behavior to "balance out" his preceding disturbed activities. Again she tried to adapt to his behavior, but finally when he chased her around the house, roaring like a lion, and was subsequently arrested by the police for creating a disturbance at a nearby church, she did conclude that he was mentally ill. Before that, she had defined him as not being normal but refused to see him as crazy or insane.

Later, after their husbands' hospitalization, many of the wives in the Yarrow and associates study reflected on their earlier attempts to avoid a definition of mental illness for their husbands. Yarrow and her associates state:

> Such reactions are almost identically described by these wives: "I put it out of my mind—I didn't want to face it—anything but a mental illness." "Maybe I was aware of it. But you know you push things away from you and keep hoping." "Now you think maybe you should have known about it. Maybe you think you should have done more than you did and that worries me."[2]

Another study by Harold Sampson, Sheldon Messinger, and Robert Towne (1961) found that husbands made a somewhat similar series of responses to their wives' abnormal behavior. First, the husband developed a pattern of accommodation to the wife's behavior. Often, a husband simply withdrew from his wife and developed new interests elsewhere—another woman, a second job, a hobby, or sports. Second, this pattern of accommodation eventually was disrupted as the pattern of withdrawal by the husband became intolerable to one or both of the parties involved. Either the husband suggested that the wife seek help, or the wife realized that she could not go on as things were. Sometimes, the husband just got rid of the "problem" by divorcing his wife. This was particularly true for men about the age of forty who looked at the future and decided they did not want to spend the remainder of their active years with their present spouse. Some husbands developed a pattern of resistance to their wives' demands for involvement. These husbands would appear indifferent if the wife sought help from a minister or a psychiatrist; or if other persons became interested in the wife's problems, they would usually respond negatively. Often, the husband did not become involved as a responsible party in the wife's mental condition until the wife was actually hospitalized, and usually this event came after some extreme act of deviance on the part of the wife, such as burning the house down, which called attention to her needs.

Sampson and his associates point out that many mental patients come to the attention of mental health professionals only during an unmanageable crisis. Without such an emergency, the patient's problem is likely to continue to

---

[2]Ibid., p. 23.

be ignored. This is consistent with Howard Becker's (1973) assertion that many people are willing to tolerate deviance or to ignore it until someone complains about it and forces society to act against the deviant.

Goffman (1961) explains that when a person begins a "career" of being a mental patient, that career will include a round of agents and agencies that marks the progress of the individual's passage from the status of "civilian" to that of mental patient. Goffman identifies the agent roles in this process as next-of-relation, complainant, and mediators. The next-of-relation, usually a relative, is the person whom the patient expects to be the last to doubt his or her sanity and the first to save the patient from being committed to a mental hospital. The complainant is the person who actually starts the patient on his or her way to the mental hospital. Because that person may also be the next-of-relation, the emotions the patient experiences during the commitment sequence are compounded. The mediators are a series of agents and agencies through which the individual is relayed until he or she is actually committed to the mental hospital. They are typically lawyers, the police, social workers, clergy, physicians, and psychiatrists. Eventually, one agent (the judge in proceedings for involuntary commitment) will have the legal mandate to sanction commitment and may exercise it. If that happens, all the mediators will retire, and the prepatient now becomes an inpatient.

Goffman observes that this passage to the mental hospital is often characterized by feelings of betrayal on the part of the patient. Goffman found that from home to hospital, the potential patient is encouraged to cooperate with others without forcing anyone to look directly at him or her or to deal with raw emotion. Upon reflection, the patient may realize that everybody else's comfort was being maintained while his or her long-range welfare was being undermined. Often, the next-of-relation will handle the patient's affairs while he or she is in the hospital. This person thus serves as a useful identity to whom the hospital can point for justification of its method of treatment. The staff's action is therefore in the patient's best interest, both because of their superior training and knowledge *and* because of the authorization by the next-of-relation (who supposedly also has the patient's best interest at heart) to work on behalf of the patient. Paradoxically, as Goffman notes, the next-of-relation is the person to whom the patient turns for support in being discharged from the hospital and also the person to whom the hospital turns for authorization to treat the patient.

Family alienation   The passage to commitment as a mental patient as described by Goffman may not apply to all potential mental patients, especially those who seek voluntary admission to a mental hospital or those who are arrested by the police and for whose commitment the state assumes responsibility. However, the import of Goffman's research is that often passage to a mental hospital is a process of alienation; the patient is removed from "normal" society to a setting in which he or she is clearly regarded as being mentally unacceptable.

The alienative nature of this situation cannot be overemphasized. Not only is the insane person likely to reject those formerly close to him or her, but also family members may come to reject the insane person. The issue here, as Goffman (1971) argues, is not that the family finds that home life is made unpleasant by the insane person (indeed, it may already be unpleasant) but that *meaningful existence is threatened.* The mentally ill person's definition of spouse and other family members is less desirable than thought and implies that the social bond between them is *more tenuous* than previously realized. Mental symptoms can be much more disruptive of social relationships than other forms of deviance can, because they distort and destroy the very core (that is, love, affection, respect, loyalty, responsibility) of what makes those relationships viable. Family members have great difficulty in coming to terms with or explaining continued insanity. It is much easier to find reasons why a family member might be a drug addict, sexually unfaithful, or a criminal than to impute insanity to him or her. The imputation of mental disorder is usually a final attempt to cope with a person whose disruptive behavior cannot otherwise be contained. It signifies that all other definitions of the questionable behavior have failed.

ACTING MENTALLY DISORDERED: THE EXAMPLE OF SCHIZOPHRENIA, ANXIETY, AND DEPRESSION

We know very little about how people conceptualize the feelings, emotions, and behaviors that cause them to be viewed as abnormal. A difficult problem in trying to analyze those perceptions is one of organizing the subject matter (insanity) into a coherent scheme for discussion. To conceptualize the insane experience in any generalizable fashion requires a systematic approach; yet insanity is a situation in which normally constituted meanings are at risk and disorder rather than order is usual. As Michel Foucault (1987) reminds us, elements of thought in mental illness are dissociated from reality as intent, time and space orientation, and sense of psychological order are freed in a style of incoherence. Therefore, a necessary first step in the sociological analysis of becoming insane is to identify common experiences among those so afflicted.

A review of patient experiences reported in sociology, psychiatry, psychology, and autobiographies suggests that the experience of becoming mentally ill can be organized into seven distinct phases: (1) alienation from "place," (2) recognizing symptoms, (3) madness as a method of coping, (4) the definitive outburst, (5) rendering of accounts, (6) the paradox of normalcy, and (7) removal from "place."[3] To illustrate these phases, examples will be drawn

---

[3]In formulating this model, the author benefited greatly from conversations with Norman K. Denzin.

from Mark Vonnegut's report of his madness in *The Eden Express* (1975) and from the accounts of schizophrenia by others. Because a distinguishing feature of schizophrenia is withdrawal from reality, we shall also focus on, for contrast, the experiences of N. S. Sutherland recorded in *Breakdown* (1977). Sutherland suffered from an anxiety disorder accompanied by severe depression but maintained a sense of reality through it all. Additionally, we will review novelist William Styron's bout with depression as depicted in his book *Darkness Visible* (1990).

Thus, we will examine schizophrenic symptoms and loss of reality (Vonnegut) as compared with anxiety symptoms (Sutherland) and a mood disorder consisting of severe depression (Styron) to demonstrate the experience of being mentally disordered. The theoretical basis of this analysis is symbolic interaction (Cockerham 1990a). It should not be presumed that all mentally ill persons pass through the phases outlined above or that all mental disorders conform to it. Rather, it is the intent here to suggest a hypothetical model, based on the self-reports of mental patients, which may account for and be used to understand the experience of mentally disordered people generally as they move toward the full-fledged expression of their disorder (see Braginsky, Braginsky, and Ring 1969; Esterson 1972; Fadiman and Kewman 1973; Goffman 1961; Grant 1963; Green 1964; Kaplan 1964; Karp 1994; Lemert 1962; Rogler and Hollingshead 1965; Sampson et al. 1961; Scheff 1984; Sutherland 1977; Styron 1990; Vonnegut 1975; Yarrow et al. 1955).

Alienation from "Place"

According to Goffman (1971) and Edwin Lemert (1972), the concept of "place" describes a person's role and status set within a particular social network or organization. Places are therefore *occasions* for social interaction based on the taken-for-granted meanings of relevant roles and statuses. Insanity in this context would be viewed as behaviors that question the normal assumptions of roles and statuses in guiding interaction. A more extensive definition of place has been constructed by Norman Denzin (1977:148–49), who maintains that places have six basic elements: (1) self-reflexive individuals, (2) physical settings, (3) social objects that exist in the setting and are acted upon by the people there, (4) a relationally specific set of rules that explicitly or tacitly guide and shape interaction, (5) a set of relationships that legitimize a person's presence in that setting, and (6) a set of definitions that indicate each person's view of self and of others relevant to the interaction. This expanded version of place allows us to view places not only as opportunities for interaction but also as the general social conditions in which harmonious interaction is possible.

Acting insane, however, is not the same as alienation from place. Alienation from place is the initial step in the experience of becoming mentally ill and represents a mental condition in which a person senses a psychological barrier between himself or herself and the social situation or "place" in which they find themselves. Troublesome feelings or interpersonal difficulties accompanied by undesirable emotional affects, like those described by Peggy Thoits (1985), appear to capture the essence of feeling alienated from place. That is, people in this situation experience feelings of despair, panic, failure, inadequacy, dread, loss, or discomfort—even in a familiar environment. Somehow they sense they are not themselves, nor are they part of their usual "place." As Denzin (1984) describes it, emotions become a wedge between the person and the world. Clearly, something is lost, and that something, as Denzin suggests, is being normal.

Schizophrenia   Let us consider, for example, the experiences of Mark Vonnegut (1975), a young college graduate in his early twenties who moved to British Columbia in 1970 to live as a hippie and start a commune. His family had a history of mental disorder, and he had put on a "schizophrenic act" to avoid being drafted into the military during the Vietnam War. Besides the stress of moving to the West to begin a new lifestyle, Vonnegut was uneasy over the breakup of his parents' marriage, the growing fame of his novelist father (Kurt Vonnegut), and the lack of warmth and understanding that characterized his relationship with his girlfriend, who stayed with him in Canada for a time. Living and working with a small circle of friends and acquaintances on a farm in the wilderness, Vonnegut nevertheless felt himself becoming extremely happy and intensely aware of his surroundings. He worked, played, and occasionally "tripped out" on drugs. He began to find everything—trees, sky, moss, people's faces, the stove, the floors—as "unbearably beautiful." People all were "charming and silly," and living was grand. But one night in early 1971, he started having hallucinations (seeing a "wrinkled, iridescent face"), hearing "voices," and feeling extremely fearful. To combat his sense of dread, he tried doing something very familiar, like pruning trees, and reports:

> Small tasks became incredibly intricate and complex. It started with pruning the fruit trees. One saw cut would take forever. I was completely absorbed in the sawdust floating gently on the ground, the feel of the saw in my hand, the incredible patterns in the bark, the muscles in my arm pulling back and then pushing forward. Everything stretched infinitely in all directions. Suddenly it seemed as if everything was slowing down and I would never finish sawing the limb. Then by some miracle that branch would be done and I'd have to rest, completely blown out. The same thing kept happening over and over. Then I found myself being unable to stick with any one tree. I'd take a branch here, a couple there. It seemed like I had been working for hours but the sun hadn't moved at all.
>
> I began to wonder if I was hurting the trees and found myself apologizing. Each tree began to take on personality. I began to wonder if any of them liked me. I became completely absorbed in looking at each tree and began to notice

that they were ever so slightly luminescent, shining with a soft inner light that played around the branches.[4]

A few days later, Vonnegut temporarily quit eating and sleeping. He continued to be fearful and sensed he was caught in a struggle going on within him. A turning point may have come when he received a letter from his girlfriend that said, among other things, that she had gone to bed with a friend of his. To add insult to injury, he had never really liked this friend. As Vonnegut described himself, he now was going to be a "new" person (the "old" person had failed somehow) and "let it all hang out. This train is bound for glory. The brakeman has resigned" (Vonnegut 1975:108). His sense of alienation from place increased:

> Time had gotten very strange. Things whizzed and whirled all about me with great speed and confusion. Then everything would stop. There was no more movement, everything was being frozen solid, life was being drained out of everything. I'd feel a scream building up deep down inside me when suddenly everything would spring to life again, violently and pointlessly. The scream would come but there'd be no sound. It was all drowned out in the frantic rush of wings beating around my head. I'd come to myself from time to time and realize I was walking, half stumbling through the woods. I'd wonder where the hell I was going, what was I doing? I'd take handfuls of snow and press them to my face, trying desperately to get some sort of hold on myself.[5]

Other accounts by schizophrenics also support the notion that alienation from place is an important component of the disorder. Aaron Esterson, for one, describes Sarah Danzig, a schizophrenic girl who is the subject of a case study in *The Leaves of Spring* (1972). Sarah Danzig began to show signs of a psychiatric problem at the age of seventeen. She would stay in bed all day—thinking, brooding, and reading the Bible—getting up only at night. She lost interest in everyday affairs and became preoccupied with religion. The root of her problem appeared to lie within the family. Her father was rigid and conservative as well as overprotective. Among other things, he took to listening in on her telephone calls and opening her mail. He wanted her to date boys but was afraid one would take advantage of her sexually. She had been taught to respect her father, yet both her mother and her brother, John, took to quarreling with him openly. When she, however, argued with her father, her mother and brother would become angry with *her*. Esterson says:

> One of the main features of her illness in the view of her parents was an unreasoned, senseless, persistent hostility to her father, but when seen alone, her

---

[4]Mark Vonnegut, *The Eden Express* (New York: Praeger, 1975), p. 99. This and all subsequent quotations reprinted by permission.
[5]Ibid., pp. 108–9.

mother, without any apparent awareness of being inconsistent, also described Sarah's hostility as a meaningful response to various things her father did. Indeed, she said he acted in the same way towards her and John, making them angry too. In fact it emerged that they were constantly quarreling. It thus became clear that Sarah's anger against her father, which her family now could not tolerate, was hardly more intense than the enmity her mother and John had directed against him for years. But they objected to Sarah acting similarly. Sarah was finally singled out by her mother, father, and brother as the one person who was *really* expected to comply with her father's wishes. This was not put to her in so many words, but each of the others privately realized that she was put in a special position, although without their being fully aware of its consequences for her. They argued that if Sarah could not get on with her father she must be ill.[6]

Actually, Sarah had a better relationship with her father than anyone else in the family did. And her father imagined himself as her protector and ally, but his support for her likewise tended to be imaginary. He did not support her either when alone with her or when she was attacked by his wife and son. Only in her absence did he tell his wife and son to leave her alone. Increasingly isolated by the family, Sarah remained in her bedroom. She was defined by her mother as being "lazy," not mentally ill, and therefore she was a "bad" person. She was trapped. Too terrified to leave the protection of her family, she had no choice in her view but to isolate herself. She tried to resolve the problem by acting like a child and using her bedroom as an area of privacy and autonomy. Shortly after her twenty-first birthday, there was a particularly important incident:

> Her bedroom was being redecorated as a birthday present from her father. The decorator failed to follow her instructions. When she protested he became insultingly familiar. She complained to her mother, but her mother failed to back her. She ran out of the house greatly distressed, and returned the following morning saying defiantly she had slept with a boy.[7]

Sarah's parents were outraged, and a doctor was called. She was committed to a mental hospital for a short time, but upon release she retired to her room, more isolated than ever, and her actions became increasingly bizarre (that is, she was hearing voices, seeing people on television talking about her). She was readmitted to the mental hospital, her alienation from "place" complete.

Vernon Grant (1963), in analyzing the experience of schizophrenia, adds to our understanding of this episode by pointing out that although it may be touched off by an event or incident, the central feature of the experience is an upheaval from within the personality. This inner upheaval absorbs the attention of the schizophrenic to the exclusion of everything else. Perceptions and emotions are distorted, and feelings of inadequacy, despair, failure, and

---

[6]Aaron Esterson, *The Leaves of Spring: A Study in the Dialectics of Madness* (Harmondsworth, England: Pelican Books, 1972), p. 7.
[7]Ibid., p. 202.

panic are common. The upheaval within the personality seems to violate the familiar boundaries of self and to arise from some unknown cause, although it is *in* the mind. Grant (1963:120) explains, "Anyone who has ever found himself, in some novel situation, acting in an impulsive way that causes him later to ask: 'What on earth made me do that?' or, 'What got into me then?' or 'That wasn't like me at all' or similar bewildered phrases, has at least a glimpse, perhaps, or the 'feel' of this behavior phenomenon."

The individual also may feel a strong sense of failure, a failure that occurs in the eyes of others and therefore invokes an intolerable loss of self-respect. (Mark Vonnegut, for instance, was going to show his girlfriend the "new" Mark as a way of compensating for her infidelity.) Overall, as Grant (1963:121) finds, the result "is a terrifying personal crisis in which thinking becomes disorganized, and in which some remarkable ideas temporarily dominate the mind." The person's scale of thinking is greatly expanded, and thoughts and sensations become vivid and quite real. Dangers imagined by that person are believed to be part of the entire world breaking down. And possibly the person senses that he or she has extraordinary powers, perhaps contact with supernatural forces, and a mission to make things better. (Vonnegut thought he had killed a lot of people and caused an earthquake in California, but he saw himself as on a mission, as being the messiah.)

But through each of these experiences runs the theme of alienation from place. As Vonnegut (1975:120) said to his friend, "Simon, I have this awful feeling I'm kissing everyone goodbye forever. It seems very sad."

Anxiety   Now let us consider a different type of mental problem in which an individual maintains a relatively firm hold on reality but nevertheless is mentally disturbed and senses alienation from place. Norman S. Sutherland (1977), a British psychologist, suffered a "nervous breakdown" around the age of forty-five. There were no hallucinations or delusions; instead, Sutherland experienced feelings of chronic anxiety and episodes of deep depression. As an adolescent he had felt somewhat inferior and had become introverted, especially around girls. To rectify this, he forced himself to act confident (even if he did not feel that way) and in doing so became aggressively outspoken. He was educated at Oxford University, one of Great Britain's most prestigious universities, where he had few friends and strongly resented what he considered to be the snobbery and pretentiousness of British university life. But, except for an occasional bout of rudeness, he kept his opinions to himself, for fear of jeopardizing his own academic career.

Once Sutherland had completed his professional training and accepted a faculty position at another British university, he plunged into a frantic routine of teaching, advising, travel, research, and writing. He was so busy he would shave in his car on the way to work in the morning. In the meantime, he had managed to get married and acquire a family, although he spent little time at home. He worked on weekends and holidays and avoided social obligations, such as dinner parties, whenever possible. In his early forties, however, he began to have doubts about the quality of his work and to worry about death and the decline of his sexual abilities that accompanied middle age. The circumstance that triggered his anxiety was sexual jealousy. Sutherland's wife began having an affair with another man, and she confided to him the most intimate details of the relationship. Sutherland states that he tolerated it because he had had a series of casual affairs with other women and felt he could not question his wife's right to do likewise. Additionally, he regarded sexual jealousy as a particularly despicable and selfish emotion. His wife had described her lover as someone whom he did not know, later revealing his identity as a man whom he did know rather well and did not especially like. Sutherland found this information "desperately upsetting." He wanted to inflict physical punishment on the man but believed that that was "uncivilized." He was so determined to be a gentleman about it that he arranged to have a drink with the man to discuss the situation and was outraged when the man stated that his wife had "thrown herself at him." "My breakdown," states Sutherland (1977:4), "dated from that moment." He drove home in a frenzy, dominated by anxiety. Clearly, the taken-for-granted meanings of his normal, everyday life were shattered, and his life was dominated by feelings of anxiety and depression that intervened between him and his normal social world.

Depression   William Styron, originally from the South but now a long-time resident of Connecticut, had written such novels as *The Confessions of Nat Turner* and *Sophie's Choice*. He experienced his alienation from place as a prelude to a depressive disorder in the summer of 1985. Styron, normally a heavy drinker, had given up alcohol. His body had reached the point that it simply rebelled against further drinking; when he tried, he felt nauseous. He dated the beginning of his depressive mood from that point. Normally, states Styron, a person would be overjoyed to give up a substance that was undermining his or her health, but instead a vague sense of malaise and that something was wrong overtook him. Styron describes his feelings at this point:

> It was not really alarming at first, since the change was subtle, but I did notice my surroundings took on a different tone at certain times: the shadow of nightfall seemed more somber, my mornings were less buoyant, walks in the woods became less zestful, and there was a moment during my working hours in the late afternoon when a kind of panic and anxiety overtook me, accompanied by a visceral queasiness—such a seizure was at least slightly alarming, after all.[8]

Styron indicates that it should have been clear to him that he was experiencing the beginning of a mood disorder, but he was ignorant of that possibility at the time.

---

[8]William Styron, *Darkness Visible: A Memoir of Madness* (New York: Random House, 1990), p. 42.

Although alienation from place constitutes the initial stage of becoming insane, it is not clear what causes it to happen, just as it is not clear what causes mental disorder. The alienation that is experienced is emotional, psychological, and social, as individuals in this situation are unable to feel normal in their social world. For these people, the ultimate cause of their estrangement may be genetic, biochemical, psychological, social, or some combination thereof. Many people who become schizophrenic, for example, have a genetic predisposition toward the disorder, which is believed triggered by some stressful situation (Weiner 1985). Yet regardless of the exact cause of a mental disorder, it is suggested that a feeling of alienation from one's usual round of daily life is the initial sign that something is wrong; that is, the trigger—whether genetic or otherwise—has been released.

Recognizing Symptoms

People can experience alienation from place, but that feeling may not necessarily mean the onset of mental disorder. Rather, a sense of alienation appears to be a first step. The second step is a recognition of symptoms. A person's understanding of his or her sanity is affected by the presence or absence of the symptoms of mental illness. Common symptoms include experiencing abnormal states of awareness, emotional reactions, mood, motor behavior, thinking, perception, memory, and intelligence (Kaplan and Sadock 1989). In recognizing the reality of having one or more of these symptoms, the person involved is moved to account for and deal with them in a way that minimizes personal costs (Whitt and Meile 1985). A number of alternative explanations are available in contemporary society for explaining bizarre feelings and abnormal behavior, such as stress, overwork, grief, and unpleasant life situations. However, if the individual finds that the situation can no longer be controlled by his or her efforts and the symptoms not only persist but become more intense, realization of being mentally disordered becomes more likely.

Thoits (1983, 1985) helps us to understand this circumstance by noting that people are most likely to label themselves mentally ill when they recognize the discrepancy between their own behavior and feeling states and what is normally expected of them. Thoits draws upon the work of George Herbert Mead (1934) to note that a person's sense of self arises from taking the role assigned by specific and then generalized others. That is, people see themselves as being a certain person (having a particular social identity), first from the perspectives of significant others (parents, family, and friends) and later from the perspective of the generalized other (groups and the wider community). Thus, they learn the cultural perspective of the wider society on normative forms of behavior. And when they violate those norms with uncontrolled, bizarre responses, they are likely to label themselves or be labeled by others as mentally ill. Therefore, individuals can recognize for themselves the symptoms of mental disorder because they are able to classify their thoughts, behavior, and feelings from the standpoint of others.

Although some people may try to deny their symptoms or consider mental disorder only as a last resort in understanding their problems, awareness of some degree of mental abnormality seems common (Thoits 1985). According to Foucault (1987), mental illness always implies a consciousness of illness. Seldom is all reference to the normal suppressed in the minds of mental patients; hence, there is a realization or an awareness of being mentally ill and what it involves. There is no escape from the evidence of one's senses.

Schizophrenia Vonnegut, for example, after he received the letter from his girlfriend describing her infidelity and began having hallucinations, knew something was wrong with him. A few weeks earlier, he had felt he could handle all his problems, but that ability was gone. He had trouble walking and, as he put it, even remembering to breathe. He knew he needed help but still had the feeling that perhaps nothing was really wrong. And, if there was something wrong with him, he wondered how he could make anyone else understand, because what was wrong was such a strange and elusive feeling that it would be easy for others to discount it. Consequently, he kept the content of his thoughts to himself as best as he could.

Anxiety Sutherland, likewise, realized that his mental state was abnormal. At first, he tried to rationalize that the affair was good for his wife, since she appeared happy. At other times, he was engulfed by hatred, jealousy, and panic attacks. He described his feelings as follows:

> The onset of my neurosis was marked by levels of physical anxiety that I would not have believed possible. If one is almost involved in a road accident, there is a delay of a second or two and then the pit of the stomach seems to fall out and one's legs go like jelly. It was this feeling multiplied a hundredfold that seized me at all hours of the day and night. My dreams were often pleasant, but as soon as I woke panic set in and it would take a few moments to work out what it was about. The realization brought anguish: an irrevocable and cataclysmic event had occurred from which I could imagine no recovery.[9]

Sutherland was also upset with himself for not being able to behave in what he considered a rational manner. He found it unbearable to be apart from his wife. He followed her around the house and even out shopping. If he lost sight of her, he would panic. He became obsessed with ideas about her affair and constantly thought about the details of the relationship that his wife had disclosed to him. His alienation from place was particularly acute at the university. He could not work and discussed his problems end-

---

[9]N. S. Sutherland, *Breakdown* (Briarcliff Manor, NY: Stein & Day, 1977), p. 2.

lessly—to the point of boredom—with his colleagues. He carried a book with him for five months, opened it several hundred times during that period, but was never able to read past the first page. The only activity that seemed satisfying was talking to others, except for two other pursuits he normally would have considered a waste of time—driving a car and doing crossword puzzles.

Depression Styron recognized his symptoms clearly in the fall of 1985 when he traveled to Paris to accept a prestigious writing award. Increasingly, he was experiencing a general sense of worthlessness and loss of self-esteem, along with insomnia. He would usually feel his best in the morning, but as the day progressed feelings of alienation, dread, and anxiety came crowding in on him, and by evening he would often be in a state of near self-paralysis. Then, in Paris, on a rainy October day, he was riding in an automobile and passed by a hotel he had stayed in as young writer some thirty-five years previously. The feeling that came over him at that moment was that his life had come full circle. He felt that when he left Paris the next day it would be forever. "I was shaken," states Styron (1990:4), "by the certainty with which I accepted the idea that I would never see France again, just as I would never recapture a lucidity that was slipping away from me with terrifying speed." Only a few days earlier, he had concluded that he was suffering from serious depression and would be unable to prevent it from continuing. Just before the Paris trip, he had made an appointment to see a psychiatrist in New York. He now wanted to leave Paris immediately and see the psychiatrist as soon as possible.

David Karp (1994), in his analysis of the subjective experience of depression, found that severely depressed individuals sense something is wrong with them but find it impossible to focus on exactly what it is. They tend initially to blame situations rather than themselves. As feelings of deep depression evolve, they feel they must must distance themselves from other people—even though they realize this has negative consequences, since it increases their social isolation. A common theme among the severely depressed is that they are aware they are on a downward emotional spiral and feel powerless to stop it. Karp finds that, in the beginning, depressed individuals may try to offset their symptoms through exercise, meditation, or experimenting with different forms of spirituality. Ultimately, these efforts fail, states Karp (1994:348), and each failure requires a reinterpretation of the cause of their depression and diminished optimism about the possibilities of a cure.

Madness as a Method of Coping

Having recognized something is wrong, the mentally disordered person will at some point find it necessary to cope with the situation. Madness, however, will likely direct the strategy employed, as it assumes greater control over the person's thoughts and feelings.

Schizophrenia   Vonnegut believed that everything would be all right if he could just see his girlfriend, Virginia. He thought that what was happening to him was caused by her desperate need for him (not his for her). He and his friend Simon went off on a trip into a nearby town to check for mail, but in Vonnegut's mind he and Simon were really going to find Virginia. He began the trip by getting dressed:

> Everything was trembling and glowing with an eerie light. One foot in front of the other, step two follows step one. Somehow I got dressed. "See, I can still function," I said to myself as I made it down the trembling ladder and into the trembling kitchen. "Everything's going to be just fine," I managed to say to Jack and Kathy. As we left I tried a reassuring smile.
>
> One foot in front of the other down to the lake in my Day-Glo boots that seemed to be walking without me—gush gush. Just put my body on automatic, everything will be fine.
>
> "Whose popsicle stand is this anyway?" Who said that? Did I say that? I didn't say that. "Simon, whose popsicle stand is this anyway? Did you say that? Zeke?"
>
> "Whose popsicle stand is this anyway, Virginia?" Can she hear me? Where is she? Did she say it?
>
> It was perfect. It was just right for our reunion. That's what I would say, "Virginia, whose popsicle stand is this anyway? Do you think it would be the sort of place we might be able to talk?"[10]

Although what Vonnegut was thinking and saying appears nonsensical, to him it made sense. He wanted a change (seeing Virginia). His view was that everything was going to be fine once he and Virginia were together. He anticipated that the popsicle stand would be the "perfect" site for their "reunion." Thus, he rehearsed what he would say to her when they met at the popsicle stand that existed only in his mind.

The phase of madness as a method of coping presumes that *there is method to madness and that insanity constitutes deliberate behavior, or at least seems so to the schizophrenic in the beginning.* Goffman (1971) notes that mental symptoms are not incidental social infractions but are specifically and pointedly offensive; that is, they are willful social deviations. *Therefore, what is being expressed as insanity is a different mental reality that does not make its expression any less deliberate.* As James Fadiman and Donald Kewman (1973:61) stated: "People who write of their own madness suggest that what appears to be disorganized, bizarre or uncontrolled is often a shrewd and consciously construed act designed to achieve a particular goal."

For example, Deborah, a sixteen-year-old girl in Hannah Green's book *I Never Promised You a Rose Garden* (1964), had her own special view of the world, which had its own complex structure of moral rules, language, and defined relationships between gods and mortals—all insane. Louis Narens (1973), who interviewed mental patients to determine their belief systems, talked to a

---

[10]Vonnegut, *Eden Express*, pp. 110–11.

woman who believed in the existence of an imaginary person she called "Oscar." Oscar had his own personality and was her companion when she needed friendship. The woman knew Oscar was not real and said so, but he seemed real to her nonetheless and was an important part of her life. Narens also interviewed a woman who believed she saw ghosts "sometimes as large as a room." He asked her to teach him to see ghosts and discovered that she "saw" ghosts by feeling temperature changes on her face. What most people would call inexplicable drafts, she called ghosts. Lara Jefferson, a mental patient writing about her madness, believed that a crazy wild woman (herself?) was in her head trying to influence her. The woman would tell her to fight fire with fire, that is, to fight madness with madness. Jefferson said of this: "She presents her idea with so much logic she makes me think that instead of losing reason in madness—and finding insanity on the other side—that in reality, I will lose insanity in madness—and find a sound mind on the other side" (Fadiman and Kewman 1973:17).

Grant (1963) agrees that there is a method in madness. He suggests that in trying to find protection from distress, the schizophrenic sacrifices much of what might be considered as normal logic. Grant states:

> What looks on the surface like a breakdown of normal thinking is, instead, a purposive flight from a reality that has become too charged with anxiety to be tolerated. There is evidence, in fact, that what appears as impaired ability to reason correctly is, instead, a *change in the method of reasoning.* The purpose of this change is not only to protect the self, but to satisfy certain other needs as well.
>
> This is to suggest that what is commonly regarded as *disorder* is, rather, *an order of a different kind,* and one very different from the thinking habits of normal people, which is undisturbed by severe emotional stresses. The normal order of human thinking is governed by the requirement of the real world, as well as by individual needs. The strangely altered "order" of schizophrenic thinking is governed less by the world as it is, and much more by individual needs.[11]

In sum, by anticipating actions and rehearsing responses, schizophrenics attempt to cope with their situation using what to them is a method that makes sense.

Anxiety   Sutherland, too, went through a phase of madness as a method of coping. "The early days of my breakdown," he (1977:6) says, "were marked by a further curious feature. I was seized by a compulsion to tell my wife not merely of every disloyal act that I had ever committed but of every disreputable thought that had ever crossed my mind." He was well aware that he should not do this, but from nowhere some incident would suddenly be remembered, and he would struggle not to reveal it. "I would even force

---

[11]Vernon W. Grant, *This Is Mental Illness* (Boston: Beacon Press, 1963), p. 121.

myself to go out and walk alone," Sutherland (1977:6) continues, "hoping that the compulsion would die away, but it never did: whilst I kept it to myself, my anxiety level would go on rising until eventually it forced me to vomit forth whatever I had on my mind." In doing so, he knew his wife would become very upset.

Another example comes from the case history of Johnny Z., a child also suffering from intense anxiety. Upon being frustrated in school, Johnny would return home and slam doors and throw his books around. When that happened, his mother made little or no attempt to deal directly with the situation. She would insist that Johnny stay in his room until he calmed down. When asked to describe how *he* felt, Johnny replied:

> Feels like I'm going to burst open and feel like I want to tear the place to pieces, then another feeling I don't like is feeling like smashing something to pieces. Then burning up the place, tearing down anything in my way, that's about all.[12]

Thus, in the minds of both Sutherland and Johnny Z. there was an anticipation of what their mental state would cause and a rehearsal of their expression of that state (that is, "vomiting" what was on one's mind, slamming doors, and throwing books).

Depression   As for Styron, he attended the ceremony in Paris at which he was presented with his award and he managed to make an acceptance speech. But as he delivered his final remarks, he felt a strong need for the day to be over. Symptoms of confusion and a lack of focus and memory swept over him. However, he was supposed to join the award committee at a lunch in his honor. He declined, stating he had made plans to lunch that day with his publisher, even though the awards luncheon had been scheduled for months. His French hosts were angry and insulted. Suddenly he realized that his unpardonable conduct and apparent confusion were the result of his illness; horrified, he apologized and then said something that he never believed he would utter. He said he had *"un problème psychiatrique"* (Styron 1990:15) The lunch was long and uncomfortable, but he got through it. At dinner with friends that evening, he could neither eat nor speak.

In the first phase of alienation from place, we see the mentally disordered sensing a barrier between themselves and their everyday environment. In the second phase, they realize they have symptoms of an abnormal mentality. Now in the third phase of madness as a method of coping, we see the mentally disturbed attempting to cope with their mental disorder in a way that threatens their normal social relationships but nonetheless is a significant expression of their insanity as a prelude to the *definitive outburst*.

---

[12]Barclay Martin, *Anxiety and Neurotic Disorders* (New York: Wiley, 1971), p. 122.

The Definitive Outburst

In this phase, the mentally disordered person clearly moves out into the open and overtly expresses his or her definition of the situation. This expression is some type of insane outburst that leaves little or no doubt about the mental disorder. As Morris Rosenberg (1984) explains, the decisive point in the attribution of mental disorder comes when the observer of the insane behavior is unable to understand the viewpoint (take the role) of the person expressing the behavior. The definitive outburst constitutes this point in the assignment of insanity to an individual. Although the mentally disordered person may display some physiological indicators of distress (for example, unusual motor or speech activity), the most obtrusive indicators will be social. They will be overt, havoc-creating behaviors that are not only pointedly offensive but also too illogical to permit definitions other than madness.

Schizophrenia   Again, we can return to the experience of Mark Vonnegut for an example. He had left the farm and gone into town with his friend Simon. After dinner in a café, they went to a nearby commune to spend the night, "crashing" on the floor with several other people. During the night, Vonnegut decided to stop being polite and quit worrying about making other people look at him oddly. He felt there was no more time.

> Thank God I screamed. I came within an ace of waiting too long but at the last moment I got my shit together and came through in the clutch. What would have happened had I not screamed out I wasn't so sure. It would have been the death of something. Maybe just the end of me and a few friends, but maybe the end of the world or worse. But I did scream. I didn't go gentle into that black night, blackly into that good night, or goodly into that gentle night.
> "STOP—FREEZE—NOBODY MOVE A MUSCLE. IT'S HAPPENING!" I reached out and grabbed Simon's arm. My eyes were closed. I was in a cold sweat. "DON'T ASK ME HOW I KNOW. THERE ISN'T TIME. JUST DO AS I SAY. I KNOW. THE RAIN HAS STOPPED." It was only fair to give out a few clues, enough so that they would know that I *knew* and do what I said. The rain's stopping definitely had something to do with it.
> It might seem strange to tell a roomful of sleeping people not to move a muscle, especially a roomful of sleeping people you don't know. But it made sense. It made more sense than anything else in my life ever had. It wasn't a night like any other night, or sleep like any other sleep.[13]

With the definitive outburst, the schizophrenic drives a wedge between himself or herself and other people. In this way, all parties experience alienation. Goffman (1971) claims that when rules of conduct are broken, two individuals run the risk of being discredited: one with an obligation to act in a certain way and the other with an expectation to be treated in a particular way.

---

[13]Vonnegut, *Eden Express*, pp. 125–26.

The result is that part of the social definition of the actor and the recipient of the action is threatened. Also threatened, but to a lesser degree, is the community that contains them both. The more insane the outburst, the more likely that there will be sanctions against the offender. In Vonnegut's case, his friends tried to comfort him, and he was taken to an apartment in Vancouver. But relationships were strained, and he was closely watched.

Anxiety   In Sutherland's case, it finally became quite obvious to him and his wife that he was mentally ill when she demanded he write letters to three women with whom he had been sexually involved. She had demanded this in apparent response to his continued confession of former infidelities. He wrote the letters, which struck him as being "unkind," with his wife watching over his shoulder. "I was in a desperate state," says Sutherland (1977:7), "and swallowed half a bottle of whiskey." He went into another room, where he addressed and stamped not three but six envelopes. Three envelopes were empty; three contained the letters. He kept the empty envelopes and gave his wife the others to mail. On the way to the mailbox, he grabbed the letters from her and put them in his pocket. She insisted on having them back, and so he handed her the three empty envelopes that he had put in another pocket. She mailed these, and Sutherland later tore up the real letters and flushed them down the toilet. But over the next few hours, his anxiety over having deceived his wife became so intolerable that he rewrote the letters as best he could and then mailed them. When he returned home, he told her what he had done. Clearly, he was unable to control his behavior.

Depression   Styron returned to his home in Connecticut and began seeing a psychiatrist, but neither conversation nor medication was helpful. In fact, the medication (Halcion) made him feel suicidal. The house he had lived in happily for thirty years now seemed ominous. The act of writing became increasingly difficult and finally he ceased doing it. On spotting a flock of geese flying overhead on a walk through the woods with his dog, he became riveted with fear and unable to move. "Going home," says Styron (1990:46), "I couldn't rid my mind of the line of Baudelaire's, dredged up from the distant past, that for several days had been skittering around at the edge of my consciousness: 'I have felt the wind of the wings of madness'."

Days later, he took a notebook full of various written observations about things he had done over a number of years and put it in the garbage. He felt that symbolically he was ending his writing career and soon would end his life as well. He did this on a day when his session with his psychiatrist was particularly useless, and he was barely able to speak during an evening dinner with friends at his home. In a few days, he saw his lawyer and rewrote his will as thoughts of taking his own life became more pronounced. Late that night, sitting alone, listening to music (a Brahms symphony), the decisive moment in Styron's mental illness occurred:

This sound, which like all music—indeed, like all pleasure—I had been numbly unresponsive to for months, pierced my heart like a dagger, and in a flood of swift recollection I thought of all the joys the house had known. . . . I drew up some last gleam of sanity to perceive the terrifying dimensions of the mortal predicament I had fallen into. I woke up my wife and soon telephone calls were made. The next day I was admitted to the hospital.[14]

Rendering of Accounts

The mentally disordered person will usually offer a tentative explanation of his or her behavior. These accounts will be excuses, justifications for misconduct, apologies, or declarations that no accounting is necessary. Accounts can be remedial or negative. *Remedial accounts* attempt to sustain the person's standing and credibility in relation to his or her place and are most likely to occur in the beginning of the insane career, when uncertainty is greatest.

Negative accounts are likely to appear later. These openly challenge the integrity of others and attempt to shift the blame from self to others.

Schizophrenia   Vonnegut, for instance, a religion major in college, found at an early stage the notion that he was going through some type of religious enlightenment to be an attractive remedial account. Another example of remedial accounts is from Mr. F, the husband in the Yarrow and associates (1955) study. Mr. F protested that he was "naturally" nervous and used his "wartime" experiences to justify his mental problems.

Vonnegut also became increasingly paranoid at one point, thinking his friends were trying to poison him, and was admitted voluntarily to a mental hospital for a short time. Upon release, he returned to the farm, but another person, named Nick, was there, whom he regarded as especially sinister and threatening. Nick thus became Vonnegut's basis for a negative account. He was upset that Simon had agreed that Nick could stay at the farm. He wondered how Simon could be so stupid as to allow Nick to live with them. Couldn't Simon see what was in Nick's eyes? Vonnegut reported:

Without Nick it might have been different. Who can say? I might have been able to relax and live happily ever after at the farm. But relaxing and feeling at home around him was about as likely as . . . ? The stream flowing up the mountain? Why not? Had to use some image and the stream did just that a few days later anyway.[15]

Anxiety   We can see the same kind of accounts and justifications in Sutherland's situation. Although recognizing that his wife was entitled to have an affair, because he had done so, he still blamed her for supplying him with so many details about her relationship. At first he felt that she had done this in

---

[14]Styron, *Darkness Visible*, pp. 66–67.
[15]Vonnegut, *Eden Express*, p. 183.

a spirit of trust, although on reflection he thought that her vivid descriptions of her sex life with her lover were a way of punishing him for his own sexual misadventures. He also offered an account of early childhood in which, at the age of two, he was not allowed to see his mother (on the advice of a nurse) for two weeks after the birth of his younger brother. He wondered if that experience had somehow predisposed him toward anxiety but had no way of really knowing.

The young schoolboy Johnny Z. likewise blamed others for his anxiety, as he sought to use their relationship with him as an excuse for his destructive tendencies. In this case, it was the parents whom Johnny blamed (Martin 1971). The mother was afraid to cope with her son's problems, and the father was openly critical of the boy. Whether that was the cause of his disorder is not known, but the boy complained about it and used it to justify his behavior.

Depression   Styron's situation was somewhat different. He kept the experience of his disturbed mind just to himself and his wife for as long as possible. His initial remedial account was that his condition was a reaction to giving up alcohol. When he became aware (especially in Paris) that he indeed had a serious depressive disorder, he finally admitted so in the apology to his hosts. He subsequently accounted for his behavior when necessary by his admission of being extremely depressed. This admission functioned as an excuse to his friends for being uncommunicative and withdrawn.

In short, the mentally disordered person seeks what he or she thinks is an acceptable explanation of his or her mental state. Once the mentally disordered person conjures up these explanations, they may be tested on others for their effectiveness. This individual may also be obliged by others to reveal these explanations as the insane career unfolds. Others will find it necessary to have some accounting from the deranged person if they are to protect, maintain, or rationalize some degree of normality in the situation. However, the longer the insanity and the more obvious its expression, the less likely it will be that any explanation will be believed. The mentally disturbed person now moves toward removal from place. But the person's attempts to prevent the final break and to restore the situation are complicated even more by another factor: the paradox of normalcy.

The Paradox of Normalcy

Should the mental disorder continue and the disordered person's accounts be rejected, the person will find that his or her madness will be normalized. It is in this context that the paradox of normalcy emerges. Human group life, being relatively arbitrary, will normalize any behavior once it is explained in some way. Consequently, a person's mental disorder, if accounted for (defined) by others as insanity, will become seen by them as normal for that particular person. That is, the person will be regarded as "mentally ill" or "crazy," and that circumstance will be viewed as normal for the person in question. Mental illness will essentially become a master status for that person. This is similar to Lemert's (1951) concept of secondary deviance, in which deviant acts become part of a person's usual social role and identity. *The paradox arises when an abnormal state (madness) is defined as normal for someone.* At that point, action to remedy the situation will be an obvious conclusion for most of the people involved in coping with the problem. For Vonnegut, Sutherland, and Styron, the point was eventually reached when mental disorder was considered normal for them.

Removal from "Place"

The removal from place occurs when it is recognized by those involved that the insane person is indeed mentally disordered. The removal itself may be made by the mentally ill person or by others, but it is the likely outcome if the madness cannot be tolerated. If it can be tolerated (perhaps viewed as harmless or eccentric) or can be treated successfully in "place" (the home or community), removal may be unnecessary or delayed. When all rationalization fails, and mental disorder is considered "normal" (the paradox of normalcy) for the person in question, removal is at hand.

The mentally disordered person may achieve the removal by simply leaving the scene and going off somewhere else to set up new relationships, perhaps even volunteering for psychiatric treatment. Or the person's associates may direct the person to leave the scene either voluntarily or involuntarily. The person may find himself or herself a mental patient, either by consent or at the direction of the state through its power to commit deranged citizens. If there is a dispute, lawyers as well as psychiatrists will be included. The mentally disordered person becomes trapped by his or her past activities and is unable at that moment to reconstruct the "place" that has been destroyed. The person's ability and capacity to reenter that place in the future, even after remedial treatment and therapy have been administered, also is problematic. In Vonnegut's case, he was returned involuntarily by his friends and the police to the mental hospital. After two exceptionally severe schizophrenic episodes, he was released and returned to the United States to start life again in a different "place."

In Sutherland's situation, he underwent psychoanalysis (which he found useless). Removal from place finally came when he admitted himself to a mental hospital, where he received tranquilizers and participated in behavior modification therapy. His anxiety slowly responded to treatment but was followed by depression. He returned home and resumed his academic career while an outpatient, and eventually the depression just disappeared. Whether it was because of the therapy he received or because depression may be self-limiting, Sutherland was not sure. He and his wife were able to stay together and work out their problems after his hospitalization, an undertaking that they tackled despite the many friends' and therapists' suggestions that they separate. Iron-ically, the pressure from other people to end their relationship had the effect of drawing them back together. Styron was hospitalized for a period of seven weeks and given a different medication. His depression vanished just as mys-teriously, in his view, as it had arrived; he never was able to determine what caused it.

An important point to recognize in all seven phases of acting mentally disordered is that insanity is not just a psychiatric or a psychological experi-ence. True, the struggle that takes place within the mind is located in the psy-chology and perhaps biochemistry of the individual, but the expression of that struggle is sociological. For *the* evidence of mental disorder is most definitely (1) the appearance of engaging in normatively meaningless events (that is, dis-rupting the usual and everyday behaviors of a particular group of people by acting so bizarre or unusual that it leaves little doubt that one is insane) and (2) the destruction of normal interpersonal relationships. This activity requires the consideration of appropriate social norms, values, and traditions if judg-ments of what is normal, as compared with what is abnormal, are to be made. To that end, sociological research on the prepatient experience is necessary for understanding that experience to its fullest extent. In this chapter, we have focused on the prepatient experiences of Vonnegut, Sutherland, and Styron to illustrate the movement toward mental patient status. This movement was a progressive deterioration of social relationships to the point of no return, that is, the final break, in which all knew and recognized the presence of madness in their midst—a madness that was no longer tolerable. Additional data from case histories are needed to pinpoint exactly how people sense alienation from place, anticipate their disorder and rehearse it as a method of coping with their problems, act mentally disordered, make excuses, and finally are caught in the paradox of normalcy en route to the removal from their usual social existence.

SUMMARY

This chapter has described the quality of the social interaction that takes place between the mentally ill and significant others in their lives. The intent was to discuss how people come to seek treatment for mental disorder and to con-sider how mentally disordered persons conceptualize their own experiences of insanity. In regard to the former, we examined the events and circumstances of both the uncoerced and the coerced efforts to obtain psychiatric care. Coer-cion and alienation appear to be particularly common in seeking help. In regard to the latter, we suggested a model to chart the phases of insane behav-ior in the schizophrenic and the person suffering from anxiety. These phases were (1) alienation from place, (2) realizing symptoms, (3) madness as a method of coping, (4) the definitive outburst, (5) rendering of accounts, (6) the paradox of normalcy, and (7) removal from place. Although not all mentally ill persons may fit this model or go through all the phases or each phase in the order presented, reports of their experiences by the mentally ill themselves and others suggest that the model is plausible. The purpose of this chapter has been to convey to the reader, at least partially, what it is like to be mentally ill and what happens in the family or among living companions when the disorder emerges.

11

The Mental Hospital Inpatient Experience

Although the use of psychiatric drugs and the increased availability of outpatient clinics and community mental health centers have significantly reduced the number of resident patients in mental hospitals, these measures have not been uniformly successful in preventing hospitalization. Increasing numbers of people are admitted to mental hospitals for short terms (a few for long terms), and mental hospitals are likely to remain a very important component of any future system of mental health care delivery. There are three reasons for the continued existence of mental hospitals, either public or private: (1) Such hospitals remove deviant and socially disruptive persons from society, thus allowing social life to continue in its usual fashion; (2) mental hospitals are set up to care for people (that is, to provide food, shelter, medical treatment) who might be mentally unable or unwilling to take care of themselves properly; (3) these institutions are established to promote the mental well-being of the patient by inducing psychological change through the use of various therapeutic techniques, such as drugs, counseling, group therapies, electroshock treatment, and so forth. Hence, mental hospitals are *incarcerative, custodial,* and, one hopes, *therapeutic.* The term "one hopes" is used in regard to therapy because some mental patients cannot be restored to a relatively normal mental state.

This chapter will discuss the inpatient experience, beginning with the admission process. Most of the discussion, however, is based on data collected by sociologists in the 1960s and 1970s. Interest in life in mental hospitals was high in sociology at that time because of the importance of the community mental health movement. Emphasizing treatment for mental patients in the community, instead of in the confines of mental hospitals, the community mental health movement was successful in changing national policy. With a majority of mental patients receiving community care, the focus of sociological research on mental health turned elsewhere, leaving behind an extensive body of research, which is reported on in this chapter.

VOLUNTARY COMMITMENT

Voluntary commitment results when individuals present themselves of their own accord for admission to a mental hospital. About 70 percent of all patients admitted to inpatient psychiatric facilities are admitted voluntarily. Elliot Mishler and Nancy Waxler (1963) studied a state and a private mental hospital and found that the most important variable in whether a mental hospital will accept a person who volunteers for treatment was a referral by a physician. Physicians' requests to admit a person were viewed as more "legitimate." Other significant factors were the presence of a relative at the admission interview, the age of the patient (younger patients were preferred), and the patient's past history of mental hospitalization (there was a low acceptance rate of ex-patients). A problem with the Mishler and Waxler study, however, is that it did not control for the severity of the disorder or the need for treatment. It may be that those patients referred for hospitalization by physicians were more readily admitted not necessarily because of the physicians' prestige but because the physicians were able to recognize that the individuals in question needed psychiatric treatment (Krohn and Akers 1977).

Nevertheless, referral by a person other than the potential patient may be an important variable in some cases. For instance, a study of admissions to a state mental hospital conducted by Werner Mendel and Samuel Rapport (1969) did control for the severity of symptoms and found that they were not especially significant in determining admission. Among those variables that seemed relevant was the presence of family or friends to support the patient's contention that hospitalization was needed. Reports by persons who had themselves admitted to mental hospitals to do research likewise confirm the need for some source of referral. Anthony Brandt (1975) gained admission to a state mental hospital in New York by claiming he heard voices over the radio telling him he was useless and a failure in life. He had a friend bring him to the hospital, explain that he had smashed his radio, and express fear he would become violent. "I had no trouble at all gaining admission and it wasn't long before I found myself being led down a corridor," says Brandt (1975:162), "by a very businesslike aide dressed in a white starched uniform."

Anne Barry (1971) tried to get herself admitted to Bellevue Hospital in New York City by taking Dexedrine, talking loudly on the street about someone following her, and hoping to attract the attention of a police officer. Passersby, including the police, ignored her or made fun of her.[1] No one took any action until a group of teenage boys took her to a police officer. Barry described the scene as follows:

Why were the police so reluctant to pick me up? I could imagine that they were only trying to be kind—who knows what hippie drug orgy they might stumble upon if they were to take me home, or what drugs they feared to find in my pocketbook. Perhaps screaming girls were now so common in New York that the jails and the hospitals were filled up with them, leaving the law to gather in only the worst cases. It might be that the hospitals, overcrowded and under-staffed, discouraged on-the-street lay diagnoses. I could see I put this policeman in a nice spot, one eye on my desperate face, he was wishing for something straightforward and clear, a burglar caught in the act, or a teenager joy-riding in a stolen car. Crazy people were out of his line. The policeman said, "What the

---

[1]According to Egon Bittner (1967), the police apprehend mentally ill persons on the basis of either a court order or their own judgment. When their judgment is the basis for apprehension, it is not enough that a case of mental illness is serious in just a psychiatric sense. It must also represent a serious police problem. To be a police problem, there must be some indication of danger to the person, other people, or property. Bittner identifies five attitudinal factors that help to explain why the police are sometimes reluctant to take action against someone on the basis of presumed mental illness. First, the police are not experts in mental disorder, and if they act on fragmentary information, there is always the possibility that their involvement could be exploited by unknown persons for unknown reasons. Therefore, they seek to avoid possible mistakes. Second, the police routinely confront people in their everyday work who, to all appearances, should be in a "booby hatch." Yet these people are able to lead lives outside mental institutions, even though they are miserable, incompetent, perverted, and disoriented. Third, although police officers recognize that dealing with mentally disturbed people is part of their work, they place much greater value upon apprehending a criminal than conveying a mental case to a hospital. Fourth, police officers sometimes complain that taking someone to a hospital for psychiatric care is a tedious, cumbersome, and uncertain job. Often they must wait for long periods while the patient is being examined, and occasionally they are asked questions by psychiatrists that place their own judgment in doubt. They are placed in an awkward position if the person they bring in is not admitted. Fifth, mental disorder is a civil rather than a criminal matter—a fact all police officers are aware of—but mentally ill people are "locked up" nonetheless. Therefore, the officer has to consider whether apprehending a mentally disturbed person warrants such confinement.

But despite their reluctance, the police in an emergency do apprehend people acting crazy and do so rather frequently. The conditions on which such apprehensions are usually made are those that (1) involve people attempting or possibly attempting suicide, (2) show evidence that a person is severely disordered, (3) suggest that a severely disordered person has committed or threatens violence, (4) occur when a disordered person becomes a public nuisance or might be harmed in some way, or (5) involve someone who stands in some sort of direct relationship (spouse, lawyer, physician, employer, landlord, or whatever) to the person who makes a complaint. These persons should have exhausted their resources in trying to deal with the situation, thus leaving no recourse but to call the police for assistance.

hell, I can't do anything, but if you want, take her down to the Ninth Precinct, on Fifth Street."[2]

The boys took her to the police station, where they discussed her situation with the desk sergeant. Barry continues:

> I was relieved the boys were with me, for I couldn't have acted out paranoia for the police. I was tearful and anxious and miserable. The boys explained about my screaming, my suicidal tendencies. . . . We went over once again that I lived alone, had neither relatives nor a job. Whenever I hesitated, Marty and Tom filled in details. I felt more withdrawn and frightened than I thought a sane person should; I didn't know whether or not I was putting on an act. . . . "I don't know what to do with her," confessed the sergeant. "You don't want us to psycho her, do you? Christ, that's horrible, the psycho ward."
> Marty said, "But what's wrong with this city, that it can't help someone who's sick and in trouble? Isn't there anybody who can help?" The question hung there, in a little pocket of silence—it was just chance that at that moment the telephone was still, the rookie [cop] was writing on a pad, the man in the Chesterfield [coat] was no longer drumming his fingers on the wooden railing; the words shifted the mood. They cut through the cigarette haze and the dust motes under the yellow light, and I was not the only one thinking of questions larger than the cost of the stolen automobile, or the facts the rookie was putting into his report. The sergeant sighed. His shoulders sagged. He said, "Let me try one more time. Miss, don't you have anyone who could look after you tonight?"[3]

No one was available, and the desk sergeant finally called for an ambulance to take her to Bellevue. At first, the examining physician at Bellevue seemed skeptical, and Barry thought she might not be admitted. But once he located her rapid pulse rate, a result of the Dexedrine, he decided to believe her story of being extremely fearful and accept her as a patient.

Research by Walter Gove and Patrick Howell (1974) argues that a person's resources affect whether one is able to gain entry to a mental hospital. Based upon data from a mental hospital in the state of Washington during a two-year period, Gove and Howell found that persons close to the patient (spouse, family physician, or psychiatrist) are more likely to initiate hospitalization for high-income persons, but that "somewhat more distant" agents (relatives other than spouse or unrelated persons) or "distant" agents (that is, police or community agencies) are more apt to initiate hospitalization for low-income patients. Gove and Howell concluded that when the severity of the disorder is controlled, upper-class and married persons are more likely to be hospitalized than persons who are from the lower class or unmarried. The reason is that they have more resources that would assist in making a correct diagno-

---

[2]Anne Barry, *Bellevue Is a State of Mind* (New York: Harcourt Brace Jovanovich, 1971), p. 10.
[3]Ibid., pp. 10–12.

sis and would therefore facilitate entrance into psychiatric treatment. Unfortunately, Gove and Howell had data on only those patients who were admitted and no data on the social class and marital status of those not admitted, so it is difficult to determine the extent to which admission was facilitated or hampered by class and marital status (Krohn and Akers 1977; Rushing 1978). Yet other research shows that younger, more motivated, communicative, and competent patients receive the most personal attention from therapists (Link and Milcarek 1980); therapists, in turn, are more highly regarded by colleagues if their patients come from more privileged social backgrounds (Link 1983).

William Rushing (1978), in an especially well designed study, tested a status resource hypothesis with data on all twenty-one- to sixty-four-year-old first admissions to all state mental hospitals in Tennessee for a ten-year period. Rushing found that the data supported the hypothesis that individuals with more rather than fewer resources are more likely to be hospitalized voluntarily, whereas individuals with fewer resources are more likely to be hospitalized involuntarily. The basic premise is that individuals with higher socioeconomic status have the greatest resources to acquire and maintain a desired social state. They are better able to purchase the goods and services that allow them to continue their lifestyle, and they are apt to be more knowledgeable about how a community's agencies operate and how these agencies can be used on one's behalf. Involuntary admissions are much more likely to be under undesirable circumstances (for example, coercion, alienation, police intervention); therefore, as Rushing posits, involuntary admissions relative to voluntary admissions would be expected to increase as socioeconomic status decreases. In other words, persons with greater resources are in a much better position to fight involuntary commitment if they so desire and are consequently more likely to be voluntary patients because it requires their cooperation. However, although socioeconomic status and resources may have important effects on the disposition of a mentally disturbed person, Rushing notes that the effect of status is modified if the disorder is particularly severe (Rushing 1978, 1979b; Rushing and Esco 1977). "Extremely disruptive persons," states Rushing (1978:525), "are apt to be dealt with coercively, *regardless* of their status characteristics. Status characteristics are more important as contingencies when the individual's behavior is less disturbing."

Erving Goffman (1961) asserts that there are no objective and universally applicable standards for admission to mental hospitals, and such studies as those by Mishler and Waxler (1963), Mendel and Rapport (1969), Gove and Howell (1974), and Rushing (1978) seem to confirm Goffman's observation. Although the extent of psychiatric impairment is important, what these studies suggest is that factors external to one's mental condition, such as referral by a physician or the presence of friends or family members, are relevant to being admitted voluntarily to a mental hospital. In a review of the literature on mental hospital admissions, Marvin Krohn and Ronald Akers (1977) found considerable support for the hypothesis that social variables influence psychiatric decisions about mental patients. "Admission to hospital treatment," explain Krohn and Akers (1977:354), "is positively related to social class and marital status among voluntary patients." Apparently, a high social status and being married are important to gaining admission, regardless of the extent of one's mental problem, unless that problem is severe and apparent.

What is suggested by David Rosenhan (1973) is that it is possible for practically anyone, sane or insane, to gain admission to a mental hospital by reporting serious symptoms that cannot be assessed definitively. The Rosenhan study was one in which eight supposedly normal persons presented themselves for admission as schizophrenics at twelve different hospitals in five states and all were admitted. Consequently, we can see that the condition may be uncertain and that social variables in psychiatric decisions may intervene. Once those decisions are made, however, and a patient is labeled in a certain way (that is, as being "schizophrenic"), that label appears to affect significantly the patient's experiences. An especially revealing finding in the Rosenhan study was that once the individual was in the hospital, what seemed to be important was not so much the patient's behavior but the general acceptance by the staff of the diagnosis given at admission. There was evidence that the history of past behavior taken during interviews was somewhat distorted to correspond to the theories of mental disorder held by the interviewer. *Thus, past circumstances did not shape the diagnosis, but instead the diagnosis appeared to shape the diagnostician's perception of past circumstances.* Rosenhan believes that the failure of the hospital staffs to discover the pseudopatients (length of hospitalization ranged from seven to fifty-two days, with an average of nineteen days) illustrates the power of labeling in psychiatric assessment. Once labeled schizophrenic, there was nothing the pseudopatients could do to change an identification that profoundly affected other people's perceptions of them and their behavior. Their release from the mental hospital was contingent upon the staff's acceptance of the idea that the nonexistent schizophrenia was in "remission."

This discussion is not intended to convey the impression that all mental hospitals are unable to tell real patients from phony ones or that factors not directly relevant to a person's mental status are always highly significant in admission procedures. In the case of Barry (1971), who faked her way into Bellevue, the staff had suspected someone might try to observe life on the ward to write about it and deduced at the time that she was the only one it could be. And certainly, extreme and bizarre expressions of behavior, especially if they are violent, result in attempts at psychiatric treatment, regardless of the patient's social background. Rather, this discussion is intended to convey the idea that without objective standards for admission, decisions made by mental hospital staffs concerning admissions are subjective and may be inaccurate—yet result in significant consequences for the person who becomes a patient. Of course, diagnoses made in other branches of medicine may also be subjective and inaccurate, but there is a greater likelihood of having conclusive and tangible evidence upon which to base a diagnosis. The Rosenhan study shows that psychiatrists, like other physicians, are biased toward treatment, even if the symptoms are uncertain. In this situation, social variables become exceptionally important.

INVOLUNTARY COMMITMENT

Involuntary commitment results when a state uses its power and authority to confine an individual to a mental hospital. Involuntary commitment proceedings are of two types: those dealing with criminal offenses, in which insanity is claimed as a defense, and those that are civil (noncriminal) in nature. Thomas Scheff (1964) observed the legal psychiatric screening procedure for civil cases in a midwestern state. There were five steps in this procedure: (1) three citizens making an application to the court, (2) an intake examination conducted by a hospital psychiatrist, (3) an examination conducted by two court-appointed psychiatrists, (4) an interview with a lawyer appointed by the court to represent the patient, and (5) a judicial hearing conducted by a judge. The primary legal rationale for depriving patients of their civil liberties was that they represented a danger to themselves, to others, or to property. Scheff found that a majority (63 percent of the patients) were not necessarily dangerous. It was his conclusion that the evidence in such cases was somewhat arbitrary (there were no objective standards for admission); that the patients were often prejudged (it was assumed that all who appeared were in need of being admitted—otherwise, they would not have been there); that the examinations were both careless and hasty (the interviews by the lawyer and the examinations by the psychiatrists lasted about ten minutes on the average); and that sometimes there was really no "evidence," but people were committed anyway (it was assumed that psychiatric treatment would either help or be neutral—it would not hurt—and that it was better to risk unnecessary hospitalization than to have the patient in a position to hurt himself or herself or others).

Other research suggests that the more diligent and thorough the petitioner is in bringing a complaint of mental disorder against a person, the more likely it is that person will be committed (Wilde 1968). But those who challenge such petitions with legal counsel of their own are less likely to be committed than others with a similar level of disturbed behavior who are not represented by a lawyer (Wenger and Fletcher 1969). In essence, it seems that factors outside a person's psychiatric condition can influence the disposition of one's case. Clearly, persons of higher social class and possessing greater personal resources are more likely to avoid involuntary commitment by fighting the proceedings.

In criminal cases, the claim of mental disorder is used as an excusing condition that relieves the individual of criminal responsibility for his or her act. The model for an excusing condition in Anglo-American law is the accident, and it defines the class of persons who fall outside the boundaries of blame (Goldstein 1967; Szasz 1968). A finding of insanity by a judge or a jury, based upon the testimony of psychiatrists as expert witnesses, is a matter of opinion, because the law, like psychiatry, does not have objective standards for ascertaining mental disorder. A verdict of insanity does not release the individual to return to society; in most jurisdictions, that person is involuntarily committed to a mental hospital.

For involuntary civil commitment, the mere designation of a mental disorder is not sufficient justification for the confinement of an individual to a mental hospital. There usually must also be a finding that the mental disorder is of such a degree or character that if the individual in question were allowed to remain at large, that person would constitute a danger to self, others, or property. Although these criteria for civil commitment are widely recognized, few concepts in the law are as elusive and undefined as dangerousness. Decisions are normally made by judges on a case-by-case basis, based upon the opinions of psychiatrists who assess the probability of the individual's committing a dangerous act. Actions ranging from murder to writing bad checks all have been found to be dangerous enough to warrant confinement on the grounds of mental illness. To determine dangerousness, courts look to the severity of the harm, the likelihood that the action will occur, and the behavior of the person who provoked the prediction of dangerousness.

As in the Mishler and Waxler study of voluntary commitment, a study by Richard Levinson and M. Zan York (1974) of the assessments used to determine dangerousness in cases of voluntary commitment also found evidence that factors outside the disorder itself were influential in the decision-making process. This study, based on the files of a large mental health program in Atlanta, found that being male, young, unmarried, with a past history of previous psychiatric treatment, and a person for whom help was solicited by a caller outside the person's household all contributed to a diagnosis of dangerousness, provided the person displayed disorderly behavior in the presence of the mental health professional making the assessment. Levinson and Zan York concluded that because standards are imprecise, criteria unrelated to the pathological condition may unduly influence the attribution of dangerousness to a particular person and the decision to commit that person to a mental hospital. More-recent research involving national and state samples of psychiatrists found a tendency among male clinicians as a group to overestimate depression among women and dangerousness among black males (Loring and Powell 1988).

Therefore, as Goffman explains, whether a person is actually launched on a career as a mental patient depends upon a number of contingencies—for example, the visibility of the offense, the socioeconomic status of the patient, the availability of treatment, the convenience of authorities, and the opinion of judges and perhaps jurors (in criminal proceedings).

According to Walter Gove (1976), one of the strongest arguments against labeling theory, as advanced by Scheff (1964), concerns the issue of *who* is most likely to be hospitalized. Labeling theory implies that the individual who is marginal to society (and least likely to be able to resist labeling) is most likely to be committed to a mental hospital. Gove suggests that, to the contrary, it is those persons with the most resources who are most likely to be mental patients. He bases his conclusion on research that indicates that lower-class persons are slower to recognize psychiatric symptoms (Hollingshead and Redlich 1958; Myers and Roberts 1959), that lower-class persons tend to delay seeking psychiatric treatment (Gove and Howell 1974; Hollingshead and Redlich 1958), and that middle-class families are less willing to tolerate mental disorder among family members (Freeman and Simmons 1961).

In rebuttal, Scheff (1974, 1975a, 1975b) points out that a majority of studies, based upon the labeling perspective, offer supportive evidence for his views over those advanced by Gove. Particularly noteworthy among the studies cited by Scheff (1974) is the work of Arnold Linsky (1970a, 1970b) and William Rushing (1971), who measured the ratio of involuntary to voluntary mental hospital admissions; both studies found a strong relationship between powerlessness (marginality) and hospital commitment. Research by Krohn and Akers (1977) further supports Scheff. This research concluded that extrapsychiatric factors (defined as social class, family influence, marital status, legal status by virtue of having a lawyer, and challenges to psychiatric decisions) were more significant than psychiatric factors (defined as the nature and severity of the mental disorder) in determining mental hospital admissions and discharges, both voluntary and involuntary. These extrapsychiatric factors generally favored more affluent persons and thus allowed them greater control over whether they were admitted or released, even though the nature and severity of their mental disorder were similar to that of less affluent or socially marginal persons. Persons with socioeconomic resources are more in control of their situation, whether it means obtaining or avoiding admission to a mental hospital. However, it seems likely that if a mental disorder is highly severe and disabling, and a case can be made that the afflicted person is a danger to self or others, that person is likely to be hospitalized regardless of who he or she is.

THE INPATIENT

The last step in being a prepatient is the recognition by the individual that he or she has been turned out by society and subjected to the restrictions of living in an institution under the authority of others. Goffman (1961:xiii) described the mental hospital as a "total institution," which he defined "as a place of residence and work where a large number of like-situated individuals, cut off from the wider society for an appreciable period of time, together lead an enclosed, formally administered round of life." The central feature of the total institution, which includes prisons, monasteries, homes for the blind, and military camps, is a breakdown of barriers normal to most people. All aspects of life are conducted in the same place under the same authority and in the immediate company of others who are treated alike and who do the same thing together. All phases of activities are scheduled to fulfill the aims of a rational plan supposedly designed to meet the official goals of the institution, which in the case of the mental hospital is therapy, custodial care, or both.

The goals of the institution, therefore, are *the* determining factors in shaping the social life that takes place within its walls. Consequently, there have been several studies by social scientists to describe and analyze the various processes that influence behavior within the context of the mental hospital ward. These studies are derived mainly from data collected in state and county mental hospitals and are not necessarily representative of what happens inside private psychiatric hospitals. In the private hospital, treatment is presumably private, humane, and more personalized, and the quality of the staff and accommodations is much better. In the public hospital, however, there are some features of ward life that are more or less common to most mental hospital living arrangements. Those features are (1) the social structure of the ward, (2) the tendency toward depersonalization, (3) the adjustment to hospital life, and (4) the possibility of institutionalization, a condition that can affect people who become dependent upon institutional living.

The Social Structure of the Ward

The social structure of the mental hospital ward generally has the following status hierarchy, ranked from top to bottom: (1) psychiatrists, (2) other physicians, (3) psychologists (with a Ph.D.), (4) registered nurses, (5) auxiliary mental health workers (that is, psychiatric social workers, occupational therapists, non-Ph.D. psychologists), (6) practical nurses and nurse's aides, (7) orderlies and attendants, (8) maintenance personnel, and (9) patients. Typically, the groups whose roles are most central to the day-to-day patterns of social interaction on the ward are the psychiatrists or other physicians, the nurses, and finally, the orderlies and the patients. First and foremost is, of course, the psychiatrist or the physician working as a psychiatrist who is in charge of the patient's therapy and who is ultimately responsible for what happens. This individual is likely to spend less time with the patient than other medical personnel do, yet will direct and manage the administration of psychiatric care. It is this person who decides if and when involuntarily admitted patients will be discharged. Obviously, the psychiatrist has a great deal of power.

The patient has considerably more contact with the nurses and the orderlies. Although the licensed registered and practical nurses and nurse's aides are generally women, the orderlies are usually men employed to care for male patients and perform whatever heavy duties are required (subduing violent patients, lifting patients out of bed, and so on). What is apparent is that nursing tasks occur in a system of social relationships that are highly stratified by sex. The registered nurse, who has the most advanced training and professional qualifications of any of the nursing workers, is generally a female who is matched occupationally with a physician, whose role is dominant and who is usually a male. The registered nurse, in turn, supervises less trained females (practical nurses and nurse's aides) and less trained males (orderlies and attendants). Thus emerges the traditional stereotype of the physician as a father figure and the nurse as a mother figure.

Although not as influential as the psychiatrist or the physician, nurses nonetheless have a great impact on the interaction that takes place on the ward. They not only see that the physician's orders are carried out but also may influence those decisions through their working relationship with the physician. Their primary role, however, is to supervise the activities of the ward, to participate in therapy, and to administer drugs as needed. The head nurse, in particular, is an extremely influential individual because the supervision of the ward is her responsibility. A stereotype of the head nurse of a mental hospital is Miss Ratched, or Big Nurse, a principal character in Ken Kesey's popular novel about life in a mental institution, *One Flew over the Cuckoo's Nest*. She ran her ward with precision and almost machinelike efficiency. Doctors who disagreed with her methods or tried to implement change were given a chilling reception and made to feel very uncomfortable until they left. The doctor Miss Ratched settles on for *her* ward is one who gives in easily to pressure. The orderlies she selects and trains over the years are picked largely on the basis of how much they hate her. The greater the hatred, the greater their efficiency is in performing her bidding. She teaches them her way of handling the ward, which is to remain calm, keep the pressure on the patients to meet the ward's schedule, and wait for an advantageous time to show who is really in charge. This is not too difficult to do, because the patients are generally powerless and the physicians reluctant to assert themselves. The novel's plot revolves around the attempts of one patient, McMurphy, to challenge the authority of Big Nurse and to reorganize life on the ward, a challenge that McMurphy eventually loses. Miss Ratched, of course, is a literary character and does not exist in reality, although some head nurses may be similar to her. Something to be learned from Kesey's novel, however, is that the social interaction on a mental hospital ward centers on how the head nurse interprets the policies of the hospital.

Gregg Wilkinson (1973) has done research on this situation that confirms that head nurses tend to be crucial in determining the attitudes and opinions of nursing personnel. Wilkinson indicates that such a finding is not surprising when it is realized that the head nurse serves as a link to the hospital world beyond the ward. She is the one who is most likely to participate regularly in meetings with the upper echelon of the hospital's staff—namely, the psychiatrists, hospital administrators, and other nursing supervisors. Hence, the head nurse is not only *the* immediate authority figure but also *the* source of information and ideas in the ward setting. She therefore is in an ideal position to influence subordinates by channeling information to them in accordance with her views. Wilkinson describes this as follows:

> Thus, by virtue of her position within the organization structure, the head nurse acts as a funneling agent and is able to filter the flow of ideas by emphasizing negative aspects of those which she disfavors and positive aspects of those with which she is in agreement. In other words a type of symbolic screening is exercised which, when combined with her influential position in the social structure, can come to have a significant effect with respect to the adoption of new ideas by subordinate personnel. Although the filtration process is not complete, and does not even have to be overt, information can be colored greatly by her views and manipulated for her purposes if she so desires. This may even occur without realization because of her prior orientation in terms of treatment practices and overall psychiatric ideology. The dependence of nursing subordinates upon the head nurse for information from outside sources enhances her prestige and overall control.[4]

The lowest level of hospital care on the ward is performed by the orderlies. As noted, orderlies are typically male; they also are usually from the lower socioeconomic class and are likely to be members of racial/ethnic minority groups. They are not especially well paid, and their job has the lowest social status of any medical position in the hospital. Although their primary duties are housekeeping, assisting with records, and maintaining order on the ward, orderlies tend to emphasize contacts with patients at the expense of these other duties (Perrucci 1974). In fact, it can be said that orderlies spend more time with the patients than anyone else does and are more likely to have intimate knowledge about them. Despite their lack of status, orderlies also have considerable power over patients because they directly control where the patients should or should not be and what they should be doing. Some orderlies are genuinely humane and responsive to patients, but as will be discussed, the very nature of the work setting requires them to be in *control* of the situation and to maintain a formal relationship with the patients. Admittedly, friendships between patients and staff do exist in total institutions (Goffman 1961). But most of the abuses of mental patients come at the hands of these psychiatric aides, who are usually the least qualified professionally yet have power over a group of people who are mentally disordered, relatively defenseless, dependent, and not particularly valued by society. In these conditions, it is not surprising that mental patients become depersonalized.

Depersonalization

Goffman (1961) explains that an important characteristic of all total institutions is the existence of some form of deference between or among its group members. In mental hospitals, that deference refers to the status of the

---

[4]Gregg S. Wilkinson, "Interaction Patterns and Staff Response to Psychiatric Innovations," *Journal of Health and Social Behavior* 14(1973), 327–28.

staff as superior and righteous and to the status of the patients as inferior and guilty of failure in the so-called normal world. This perspective lends itself to a process of dehumanization that makes it easier for the staff to disregard the inmates to achieve greater efficiency without a great expenditure of personal energy and emotional involvement. Although not all mental patients in all mental hospitals become depersonalized, the dependent status of the patient does open itself to the possibility. Furthermore, Goffman states that the ease with which an inmate can be managed by the staff is likely to increase the degree to which that inmate is dehumanized.

Brandt (1975) comments that reducing patients to the status of an impersonal "object" is an inherent feature of the work situation. Upon being admitted to a mental hospital, Brandt was searched by two male orderlies who did not speak to him except to give orders. He was stripped, his body was examined, and then he was told to take a shower. While he showered, the belongings he had brought to the hospital were searched. He was given a towel, he dried himself, and next he was handed a pair of hospital pajamas, a bathrobe, and slippers. Brandt continues:

> During all this procedure the two aides said very little to me and later I came to see why. It wasn't because they disliked me or were trying to frighten me, although they did. It was simply that they were working. This was obviously routine procedure, a precaution they were required to take with every incoming patient to make sure he carried no drugs or weapons or other forbidden objects on his person. I was part of their work, the object they were working on, the thing to be processed. You don't normally talk to your work; if the work is routine, you don't even talk about it. You just do it.
> The effect on me of what they took for granted however, was startling. I did not understand it at the time, but the meaning of the process must have been sinking in regardless. I was an object, possibly dangerous, which had to be inspected; it might be concealing something, it could not be trusted and in any case it had to be described. So they searched it. It never occurred to them to explain to the object what they were doing; you don't explain things to objects, you give them orders.[5]

Brandt felt that in the span of about fifteen minutes, the two aides had "colonized" him. That is, he had been integrated almost completely into the social structure of the hospital. In a few more minutes, he felt the process was indeed completed when he was taken to a nurses' station. Two other aides carried on a conversation in front of him as if he did not exist. He was given an injection in the buttocks to help him sleep and then was led to his bed. The entire sequence of events was totally impersonal. In asking himself why he allowed himself to submit to this, he felt it was natural that he just fall in with the work and not ask questions or protest. This was so because he believed that

---

[5]Anthony Brandt, *Reality Police: The Experience of Insanity in America* (New York: Morrow, 1975), p. 164.

he, like other people, had been trained from childhood to submit to authority and that in a stressful situation there is a tendency to allow others—who are in authoritative positions—to make decisions on one's behalf. In fact, Brandt was thankful he had not been brutalized in some way.

Although the process of dehumanization is greatly influenced by the low social status of the patients, its basis is ultimately found in the work situation, as Brandt observes. This condition can be present in any large organization where it is necessary to take groups of people and direct them collectively toward the goals of the organization—especially if the people involved have a highly dependent status. Consider, for example, the situation occurring on bath day at a large mental hospital, created by the requirement to bathe the patients. According to a staff member, the patients suffered through a dehumanizing experience in one particular building because the shower facilities were not adequate for mass bathing, even though it was necessary (because of the staff's allocation of time) to supervise large numbers of patients bathing simultaneously. The staff member, a young woman, describes the scene:

> Bath day in the hospital was like branding day on a cattle ranch. I used to hope that some of the less ill patients weren't too bashful, for there was no such thing as modesty allowed in this mental institution. The patients were literally herded to the tile section and stripped of their clothes. There was a school of nursing at Willard, and the student nurses, who always got the hardest and dirtiest jobs, usually did the bathing. The showers were large at Sampson Hall, so many patients could get in at one time. However, at Elliott Hall the showers were smaller and only one patient could shower at a time. The others waited in line for their turn. I hated bath day because of the lack of privacy. There were a few young patients about my age, and I knew how they must feel to strip in front of everybody. Most of the patients hated bath day, and I didn't blame them.[6]

The mental hospital employees who spend the most time with the patients, as mentioned previously, are the psychiatric orderlies or aides who are charged with maintaining control over the patients and the ward housekeeping. Although these aides have little status in the overall social hierarchy of the hospital, they nonetheless rank well above the patients and can exercise considerable power over the patients in maintaining social control. Research by Bernard Berk and Victor Goertzel (1975) on the work-related attitudes of psychiatric aides suggests that "custodial" (most authoritarian, most restrictive, and least benevolent) attitudes among these mental hospital employees tend to strengthen over time. Berk and Goertzel studied a group of psychiatric aides at a large mental hospital in the western United States over a one-year period in which the aides (all of whom had been hired within the last five months) were tested on the first day of employment, then six months after that when

---

[6]Louella Sturm, *The Mental Hospital Nightmare* (New York: Exposition Press, 1973), p. 57.

they were working in their regular ward assignments. The aides tended to be young (median age twenty-four), male, not well educated, from small communities in the area, and from the lower class. During the study, some 35 percent of the "humanitarian" (least authoritarian, least restrictive, and most benevolent) aides had terminated their employment, compared with only 6 percent of the custodial aides. Younger and better-educated aides tended to quit sooner. Although social selection out of the organization had left somewhat more custodial aides, there was a striking change in attitude generally once the aides began to work in their regular role assignments. Berk and Goertzel explain what happened:

> Approximately 54 percent of the aides became more authoritarian, 83 percent became less benevolent, and 58 percent became more restrictive during the period of regular work assignments to hospital wards. This trend plainly indicates that the overall direction of attitude change, as a consequence of regular role occupancy, was toward increased custodial orientations.[7]

Berk and Goertzel believe that the change in attitudes was influenced by other staff members on the ward to which the new aide was assigned. Once working in their jobs, these aides tended to conform to the subculture of the institution. And in this subculture, a custodial orientation seemed to produce the greatest organizational efficiency. Hence, the aides tended to adopt it. Since the higher job performance ratings on the wards usually went to the more restrictive aides, the custodial orientation was reinforced.

Because the aides are required to control difficult and perhaps violent patients, they tend to adopt a forceful manner. As Frank LeBar (1973:227) observed in his study of a mental hospital, a normative belief among the aides is that "patients will take advantage of you if they know you are afraid of them." New aides are taught this attitude by the older aides as they begin working on their ward assignments. Although the newer aides, fresh from their training course, tended at first to manifest a "caring" attitude toward the patients, the older aides strove to socialize the newcomers into believing that "experience was the best teacher" and that firmness was the best method of handling the patients. LeBar reports:

> The aide subculture supported the idea that to express fear of a patient was to lose one's control over him. Patients were presumed to have the animal-like ability to detect the presence of fear in those entrusted with their supervision. A favorite aphorism was to the effect "that there is no place on a mental hospital ward for anybody who is afraid of mental patients." Thus, the quality of fearlessness, and expressions of fearlessness, were sought after and highly-approved attributes within the informal aide subculture.

---

[7]Bernard B. Berk and Victor Goertzel, "Selection versus Role Occupancy as Determinants of Role-Related Attitudes among Psychiatric Aides," *Journal of Health and Social Behavior* 16 (1975), 188.

Allied to fearlessness as a desirable quality was toughness. The traditional aide subculture held firmly to the idea that "you have to show 'em who's boss." To show tenderness or concern—to "give in" to a patient's demands—was to lose control over patients.[8]

Even though the aides were reminded by the nurses to be "therapeutic" in their interaction with the patients, the male aides often resented the dominance of the female nursing supervisors. Consequently, the aides emphasized attitudes of "manliness" to compensate for their lack of prestige and social inferiority in the hospital. The aides saw themselves as engaging in a dangerous and hazardous occupation that only "real men" could handle. To be sure, at times patients were violent and in need of being subdued, but the aides overemphasized the extent to which that was necessary, to feel better about their roles.

LeBar observes that in a very real sense the aides were caught in a dilemma. They were supposed to maintain social control, but the hospital also was expected to be "easy" on patients and to provide "tender loving care." From the point of view of the aides, the two goals were incompatible and the hospital offered no solution that made sense to the aides. The aides were encouraged by hospital ideology to expand their role in a therapeutic direction but sometimes were discouraged by the nurses from putting those ideas into practice. The nurses required the aides to "supervise" the patients and to act formally toward them. As a result, says LeBar (1973:251), it was not uncommon "to see an aide playing cards with a patient while standing and with one eye on the door to the dayroom—behavior which reflected the fact that aides were liable to be reprimanded for playing cards with patients."

In his study of normal people posing as patients, Rosenhan found that being a mental patient required the recognition that powerlessness was evident everywhere. What mental patients said was not believed because of their mental disorder. They could not initiate contact with the staff but could only respond to overtures from them. Furthermore, there was only minimal personal privacy, and personal thoughts and history were open to inspection by any staff member, no matter what the reason. Rosenhan stated:

> At times, depersonalization reached such proportions that pseudopatients had the sense they were invisible, or at least unworthy of account. Upon being admitted, I and other pseudopatients took the initial physical examinations in a semipublic room, where staff members went about their own business as if we were not there.
> On the ward, attendants delivered verbal and occasionally serious physical abuse to patients in the presence of other observing patients, some of whom (the pseudopatients) were writing it all down. Abusive behavior, on the other hand, terminated quite abruptly when other staff members were known to be coming. Staff were credible witnesses. Patients are not.

---

[8]Frank M. LeBar, *Segregative Care in an Institutional Setting: The Ethnography of a Psychiatric Hospital* (New Haven, CT: Human Relations Area Files, 1973), pp. 239–40.

A nurse unbuttoned her uniform to adjust her brassiere in the presence of an entire ward of viewing men. One did not have the sense she was being seductive. Rather, she didn't notice us. A group of staff persons might point to a patient in the dayroom and discuss him animatedly, as if he were not there.[9]

Rosenhan attributed the origins of depersonalization to two factors: (1) the attitudes held by society toward the mentally ill, including those who treat them, as *"something* that is unattractive" despite benevolent intentions toward them; and (2) the hierarchical structure of the mental hospital, which facilitated depersonalization in that those at the top had the least contact with patients and their behavior was a model for the rest of the staff. Rosenhan found that patients spent very little time with hospital physicians (an average of 6.8 minutes a day for six pseudopatients over a total of 129 days of hospitalization) and that the physicians, in turn, influenced the behavior of the nurses and ward attendants, who likewise tended to reduce the time they spent with patients. Heavy reliance upon drug therapy also seemed to contribute to the process of depersonalization, by allowing the staff to rationalize that treatment was being given and that additional contact with the patient was not needed.

It would seem, therefore, that life in mental hospitals is generally a dehumanizing and oppressive experience for the patients. Raymond Weinstein (1979, 1981, 1983) tells us that this is not necessarily the case, however. Weinstein notes that reports of what it is like to be a patient in a mental hospital have usually been derived from qualitative data: participant observation, interviewing, or masquerading as patients. "The hospital is generally pictured," says Weinstein (1979:239), "as an authoritarian system that forces patients to define themselves as mentally ill, change their thinking and behavior, suffer humiliations, accept restrictions, and adjust to institutional life." Weinstein challenges this conclusion and argues that most mental patients have relatively positive attitudes toward the hospital. He comments, for example, on the experiences of one sociologist who became mentally ill and entered a mental hospital fearful of what was going to happen because of his knowledge of past studies on the subject. Yet on release he felt—to the contrary—that his experience had been a pleasant one and that the culture and structure of the hospital had facilitated his recovery (Killian and Bloomberg 1975).

Weinstein's argument is based upon a review of quantitative studies of mental patients, employing objective tests and questionnaire scales. According to these studies, a large majority of patients indicated favorable attitudes toward mental hospitals in general and toward their own institution as well. Weinstein (1979:251) states: "Patients often claim that they (or other patients) benefit from treatment, are not bothered by restrictions, enjoy the comforts of the hospital, are helped by the staff, gain insight into their problems, and are satisfied with ward activities." Weinstein complains that qualitative

---

[9]David L. Rosenhan, "On Being Sane in Insane Places," *Science* 179 (1973), 256.

researchers have tended to identify themselves with disadvantaged patients, have not tested patient attitudes systematically, and have not focused on the patients but rather on the effects of hospitalization on the patients. He is particularly suspicious of researchers posing as patients because he feels that pseudopatients are not mentally ill and thus are not in a position either to benefit from treatment or to perceive their experiences in the same manner as do actual patients. He reasons that mental patients may be favorably disposed to hospitalization because (1) the hospital can be a "temporary haven"; (2) the environment of the hospital may be more attractive than living in conditions of poverty, deprivation, and inactivity; and (3) hospitalization represents an opportunity for self-improvement.

The answer to whether mental patients generally perceive hospitalization as either positive or negative probably lies somewhere between the two extremes of "good" and "bad." For some patients, the experience is no doubt positive, especially for those who, as noted by Weinstein, have severe mental problems. The mental hospital can provide a better environment than some alternative living situations, particularly if the facilities are good and adequately staffed and if the staff is generally supportive of the patients. For other patients, the experience may be unpleasant, since they must cope with depersonalization, restrictive rules, lack of privacy, confinement, unpleasant associates, and a schedule of activities that is not of their own choosing. Moreover, they may have been alienated from friends and family on the way to being hospitalized, have had their identity placed in circumstances in which they are viewed by others as less than desirable, and have been forced to exhibit their most private thoughts in the attempt to treat them. For most people, there is a better way to live than being a patient in a mental hospital.

Adjustment to Hospital Life

Regardless of whether individual mental patients have a positive or a negative view of their situation, Goffman observes that mental patients actually have very little choice but to adapt to the social environment of the hospital. He identifies four types of adjustment to the total institution: (1) situational withdrawal, (2) intransigence (rebellion), (3) colonization (using the experiences of the life in the outside world to demonstrate the desirability of life on the inside), and (4) conversion (living up to the staff-sponsored, ideal model). Goffman tells us that typically the inmates will not follow completely any one particular mode of adaptation but will most likely adopt a somewhat opportunistic combination of conversion, colonization, and loyalty to the inmate group. Instead of making what Goffman calls a primary adjustment of "giving in" to the system, the patient will make a secondary adjustment, which is to appear to conform to the system while gaining hidden satisfactions whenever possible.

Hidden satisfactions were usually obtained in such ways as sneaking food out of the cafeteria for a midnight snack, becoming romantically involved with someone else, or acquiring a job in the hospital that gave one the opportunity of gaining advantages. The last would include jobs in the kitchen, laundry, shoe-repair shop, or recreation facilities, or in gardening, repair work, baby-sitting, or running errands for the orderlies—all functions that gave the patients access to goods or services that could be exchanged for money, privileges, or similar goods and services. The most important way to "work the system," as Goffman relates, was to secure a "workable" job as described above. Such an assignment during the day not only helped the patient obtain resources to use to his or her personal advantage but also allowed that patient temporarily to escape the ward and the supervisory control and discomfort that might be there. If nothing else, it gave the patient something to do.

Another source of satisfaction from secondary modes of adjustment was the use of space. Goffman notes that the underlife of a mental institution takes place in a world consisting of three parts. First is *off-limits space* or *out-of-bounds space*. This is an area (for example, doctor's office, administrative offices, nursing stations) that a patient is not allowed to enter and is actively prohibited from doing so. Second is *surveillance space,* an area the patient may enter but where he or she is clearly subject to the authority of the institution. This area includes most of the hospital, even for those patients on parole and allowed to move about the institution somewhat freely. Third is the area of *free places,* which are ruled with less than usual staff authority. Examples of free places given by Goffman were a patch of woods behind the hospital building that could be used for drinking smuggled whiskey, an area behind the recreation building and the shade of a large tree that could be used for playing poker. Or there might be seldom-used rooms in the hospital, perhaps discovered and used by patients with special work assignments, where patients could disappear for a short time to have sex or perhaps simply to get away from the staff or a noisy, crowded ward. Sometimes, free places were spaces out in the general public view that nonetheless afforded a psychological respite, such as benches in a hall by a soft drink machine where the staff typically left patients alone, or a bench close to an outside fence where the patients could sun themselves and gaze at people outside the hospital going about their usual lives. Patients might even press their faces against a special window in such a way as to seal themselves off from the ward life behind their backs.

Within the space allocated to them, patients might also establish what Goffman calls *group territories* and *private territories.* Group territories were particular spaces used by a select group of patients who would be allowed to enter, but where others would be unwelcome. Here a patient might relax with comrades in a special relationship signified by free use of a territory, such as a corner of the dayroom, certain chairs in front of the television, and the like. Usually it was the strongest who secured this type of privilege. Private territory was best because it was shut to all other patients except by invitation. The most basic private situation was the private sleeping room, available to few patients, which could be made into a refuge and stocked with the patient's own belongings. Or a patient might have a special chair or spot by the radiator to which he or she had first claim. At the very minimum, a patient had his or her own blanket.

The ultimate aim of these secondary adjustments, says Goffman, is to put some distance, some elbowroom, between the patient and others. In establishing a barrier, the mental hospital patient may be "rejecting one's rejectors" and gaining some modicum of self-presentation. As Goffman points out, it is thus against *something* that the self can emerge. This is a process that happens in any kind of social organization as people develop a sense of themselves. Furthermore, attempts to preserve something of one's self from an institution are not uncommon. They are particularly obvious in a mental hospital and indicate one's desire to maintain some private sense of self in an unprivate place.

One of the primary functions of inmate society is to help maintain a sympathetic and supportive atmosphere in the hospital ward and to serve as a vehicle by which the patient can assert a self-identity and perhaps some independence within an overall context of dependence and forced association. Apparently, one of the prominent activities in these patient "societies" is the expression of face-saving rationalizations for one another's presence in the hospital. Goffman explains that such stories as the following are given:

> I was going to night school to get an M.A. degree and holding down a job in addition, and the load got too much for me.
> I got here by mistake because of a diabetes diagnosis and I'll leave in a couple of days. (The patient had been in seven weeks.)
> The others here are sick mentally but I'm suffering from a bad nervous system and that is what is giving me these phobias.[10]

As Goffman notes, an entire social role in the patient community may be constructed from these fictions; thus, what we see in these exchanges is the classic function of a network of equals to serve as audiences for one another's self-supportive statements. But although the patient may be denying that he or she is mentally ill, that same patient may at other times show evidence of mental disorder. And, as Goffman indicates, there is still that official sheet of paper to confirm the patient's illness. Regardless of the patient's attempts to rationalize his or her fate, being admitted as a mental patient seriously inhibits the credibility of the rationalizations. Goffman states:

> Certainly the degrading conditions of the hospital setting belie many of the self-stories that are presented by patients, and the very fact of being in the mental hospital is evidence against these tales. And of course there is not always suffi-

---

[10]Erving Goffman, *Asylums* (Garden City, NY: Doubleday, Anchor Books, 1961), pp. 152–53.

cient patient solidarity to prevent patient discrediting patient, just as there is not always a sufficient number of "professionalized" attendants to prevent attendant discrediting patient. As one patient informant repeatedly suggested to a fellow patient: If you're so smart, how come you got your ass in here?[11]

Thus, despite the possible supports provided by inmate society, the influence and power of the hospital staff are pervasive. Sometimes the staff will even deliberately discredit a patient's story so that the patient will be encouraged to adopt the hospital's view of himself or herself. What is that view? Generally, the "good" patient is expected to (1) believe that recovery is possible, (2) recognize that he or she is mentally ill and needs treatment, (3) trust and have faith in the therapist, (4) conform willingly to hospital life, and (5) accept the treatment that is prescribed (Denzin 1968). If a patient follows this prescription, then that patient is "converted," to use Goffman's terminology. And because the patient's release from the hospital (in cases of noncriminal confinement) is dependent upon the staff's assessment of how well he or she conforms to the staff's expectations of behavior, the staff has tremendous leverage in their influence over the patient.

Recent studies, however, indicate that many mental patients do not necessarily think of themselves as mentally ill and that conversion is mostly an acceptance of hospital life and the status of mental patient—not necessarily an acceptance of the institution's definition of themselves (Braginsky et al. 1969; Townsend 1976). As Goffman explains in his general approach to institutionalization, inmates, over time, will make opportunistic adjustments to the institution. Townsend (1976) notes that mental patients are in a special situation. They know that their subjective and personal feelings are under observation and that the outcome of that observation will help determine their fate. Thus, they adjust their behavior to the situation, depending on what they perceive its purpose to be. Townsend states:

> Given the mental patient's special situation, it may not be a meaningful question to ask what he "really" thinks of himself. His responses will not necessarily match his actual feelings at the moment and, in any case, both feelings and responses tend to vary with context. At times the patient may feel good about himself; at other times, bad. Some may suspect at times that they are insane and yet not admit these suspicions. At other times, things may be going well and they consequently feel healthy. Even so, they might still fear leaving the hospital, and, as a result, do poorly during a staff evaluation. Patients, like anyone, are also capable of deceiving themselves. They may inwardly suspect they are insane, yet ward off confrontation with these feelings by rationalizing their presence in the hospital and denying that they are mentally ill.

It thus appears that it is difficult to define exactly what a patient thinks of his

---

[11]Ibid., p. 154.

condition at any one time, and it may be that this is not an empirically useful question.[12]

Institutionalization

A number of medical sociologists and other persons interested in the treatment of mental patients have expressed concern about the effects of the mental hospital as a total institution on the attitudes and self-concepts of the inmates. The primary focus of their concern is the effect of prolonged living in a state of enforced dependency. It is feared that this process may influence the patient to become so dependent on the hospital and its routines that it becomes nearly impossible for the patient to leave. As William Eaton (1974a:252) describes it, the patient "gradually learns to play the chronic sick role, to reduce aspirations, and to find friends within the hospital instead of outside." From the literature, it is clear that the longer a person stays at a mental hospital, the less likely it is that he or she will leave (Eaton 1974a; Townsend 1976). One of the main themes of Kesey's *One Flew over the Cuckoo's Nest* is the effort of the patient McMurphy to organize inmate society and to force it to recognize that life outside the hospital is much more attractive. Two of the studies most often cited as depicting the effects of institutionalization are those by Ailon Shiloh (1971) and John Wing (1967). Shiloh investigated the attitudes of mental patients toward the outside world in a veterans' hospital in Illinois and found two main groups, whose goals were diametrically opposed. He classified about 40 percent of the patients as being "institutionalized" and not wanting to leave the hospital and 25 percent as "noninstitutionalized" and having a reasonable expectation of getting out. The remaining 35 percent of the patients could not be classified in either group. The key difference between the institutionalized and noninstitutionalized patients was that the former group was generally poorly educated, single or divorced, and from the lower class; the noninstitutionalized patients were mostly from the middle class, married, and well educated. Noninstitutionalized patients saw being hospitalized as a temporary but unfortunate state. In contrast, the institutionalized patients considered themselves as simply cut off from the outside world but were well aware of the hospital's comforts—food, warm beds, television, movies. The goal of the institutionalized inmates was very plainly that of security.

Wing studied the patients in two mental hospitals in London and found that the syndrome of institutionalization is dependent upon three factors. First is the social perspective of the patient. Patients who lacked strong family and community ties were usually not too concerned with restrictions on personal

[12]J. Marshall Townsend, "Self-Concept and the Institutionalization of Mental Patients: An Overview and Critique," *Journal of Health and Social Behavior* 17 (1976), 269.

liberty. Second, the disease process itself may be significant, because many mental disorders promote social withdrawal. And third, the influence of the institution itself, particularly over a long period of time, may gradually affect the patient by making him or her more dependent upon institutional life and unable to adapt to other living situations.

Eaton (1974a) has investigated the influence of the mental hospital upon institutionalization by proposing four theoretical models to account for the number of times a person is hospitalized for schizophrenia. The positive reinforcement model holds that the hospital positively reinforces the individual at each episode and is consonant with institutionalization. The negative reinforcement model takes the opposite position, that the hospital experience causes individuals not to want to return. The heterogeneity model proposes that individual differences between people explain the variation, and the pure random model assigns a strictly random cause for recurrent stays in mental hospitals. Eaton suggested that all four models represent processes that occur to some degree; however, the heterogeneity model was found to be the most satisfactory in explaining the data.

Although institutions may be able in some cases to reinforce positively an individual's attitude toward accepting hospital life, the most relevant factor, as suggested by Eaton's work, is apparently that people exhibit psychological and social characteristics that lend themselves, to different degrees, to accept enforced dependency. Some people are apparently very attracted to situations in which their needs are provided for with little effort or risk on their part.

As for duration of stay in the mental hospital, those who have the shortest stays are usually individuals with the least severe mental problems, the highest level of social competence, and the most personal resources. Extrapsychiatric variables such as social class, marital status, work performance, family influence, having a lawyer, and challenging psychiatric decisions seem to be relevant to gaining release, even when the severity of the psychiatric disorder is controlled (Krohn and Akers 1977; Linsky 1970b, Rushing 1971, 1978; Turner and Gartrell 1978).

A great problem faced by many mental patients is that the day of discharge from a mental hospital is not a particularly happy one. As Joy Query (1980) noted in a ten-year study of sixty-seven chronically disturbed mental patients in Great Britain, discharge often meant a return to an outside world that had long ago lost any real meaning. After a decade, many family members were dead or aged, or had developed a life quite different from that known by the patient before he or she was committed to a mental hospital. The majority of these patients were in late middle age—in their late forties or early fifties—and the difficulties in starting life over again were considerable. Yet about 70 percent of the patients were eventually able to maintain themselves in a "halfway" situation. Some patients both lived and worked at the hospital, although they were in a "discharged" status; others lived on the hospital grounds but worked in a nearby town; and the remainder were able to live and work in the town. What had allowed this situation to occur was a program of "resocialization" before discharge in which the patients and the staff worked together to reproduce the "real society." The patients were given jobs, for which they were paid a salary, and their working hours were gradually increased. Typical jobs were those of gardeners, pipe fitters, carpenters, upholsterers, bricklayers, cooks, hospital orderlies, and clerks. The patients were free to leave the hospital grounds to go into town—sometimes with staff members, other times on their own—and to shop, go to movies, and go to restaurants. Eventually (the program usually lasted about two years), most of these chronically disturbed patients were able to earn a living and become less dependent upon the hospital.

SUMMARY

This chapter has examined the experience of being hospitalized in a mental hospital and has reviewed those factors thought to be relevant to both voluntary and involuntary commitment, inpatient status, and the problem of institutionalization. For some mental patients, hospitalization is a positive experience; for others it is negatively associated with alienation, loss of status, depersonalization, and restriction. Some support is offered by the patients themselves in the form of an inmate society. But regardless of whether the patient sees his or her experience as negative or positive, the patient is required to make some type of adjustment to the situation. According to Goffman, the principal adjustment is likely to be some combination of conversion, colonization, and loyalty to the inmate group.

Even though hospitalization may encourage dependency and expose the patient to a living situation that is controlled, lacks privacy, and may be dehumanizing, it does not mean that all mental hospitals should be closed and the patients released to live in the community. One of mental hospitals' main goals is to provide a therapeutic environment; that is, to help the patient recover in a protected surrounding. Whether community treatment or hospital care is best for the patients depends upon the individual patient and his or her condition. David Mechanic (1989) has observed that when mental patients do show impressive signs of remission during hospitalization, the symptoms often reappear when the patient returns home. This would seem to indicate difficulties in the home environment, which may remain unchanged. Also, one of the benefits of hospitalization is that it affords a respite—both to the patient and to the family—from the turmoil that may have been a main cause of the onset and progress of the disorder. That respite can provide a period of reassessment and redefinition leading to a hopeful outlook (Clausen and Huffine 1975). Sampson and his associates (1961) have found that a significant effect of hospitalization on marital ties is to separate the disputants, block final action, and defer formalization of the end of the marriage so that other solutions can be attempted. Often, hospitalization may create conditions under which a relationship can be resumed.

The decision whether to opt for hospital care or community (home) care, therefore, seems to depend on the particular situation. Merely to conclude that institutional life is dehumanizing and necessarily bad is to overlook those situations for which it may be the better alternative.

12

The Postpatient Experience

An important part of being a former mental patient is the social responses of other people to that experience. Much of the research on postpatient phase has been concerned with the effect of stigma on these individuals. Therefore, before discussing family and community reactions to mental patients, this chapter will first define and then briefly describe the social phenomenon of stigma. The problem of stigma can be real not only for former mental patients but also for outpatients currently being cared for in the community. Chapter 13 contains a discussion of community care and the policy of deinstitutionalization. This chapter will focus on the responses of families and communities to former mental patients as they attempt to reestablish their lives in the community.

STIGMA

According to Erving Goffman (1963:3), stigma can be defined as "an attribute that is deeply discrediting." Goffman reminds us that the term *stigma* apparently originated with the ancient Greeks, who used it to refer to marks on the body. These marks were intended to represent something unusual and morally bad about the people having them. Usually, the marks were brands cut or burned into the body to identify the bearer as a criminal, a slave, or a traitor. Thus, any citizen encountering the stigmatized person was entitled to treat him or her badly or, once aware of the mark, was expected to avoid contact altogether with that person. In contemporary society, Goffman explains, there are three main forms of stigma: (1) abominations of the body, such as various types of physical deformities; (2) blemishes of individual character—that is, mental disorder, sexual deviance, dishonesty, criminality, addiction to drugs, alcoholism, suicidal tendency, political radicalism, and so forth; and (3) the stigma of race, religion, and nationality. The person with such attributes is therefore someone who is different from most other people, but different in a negative (supposedly less human) way. "On this assumption," says Goffman (1963:5), "we exercise varieties of discrimination, through which we effectively, if often unthinkingly, reduce his life chances."

Consequently, we see in Goffman's scheme that the former mental patient is someone who may be discredited because of a blemish of character, that blemish being, of course, past residence in a mental hospital. The popular stereotype is a person who is "unsound," "unpredictable," and maybe even "violent." At any rate, such a person is stigmatized as being "not quite right" and is subject to exclusion from the close company of "normals."

FAMILY RESPONSES TO FORMER MENTAL PATIENTS

Having a mentally ill family member is a disturbing circumstance. The experience may draw the family closer together, reinforcing and strengthening their ties of affection. But when mental disorder is present in the family, it is more likely that the experience for all concerned will be negative. Mental disorder can tear at the very bonds that make family life significant and worthwhile. Mental disorder can also bring fear, violence, discord, anxiety, and other stresses into the family circle. The bizarre behavior of the deranged family member can produce an intolerable situation in which not only treatment but also hospitalization is a welcome respite. In the aftermath of the experience, the remaining family members may feel a strong sense of embarrassment, guilt, and shame about what happened. In fact, the family itself may feel stigmatized. As Dolores Kreisman and Virginia Joy (1974) explain, being associated with a mentally disordered person has its own dilemma. "Since a close relationship results in being 'tainted' oneself," state Kreisman and Joy (1974:39), "a relative can choose either to embrace the fate of the stigmatized person and identify with him or to reject sharing the discredit of the stigmatized person by avoiding or terminating the relationship."

Few studies suggest that families attempt to terminate their relationship with an insane family member, but it does happen. For instance, Elaine and John Cumming (1957) report on a woman who was shunned by her sister after she had been hospitalized in a mental institution for only a brief period of time. Even though the two women had lived together for a number of years, during which the patient had repeatedly complained of being subjected to "sex-rays," the "normal" sister refused to allow the "crazy" sister to come back home after being hospitalized. "Mental illness, it seems," remark Cumming and Cumming (1957:101) somewhat sarcastically, "is a condition which afflicts people who must go to a mental institution, but up until they go almost anything they do is fairly normal."

In other research, Oscar Grusky and his colleagues (1985) found in a study of chronically mentally ill adults in eleven states and the District of Columbia that long periods of hospitalization had negative effects on family ties. Persons who had been hospitalized many times or for long periods had less opportunity to develop and strengthen close family relationships. If a family member is completely rejected, it is more likely to be a spouse than a child, sibling, or parent. Divorce rates for mental patients tend to be higher than those for the general public (Brown et al. 1966; Kreisman and Joy 1974). However, sometimes mental hospitalization has the opposite effect, of preventing divorce. A study by Harold Sampson and colleagues (1961) of seventeen families in California that included a mentally disturbed wife with young children found that hospitalization (all were first admissions) tended to halt disintegration of the marriage. In each of the cases, the wife had been unable to assume responsibility and had reached the point at which she was unable to carry on without help. These women were severely disturbed, and the husbands were unable to cope with the situation, short of divorce or hospitalization. Although they recognized that hospitalization, especially if it was prolonged, could weaken the marriage and further encourage them to get a divorce, that did not happen. Sampson and his associates point out that hospitalization thus interrupted a situation that was thought of as "impossible" by one or both of the marriage partners. Any definitive action to end the marriage was suspended while the wife underwent treatment. After the wife returned home, efforts to resume the marriage were typical.

Generally, it seems that people who have had close relationships with former mental patients are less prejudiced against them than those who have not had such contact. Research by Howard Freeman and Ozzie Simmons (1961), for instance, found that although some upper-class and middle-class families tended to be sensitive about having a former mental patient in the family, those feelings were not strong among most of the families. In another study, Freeman and Simmons (1963) investigated the experiences of 649 adults in Massachusetts over a one-year period after hospitalization. A close relative, usually the spouse or the mother, was interviewed twice after the patient returned home from the hospital. The first interview came about six weeks after discharge, and the second followed one year later. The relatives had rather high expectations of how well the former patients would do socially and on the job. And there was little change in these expectations over the year. Although research shows that family expectations of the mental patient do not necessarily influence the expressions of psychiatric symptoms (Greenley 1979), such studies also suggest that often families initially regard the family member as more or less cured after hospitalization and give that person the benefit of the doubt until there is evidence to the contrary.

COMMUNITY RESPONSES TO FORMER MENTAL PATIENTS

The family's attempts to cope with stigma are influenced to a certain extent by the community's responses to former mental patients. If the attitudes of a particular community or perhaps even a neighborhood are relatively open and unprejudiced toward former mental patients, then it seems likely the family of an ex-patient will sense little stigma. Conversely, stigmatization may make the family feel that it is difficult living where they do, and they may move away or avoid contacts with others. Therefore, knowledge of how a particular community feels about mental illness is an important indicator of what kinds of situations ex-patients and those associated with them will be required to contend with as the former patients attempt to return to their lives there. Knowledge of community attitudes is also important to community mental health workers charged with planning and implementing community mental health programs. However, like many issues in the field of mental health, the question of community attitudes toward the mentally disordered is controversial. The current literature generally reflects two opposing positions. One position, supportive of labeling theory, holds that former patients are feared and avoided by the public at large; the other maintains that attitudes have become more tolerant in recent years. We shall now explore the issues in this controversy.

Public Opinion and the Mentally Ill

Although the devaluation of the mentally ill and their treatment as objects of contempt, abuse, and ridicule in human societies have been documented since biblical times and ancient Greece (Clausen and Huffine 1975; Mora 1985), the first systematic studies of community attitudes toward former patients and, for that matter, toward the mentally ill in general were not made until the 1950s. These early studies, conducted by Shirley Star (1952, 1955), Cumming and Cumming (1957), Charles Whatley (1959), J. C. Nunnally (1961), and others, provided evidence based on scientific methods that public attitudes toward the mentally ill were characteristically negative and rejecting. An initial study was Star's nationwide survey of thirty-five hundred persons. Star used a series of vignettes depicting individuals expressing various symptoms to test how people felt about the mentally ill. She not only contributed a case history methodology used in many subsequent studies, but also found that the general public held negative views about mentally disturbed people and were rather poorly informed about the nature of mental disorder. A few years later, Cumming and Cumming (1957) used Star's techniques in studying attitudes in a small, rural, middle-class Canadian community both before and after a six-month publicity campaign designed to promote tolerant attitudes toward mental illness. Although the campaign had some success in broadening the definitions of normal behavior and in disseminating the idea that mental disorder was treatable, it failed to change negative feelings about the mentally ill as people.

Whatley (1959), in turn, focused upon the concept of social distance and found that strong tendencies to shun former mental patients were most prevalent in intimate situations (for example, those associated with courtship, immediate friends or neighbors, close work associates), although there was some tolerance in relatively impersonal circumstances. Finally, in a survey of Illinois residents living in or around Urbana-Champaign, Nunnally (1961) found a strong association between stigma and mental illness, regardless of the social background of the respondents. Nunnally (1961:51) described the responses this way: "Old people and young people, highly educated people and people with little formal training—all tend to regard the mentally ill as relatively dangerous, dirty, unpredictable and worthless."

Consequently, by the 1960s it seemed that the public generally believed the mentally ill were rather hopelessly disturbed people who could not respond to treatment, who were probably not very worthwhile people to begin with, and whose social status was irreversibly lowered (Rabkin 1974:28). Moreover, being a former mental patient was a distinct liability in obtaining friends, housing, and employment (Rabkin 1974; Whatley 1959).

Similar findings of negative attitudes toward both mental patients and ex-patients continued to be reported in many studies after 1960, thereby reinforcing the dominant direction of the literature (Armstrong 1976; Aviram and Segal 1973; Cumming and Cumming 1965; Fracchia et al. 1976; Miller 1971; Mulford 1968; Phillips 1963, 1964, 1966, 1967; Townsend 1978; Whatley 1964). But during this period, other findings emerged that claimed public attitudes toward the mentally ill were not necessarily adverse. These findings were presumably influenced by the public's being made more aware of mental disorder through mass media presentations, academic education, mental health legislation, and community mental health programs (Dohrenwend and Chin-Song 1967; Halpert 1969; Rabkin 1974; Spiro, Siassi, and Crocetti 1973). Some community mental health professionals were, in fact, depicted as engaging in a "moral crusade" to convince the public that mental illnesses were little or no different from other illnesses (Sarbin and Mancuso 1970). Although there is some question as to the extent and nature of the change in public recognition of mental illness (Clausen and Huffine 1975; D'Arcy and Brockman 1976), in the 1970s, most investigators agreed that there had been a change and that the public generally knew more about mental disorder than it had in the 1950s and early 1960s (Bentz, Edgerton, and Kherlopian 1969; Bentz, Edgerton, and Miller 1969; Dohrenwend and Chin-Song 1967; Myers 1964; Rabkin 1974).

Among the studies conducted during this period of reportedly greater public knowledge of mental disorder, that by Walter Gove and Terry Fain (1973) suggests that even though negative stereotypes of the mentally ill persist, actual behavior toward them is supportive. Other research suggests that many people view mental patients negatively but do not overtly discriminate against them. This is the position taken by Carol Huffine and John Clausen (1979), who believe that the intensity of the negative stereotype possibly deters its application in actual practice.

Huffine and Clausen argue, in line with the theory of cognitive consistency, that the human mind has a strong need for consistency and that often attitudes are changed to eliminate some inconsistency in thinking. Since the stereotype of mental patients (that is, as being dirty, worthless, unpredictable, dangerous) tends to be extremely negative and to be the attitudinal basis for rejecting the mentally ill, Huffine and Clausen are suggesting that once people observe former mental patients acting relatively normal, they are likely to adjust their thinking about them to be more positive.

Huffine and Clausen explain that this is particularly true for employment. When deciding whether to employ former patients, employers have to balance their information about the ex-patient's appearance, communication skills, personality, and past work history with whatever stereotypes they hold of the mentally ill. There is research that indicates employers are less likely to reject former mental patients applying for jobs whom they have personally interviewed (Farina, Felner, and Boudreau 1973). Also, employers tend to rehire former employees who have had an episode of mental illness because they already know the former patient (Brown et al. 1966; Clausen and Huffine 1975). In the latter case, the label "mental patient" may be inconsistent with what the employer knows through personal experience—especially if the former patient had held his or her job for a long time before becoming ill. Moreover, other research, such as that by Donald Olmsted and Katherine Durham (1976), suggests that although Americans tend to reject persons classified as mental patients, they also tend to accept the authoritative judgments of psychiatrists that a person has recovered and is "normal."

Many of the remaining studies reject altogether the notion of negative stereotypes for former mental patients. These studies indicate relatively optimistic assessments by the public of former mental patients. In Baltimore, for example, Guido Crocetti and his colleagues (Crocetti and Lemkau 1963; Crocetti, Spiro, and Siassi 1974; Lemkau and Crocetti 1962) conducted a series of studies that found, contrary to most previous work, that the public generally is understanding and tolerant of the mentally disordered. Outside Baltimore, in a rural Maryland county, further research replicated the work of Crocetti and his associates and confirmed their findings (Myers 1964). Other research in different locales has likewise noted the prevalence of relatively tolerant public attitudes (Dohrenwend 1966; Dohrenwend, Bernard, and Kolb 1962; Edgerton and Bentz 1969; Fracchia et al. 1975; Freeman and Simmons 1961; Lehmann, Kreisman, and Simmens 1976; Ridenour 1961).

Furthermore, the existing research suggests that certain variables are more important than others in determining who is and who is not likely to hold negative attitudes toward the mentally disturbed. For instance, several studies agree that older people are more likely to reject the mentally ill than younger people are (Crocetti and Lemkau 1963; Cumming and Cumming 1957; Phillips 1964; Whatley 1959). Blacks appear more rejecting than whites (Crocetti and Lemkau 1963; Whatley 1959). Lower-class people and those with less education seem to be more rejecting than middle- or upper-class people and the better educated (Cumming and Cumming 1957; Dohrenwend and Chin-Song 1967; Lemkau and Crocetti 1962; Whatley 1959). Research on differences in attitudes by sex is very sketchy and inconclusive. Some findings suggest that women are more rejecting than men (LeTorre 1975), but other research states the opposite (Farina et al. 1973).

A primary reason for measuring attitudes toward former mental patients has been to determine the overall pattern of attitudes. Here we find the literature firmly divided. Much evidence supports the view that people who are or who have been mental patients are generally subject to stigma and discrimination. Yet we also find a sizable body of research that supports the view that more tolerant attitudes are emerging. And there is a third position, which maintains that the public does define former mental patients negatively but does not openly discriminate against them and may come, through close association, to view them more positively.

Which view is correct? The best answer seems to be that although the stereotype of former mental patients is still negative, attitudes toward them have become *somewhat* more liberal. Most likely, this change is due to Americans' increased knowledge of mental disorder and more liberal attitudes generally toward the disadvantaged, as evidenced by the gains made by the civil rights and community mental health movements during the 1960s and early 1970s. However, even though there is enough evidence to suggest that public attitudes toward former mental patients have become somewhat more tolerant in America since the 1950s, social rejection of such people still persists. Bruce Link (1982), for example, found in a study of New York City residents that former mental patients tended to have less well paying jobs and that they felt that the perceptions of others about their former status were an important factor in that situation. Link concluded that the label of former mental patient still had important consequences for individuals. The label still makes some people uncomfortable and reduces employment opportunities. In another study, Link and his associates (Link et al. 1987) determined that the label "previous mental patient" fostered social distance among those persons who perceived mental patients to be dangerous, but not among those who do not see such persons as a threat. The significance of this study is that it demonstrates that labels matter. If people are uncomfortable about mental patients, they will tend to distance themselves from people who carry the label of former mental patient as part of their identity.

Implications for Labeling Theory

Studies showing relatively positive attitudes toward former mental patients have definite implications for labeling theory. Thomas Scheff's (1975a, 1984) work implies that in the minds of others in the community, once a mental patient, always a mental patient. That is, once labeled a "mental patient," the person begins a long-term (chronic) career as a mental patient because it is exceedingly difficult ever to shed the label once applied. Thus, the deviance becomes stabilized and more or less permanently part of the person's identity. As Scheff (1975a:10) states, "The offender, through the agency of labeling is launched on a career of 'chronic mental illness.' "

However, as the number of studies finding little stigma attached to former mental patients increases, the labeling theory position advocating the idea that the status of a mental patient is an irreversible master status weakens. That is not to claim that labeling does not have serious negative consequences for mental patients, including varying degrees of stigma, discrimination, abuse, ridicule, rejection, and impaired social interaction. The work of Goffman (1961), David Rosenhan (1973), and Link (1982; Link et al. 1987) is particularly illustrative in this regard.

But it does seem likely that the label "mental patient" does not necessarily carry over into the future of former mental patients if over time their behavior does not correspond to the label. Evidence that it is possible for a former mental patient to resume his or her past role in the community without irreversible stigma is found in the study of a small group of thirty-six married men whose occupational careers were followed by Huffine and Clausen (1979) over a twenty-year period. Because all these males were married, they are not typical of all male ex-patients, because the ability to sustain a marital relationship is an important indicator of a positive outcome for the mentally disturbed person. Yet, as Huffine and Clausen (1979:1052) note, "The stigmatizing aspect of confinement to a mental hospital should be no less for a married man than for a single one." Hence, examining the occupational careers of this group of males (most of whom were under the age of forty at the time of admission to a mental hospital, and all of whom were first admissions and suffering from a severe disorder—schizophrenia) can provide useful information about the posthospitalization experience.

Of the original thirty-six men, twenty-nine survived until the end of the study. Nine men had been symptom free for at least five years before the follow-up, and most had been symptom free since their initial hospitalization. All nine were working at jobs of equal status with or higher status than those they held before their hospitalization. Nine others had been mildly symptomatic over the years or had experienced infrequent recurrences of serious symptoms. Five of these men worked at jobs equal to or higher than their jobs before admission to a mental hospital, and four had slipped to lesser jobs. There were sufficient data to assess the outcome for an additional nine men. These men had suffered serious symptoms and had been rehospitalized frequently (the average number of readmissions was four) following their initial admission. Interestingly, all these last nine men, despite the severity of their problems, had worked at jobs during the period of the study. Four of them had kept jobs equal to or better than those held at first admission, but the remaining five men had had lesser jobs. Of the four men who had maintained or improved their job status, Huffine and Clausen (1979:1059) comment that their ability "to continue to work effectively and to retain their jobs in spite of recurrent or persistent severe symptomatology is impressive indeed." Two of these men, in fact, had jobs requiring considerable skill. However, among the men who worked at lesser jobs after hospitalization, most were unable to work at all by the time of the follow-up interview.

Because all these men had returned to work (some much sooner than others) after their initial admission to a mental hospital, Huffine and Clausen report that they and their wives tended to be sensitive to the possibility of stigmatization. But they had few direct experiences with it. Most of the men either perceived no change in their relationships with coworkers or found expressions of sympathy and reconciliation. Only two of the men experienced any overt hostility. The men tended to be apprehensive and to lack confidence upon returning to work, but self-doubt usually disappeared after they demonstrated their ability to perform on the job. Their wives also were interviewed:

> Wives described a variety of effects they thought their husbands' illnesses and hospitalizations had exerted on their careers. Only two, however, reported feeling that hospitalization, in and of itself, had created problems. One thought her husband might have been promoted further and faster had it not been for the hospitalization and another felt that her husband had been barred from federal employment because of his history of mental illness.[1]

Therefore, what seems to be significant to the occupational histories of these men was not that they had once been mental patients but the degree of severity and the persistence of symptoms of mental abnormality. Those men with long-term employment and short-term symptoms before hospitalization were able to have stable or upwardly mobile careers, but the others with short-term employment and long-term symptoms before their initial hospital admission were downwardly mobile. Older men were also downwardly mobile. These men thus failed in trying to keep the same jobs after their hospitalization as a mental patient, but the others who were able to establish their work competence before going into the mental hospital generally maintained their careers,

---

[1]Carol L. Huffine and John A. Clausen, "Madness and Work: Short- and Long-Term Effects of Mental Illness on Occupational Careers," *Social Forces* 57 (1979), 1059.

despite severe symptoms. Huffine and Clausen conclude that being labeled mentally ill does not itself determine the direction of a person's career, even though he or she has been confined for months in a public mental hospital.

Studies such as those by Huffine and Clausen (1979) and others (Greenley 1979) provide strong evidence that labeling does not stabilize people's symptoms of mental disorder or "launch" them on a career of chronic mental disorder. Gove (1976), for one, has seriously questioned whether labeling results in being accorded a permanent deviant status, subsequently stabilizing the deviance as a routine behavior for the deviant person. Consequently, Gove suggests that most deviance is transitory and indicates that it is quite possible for a person labeled deviant to return to a normal status. Clausen and Huffine summarize this as follows:

> . . . it is apparent that getting the patient to treatment tends far more often to lead to loss of symptoms than to their exacerbation or stabilization. Admission to a psychiatric service constitutes a crisis for patient and family and may sometimes be followed by more acute symptomatology for a short period but more often it seems to afford patient and family not only a respite from intense interpersonal turmoil and a redefinition of past behaviors but a hopeful outlook.
>
> The assumption that once labeled mentally ill a person has been irreparably stigmatized will simply not stand up when one studies patients and families over time. If a former mental patient manages to function well on the job and in the family—and many do—such feelings of stigma as were originally engendered will diminish and neither patient, family, nor friends will be disposed to think in terms of former patienthood or mental disorder.[2]

Based upon the literature of the 1960s when Scheff formulated his influential version of the labeling approach to mental disorder, one can readily see why he developed the notion that labeling leads to the stabilization of psychiatric symptoms and to careers of chronic mental patient status. Almost all the literature of that time strongly agreed that the public viewed former mental patients negatively and responded to them accordingly. But it can now be argued that times have changed and that studies showing increased tolerance reflect that change, thereby suggesting further that the dominant direction of the literature itself may be changing somewhat. If former mental patients can act relatively normal, they probably can shed their label and live a normal life. Yet labels can still be powerful influences on how people are perceived, and former mental patients can find that being considered normal is difficult. Consequently, labeling theory remains an important concept.

---

[2]John A. Clausen and Carol L. Huffine, "Sociocultural and Social-Psychological Factors Affecting Social Responses to Mental Disorder," *Journal of Health and Social Behavior* 16 (1975), 414–15.

ADJUSTMENT TO THE OUTSIDE WORLD

Many former mental patients, principally those who have families who care for them and jobs either awaiting them or readily available, are able to make a relatively smooth transition from the mental hospital to life in the outside world—providing their symptoms are not too severe. And if a good family life and job are available, the former patient may still be able to have a satisfactory life outside the hospital even if severe symptoms recur, according to the Huffine and Clausen (1979) study. Yet many mental patients face an uncertain and bleak existence in the outside community, particularly if they have been hospitalized for a long time. These patients may have become elderly, have seen their family likewise grow old or die, or perhaps have lost contact with them. Thus, they are alone in facing their problems, except for help from community mental health programs and social welfare agencies. It is this group of patients that has particular difficulty in getting reestablished in a community. Often they end up living meagerly in slum-area housing, and their mental condition is compounded by living in poverty. Therefore, although public attitudes in general may be "easing up" or becoming less negative, many ex-patients are nonetheless condemned to live in unpleasant circumstances because of their symptoms and lack of family, friends, and income.

Another problem in coping with life outside a mental hospital is a lack of self-confidence in rebuilding or reestablishing a relatively independent social life. As Dorothy Miller and William Dawson (1965) explain, feelings of stigma and shame are highly subjective and therefore difficult to measure among mental patients, as well as anybody else. Yet such feelings do adversely affect an individual's self-image and personal confidence. Goffman (1961) reminds us, for instance, that being admitted to a mental hospital often means being "turned out" by society on the grounds of being socially unacceptable. Hence, it is not difficult to see that a former mental patient recognizes that he or she has been the occupant of an undesirable social position and is devalued by many other people because of that experience. Miller and Dawson studied the effects of stigma on reemployment after discharge from a mental hospital and found that problems of gaining employment were common for about one-third of 1,082 mental patients in California released to go back into the community. Some of the patients were unable to work because of their mental condition, and of 156 patients interviewed after readmission, 35 percent indicated that they felt such low self-esteem that they made little or no effort to seek employment or reemployment. Miller and Dawson recommended both psychiatric therapy and vocational guidance before release to help self-disparaging patients build up sufficient ego strength to obtain and maintain a productive job.

The key to adequate readjustment to the outside world for most former mental patients is probably being able to construct a social-psychological framework in which they can be competent. Miller (1971) identified four elements as being significant to the patient's ability to stay out of the mental hospital. First, an adequate source of material support was needed. Second, it was important to have someone who cared about the patient and supported the patient's attempts to cope with the outside world. Third, the patient needed to have a series of spontaneous, positive relationships with other people. And fourth, it was helpful for the patient to have some control over new situations. If any of those four elements were missing, Miller believes that ex-patients were likely to fail to develop a satisfying life outside the hospital.

In over one thousand case histories examined by Miller, she found that a majority of released patients did not have the jobs, the indications from others that they were competent and respected, and the positive self-image required to maintain themselves; most were readmitted and released, readmitted and released, time and time again. The most successful patients were those able to go back into families as a wife or a husband. Miller states:

> World-building seems to require support from someone close, a partner in life— in other words, usually a spouse. This is especially true if the patient is still so disturbed that he cannot rebuild his own world without help. If he must, like Cinderella, exist on the edge of someone else's family (or even in his own), reduced until he has little power or importance, then he will fail to construct (or reconstruct) his world outside the hospital walls. (At least inside the walls he had *some* sort of place and support.)
>
> To drive the point home, we found a definite significant relationship between the positive feelings the spouse had for the returning patient and his chances of remaining out. The spouse's confidence that he could stay out, while helpful, was actually not as important as regard and support. Affection, apparently, is more therapeutic than optimism.[3]

Only about half of the patients in the Miller study were married, however. The remainder either lived with their parents after release from the mental hospital or lived alone. As Miller (1971:105) describes them, "Generally they were important to nobody."

There now are, however, more facilities available in most communities for helping discharged mental patients either with or without families than there were in the 1960s when Miller collected her data. Even though many ex-patients still have serious difficulties in coping with life outside an institution, some communities have an established system of halfway houses, community mental health centers, day-care treatment programs, crisis intervention services, and social welfare agencies designed to assist the former patient in handling his or her problem in day-to-day living. The workings of this system will be examined in the next chapter ("Community Care and Public Policy"), and

---

[3]Dorothy H. Miller, "Worlds that Fail," in *Total Institutions,* ed. S. Wallace (Chicago: Aldine, 1971), pp. 110–11.

accounts of ex-patients' posthospitalization experiences will be discussed to show how those experiences have been shaped by policy decisions—especially the decision to deinstitutionalize.

There are also various self-help organizations and clubs developed by ex–mental patients to assist others like them. Some of these organizations employ mental health professionals to provide psychological support and therapy; others are forums for self-help. Over one hundred former mental patient groups exist in the United States (Emerick 1991).

One self-help group is Recovery, Inc., a nationwide organization for ex–mental patients and "nervous" people. Members are asked to use the "power of positive thinking" to handle their emotional problems and to give examples at group meetings of how they accomplish that. Because the group has no special goals, membership and participation are more or less indefinite (Omark 1979, 1982). Essentially, Recovery, Inc., is an organization like Alcoholics Anonymous, Overeaters Anonymous, and Gamblers Anonymous, in which people with a particular problem can meet to discuss their difficulties and participate in a program designed to help them handle their problems better. Most ex-patients' clubs are small (usually about six to twenty members) and appeal to people who like to talk out their situations and who need reinforcement and the companionship of others like themselves.

Oscar Grusky and Melvin Pollner (1981) summarize research findings on the treatment of mental patients in the community by noting that many patients who otherwise might have been institutionalized in mental hospitals are probably better off being treated in the community. They also find that former mental hospital patients with satisfactory social support systems, such as family and friends, cope reasonably well outside a mental hospital in comparison with those lacking such support. However, a substantial portion of mental patients lack this support and probably experience care in the community that is no better and, for some, even worse than that available in state and county mental hospitals. Community care is not the answer in all cases.

It is also apparent, despite the research discussed here, that future studies of the day-to-day life of mental patients coping with mental disorder in a noninstitutionalized environment are needed. A serious deficiency in the research literature on this topic is that there is a lack of research in sociology of mental patients who have the option of community care. Future work needs to address this situation.

SUMMARY

This chapter has focused on the problem of stigma that many former mental hospital patients are believed to have to confront after discharge from the hospital. A review of the literature on this topic discloses that most studies conducted during the 1950s and early 1960s found strong evidence in American society of negative attitudes toward former patients. However, improved education by a variety of sources (for example, mass media, community mental health programs, government legislation) has apparently produced greater public knowledge and awareness of mental disorder. Most current studies indicate that attitudes toward ex-patients, beginning in the 1960s and continuing until the present time, are becoming increasingly tolerant and that the mentally ill are not always stigmatized in the eyes of others. Having a family, particularly a caring spouse, seems to be a very important variable in out of a mental hospital. Other factors are also important, such as the severity and persistence of symptoms, which ultimately are most responsible for an ex-patient's fate.

13

Community Care and Public Policy

This chapter will present an overview of the delivery of mental health services in the United States and will describe the various types of contemporary mental health facilities. Most important, it will review current trends in mental health policy, with an emphasis on the state of community care as the most salient policy issue facing the American public.

DELIVERY OF MENTAL HEALTH SERVICES

The actual number of people in the United States who have some type of mental disorder is not known; however, one authoritative nationwide study estimates that 52 million Americans may suffer from a psychological affliction or a substance abuse problem (Narrow et al. 1993). These disorders range from extremely serious disorders like schizophrenia to relatively minor problems like simple phobias, such as fear of heights, or adjustment disorders with depressed mood. Alcoholism and drug addiction are also included. It is further estimated that only 28 percent of all people with mental or addictive illnesses receive treatment from a mental health specialist, a physician other than a psychiatrist, or a self-help group such as Alcoholics Anonymous (Narrow et al. 1993). Clearly, most people who are psychologically distressed do not seek professional help or receive it. For those persons who turn to the health care professionals and institutions for help, treatment is available in (1) the primary care and outpatient medical sector, (2) the general hospital inpatient and nursing home sector, or (3) the specialty mental health sector. Each of these sectors will be described below.

The Primary Care and Outpatient Medical Sector

The largest percentage of mentally disturbed people who receive professional help, about 70 percent, are treated in the primary medical care and outpatient medical sector. Most are seen by office-based primary care physicians or in general hospital outpatient clinics and emergency rooms. Others are treated in the offices of nonprimary care physicians, usually specialists in family practice or internal medicine. What is indicated here is that the majority of people with mental difficulties are not treated by psychiatrists, nor are they treated in the specialty mental health sector. Instead, they are treated mostly by physicians other than psychiatrists.

The professional treating the largest percentage of all mentally disturbed people is the office-based primary care physician. The reason for that is understandable. The primary care physician is generally accessible, needs no referral, and is often initially contacted by distressed persons who are not aware of the nature of their problem. The person then may be referred to a psychiatrist or another specialist or may be treated by the primary care physician.

The disorders most likely to be treated in the offices of primary care physicians and other medical specialists are depression, anxiety disorders, disorders of childhood and adolescence, sleep disorders, and substance- and alcohol-related disorders. Also, the factitious, somatoform, psychosexual, and impulse control disorders are commonly treated by physicians other than psychiatrists.

Other principal providers of mental health care are general hospital outpatient and emergency room services. The use of general hospital outpatient services is related to the nationwide growth since the 1950s in outpatient services for psychiatric care. The emergency room is a unique setting in that the medical or psychiatric practitioner must make a rapid diagnosis, give immediate treatment, and quickly complete the disposition of the mentally ill patient—procedures that are not usually required in most other practices. Here the practitioner must often control violent and disorderly behavior and deal with people who are alcoholics or drug addicts, who are depressed, manic, anxious, or suicidal, or who show psychotic symptoms. The most common mental disorders seen in hospital emergency rooms are substance- and alcohol-related disorders, schizophrenia, and manic phases of mood disorders.

The General Hospital Inpatient and Nursing Home Sector

The general hospital inpatient and nursing home sector handles about 5 percent of all mental patients. But the increasing numbers of these units developed since the 1950s have had a significant impact on the delivery of mental health services. The importance of general hospitals with psychiatric inpatient units is that they are able to admit and treat patients for extended periods who might otherwise be committed some distance away in state or county mental hospitals or be released altogether. Increased numbers of nursing homes with psychiatric units have helped to remove many elderly mental patients from state and county mental hospitals, thereby reducing the number of resident patients in those facilities and transferring elderly patients to a setting that specializes in the care of the aged.

The Speciality Mental Health Sector

The specialty mental health sector treats about 25 percent of all persons with a mental disorder. These persons are treated either in freestanding outpatient or multiservice clinics or in community mental health centers. Others are patients in state and county mental hospitals or are treated by office-based private practice psychiatrists. What is apparent is that about only one-fourth of all persons with a mental disorder are treated by specialists trained in mental health. These persons receive the most extensive and expensive services, but since they represent a minority of persons with mental problems, it is obvious that not all mental health needs have to be met by mental health specialists.

Specialty Mental Health Facilities

Table 13–1 shows the total number of mental health facilities and institutions in the United States as of 1990. The total number of all facilities is 5,284, with the 1,674 nonfederal general hospital psychiatric wards constituting the largest type of facility. Freestanding outpatient clinics (743) are administratively separate facilities whose basic purpose is to provide nonresident mental health services under the direction of a psychiatrist who assumes medical responsibility for all patients. Next are residential treatment centers for emotionally disturbed children (501), state and county hospitals (273), private hospitals (462), and Veterans Administration psychiatric services (141). Most of the mental health facilities are oriented toward outpatient care, that is, freestanding clinics and general hospital outpatient services.

In 1990, there were 416,282 patient care staff positions in mental health

Table 13–1   Number of mental health facilities in the United States, 1990

TYPE OF FACILITY	NUMBER OF FACILITIES
Total, all facilities	5,284
State and county mental hospitals	273
Private psychiatric hospitals	462
VA psychiatric services	141
Nonfederal general hospitals	1,674
Residential treatment centers for emotionally disturbed children	501
Freestanding psychiatric outpatient clinics	743
Freestanding psychiatric partial care organizations	93
Multiservice mental health organizations	1,397

Source: Center for Mental Health Services, *Mental Health, United States,* 1994 (Washington, DC: U.S. Government Printing Office, 1994).

organizations. These staff members can be divided into two groups: those with professional training and expertise and those with vocational training. The professional staff consisted of registered nurses (18.7 percent), social workers (12.8 percent), psychiatrists (4.5 percent), psychologists (5.5 percent), other professional staff (24.2 percent), and other mental health workers (34.2 percent). About one-third of all professional staff members worked in state and county mental hospitals, compared with more than one-half of the other staff members. Most of these persons worked in urban rather than rural areas; this was especially true of psychiatrists, social workers, and registered nurses. Others, including psychologists, seem to be more evenly distributed geographically.

Office-based private practice psychiatrists   Office-based private practice psychiatrists tend to be concentrated in metropolitan areas. About 95 percent of all office visits to psychiatrists were to those situated in urban areas, which is a higher proportion than that for all other physician specialists. The concentration of psychiatrists in large cities is undoubtedly one factor affecting their nationwide availability. Another factor is the number of psychiatrists. In 1992, there were 21,826 psychiatrists in active practice in the United States; most were in patient care. The ratio of psychiatrists providing patient services in various settings is approximately 9 to every 100,000 persons in the general population. Psychiatric assistance is thus limited because of both geographical setting (accessibility) and actual number (availability). The disorders most likely to prompt visits to psychiatrists working in office-based practices (about one-half of all active psychiatrists) are depression (some 28 percent of all office visits) and anxiety (16 percent).

THE CHANGING FOCUS OF MENTAL
HEALTH CARE DELIVERY

Today, the majority of mental health care is on an outpatient basis, as opposed to inpatient services. This was not always the case. In the 1950s, emphasis was upon inpatient care. The events in the United States during the 1950s and 1960s that caused this change were (1) the passage of the National Mental Health Act of 1946, which promoted a significant increase in basic, clinical, and administrative research, in planning and implementing community programs, and in training mental health practitioners and workers; (2) the increase in numbers of outpatient clinics, general hospital inpatient services, and nursing home beds for the mentally ill; (3) the increasingly widespread use of psychoactive drugs to treat mental patients; (4) the enactment of the Mental Health Study Act in 1955, which established the Joint Commission on Mental Illness and Mental Health, whose purpose is to analyze and evaluate the needs of the mentally ill; and (5) the passage of the Mental Retardation Facilities and Community Mental Health Centers Construction Act in 1963, which stimulated programs designed to provide community mental health services.

Although the development and use of psychotropic drugs are the most important source of change, all these factors helped reorient the delivery of mental health services in the United States toward outpatient facilities. The effects of this trend were most pronounced in state and county mental hospitals. In 1954, there were 352 state and county mental hospitals; by 1990, the number of such hospitals had been reduced to 273. This decrease in the number of public mental hospitals is reflected in the significant decline in the number of resident patients from 558,922 in 1955 to 83,320 in 1992. These decreases took place in relation to increases in general hospital outpatient clinics and community mental health centers. Clearly, mental disorder has come to be treated in such a way that it is common for the mentally disturbed person to remain in the community. When institutionalization in a mental hospital is needed, the length of stay is usually less than a month. For example, in 1970 the average stay in a state or county mental hospital was forty-one days; in 1990, the average length of stay had dropped to fifteen days. The time spent in the hospital is, on the average, shorter than ever before, and treatment is likely to be continued in the community.

COMMUNITY MENTAL HEALTH CENTERS

By any measure, the most significant recent change in mental health policy for the specialized mental health sector has been the shift to outpatient services. The Mental Retardation Facilities and Community Mental Health Centers Construction Act of 1963, a commitment by the federal government to help support easily accessible and locally controlled mental health centers, reflected the objective of modern treatment to support mental patients in their own communities. This break with the past was in response to President John F. Kennedy's call for a "bold new approach" to helping the mentally ill. As we have seen, there has been a substantial reduction in the number of resident mental hospital patients since the mid-1950s. But this achievement is offset by a large increase in mental hospital admissions—indicating a high turnover of patients through shorter periods of hospitalization—and in the number of discharged patients relegated to living in nursing homes, single rooms in low-cost hotels, and slum-area rooming houses. Thus, there is debate as to whether the community mental health movement has achieved its promise of providing more effective and humane care for the mentally disturbed than that available in mental hospitals. The remainder of this section will explore this issue.

Community Mental Health: Developmental Issues

The community mental health movement in the 1960s was both a political and a social movement. It was not entirely unlike the civil rights movement, which took place at the same time and also caught the imagination of similar, well-meaning people while actively stimulating liberal tendencies in the direction of changing society for the better. According to David Mechanic (1989), the influential report *Action for Mental Health*, issued by the Joint Commission on Mental Illness in 1961, was essentially an ideological document. It strongly attacked the methods of handling patients in large state mental hospitals and argued that such institutions be converted into smaller regional centers for the most serious cases. Otherwise, the bulk of all mental patients were to be cared for in the community among family and friends, to facilitate humane treatment and recovery. In this context, depersonalizing and dehumanizing aspects of mental hospitalization would, one hoped, be avoided. Although this report was advisory, it was influential in the 1963 legislation that led to the development of the community mental health system.

This development was made possible by other favorable conditions as well. First, as Mechanic notes, the economy was in good condition and funds were available to support the program. Second, President Kennedy was committed to the idea and there were no strong opposition groups. Third, the use and success of psychoactive drugs had changed the climate of mental health care and had influenced the attitudes of mental health administrators and the general public toward community care. Fourth, many people were aware of the abuses and dehumanization that often attended the custodial care provided in state mental hospitals. Fifth, deinstitutionalization and removal of mental patients to community centers allowed many state governments to conserve funds intended for mental health and to use them elsewhere. Community mental health centers were less expensive to staff, equip, and maintain than mental hospitals and were heavily subsidized by the federal government. This whole situation was permeated by the rather naive belief that the community environment was "good" and the hospital environment was inherently "bad."

Morton Wagenfeld and Stanley Robin (1976) also observed that the community mental health movement departed from the traditional system of mental health care, not only because it sought to reduce the impatient population of mental hospitals, but also because it was intended to deliver mental health services to all segments of the population—not just to affluent urban dwellers. Because the movement was based upon a public health approach, community mental health programs were designed for the *primary prevention* of mental disorder. This meant that although the community was regarded as a therapeutic tool, certain aspects of community life—for example, poverty, racism, inequality—were seen as pathogenic and contributing factors in the onset of mental disorder. Thus, the community and its institutions were regarded as appropriate sites for intervention. The result was to extend mental health programs into public schools, social service agencies, nursery and day-care programs, church programs, law enforcement agencies, youth organizations, and the like. Special target groups were children and the poor.

Consequently, some community mental health workers engaged in a certain amount of "boundary busting"; that is, the scope of their efforts tended to be very broad and to extend beyond the boundaries of traditional psychiatry (Robin and Wagenfeld 1977; Wagenfeld and Robin 1976). These efforts not only placed community mental health workers in the position of providing services to psychologically distressed individuals but also oriented them toward social activism. The range of activism varies from consulting with established agencies to organizing the poor and other disadvantaged people for militant social action—all intended to bear some relation to improved mental health in the community.

However, a particularly important constraint on the development of community mental health programs and centers was a curtailment of funds after the end of the Kennedy administration. The ambitions of President Lyndon Johnson and his programs for the "Great Society" were adversely affected by the economic drain of the Vietnam War, and the administration of President Richard Nixon was openly unsupportive of community mental health. In 1972, the Nixon administration announced plans to phase out the federal grants that supported the centers and then attempted to impound the funds already appropriated for that purpose by Congress. The National Council of Community Mental Health Centers sued and won its money back, but the political climate suggested that the community mental health movement would face severe budget cuts in the future. And that is precisely what happened during the 1980–92 period of the Reagan and Bush administrations.

Moreover, as Mechanic (1989) explains, it was evident that many, if not most, community mental health centers were dealing primarily with day-to-day problems of living, rather than the problems of chronic mental patients who had been released to return to the community. Harsh criticism of community mental health programs ensued, and a reassessment was made. Subsequently, outpatient care and psychiatric services were emphasized, although primary prevention programs, needs assessments, and coordination of services with other helping agencies remain important.

The most significant public role of community mental health centers is deinstitutionalization—assisting the chronically disturbed to live outside mental hospitals. In line with this, the 1975 amendments to the Community Mental Health Centers Act required that comprehensive community care include halfway houses to provide both short-term and long-term living arrangements for former mental patients making the transition from the mental hospital to the community mental health center. The halfway house, originally conceived as an aftercare facility for discharged patients, has increasingly become a temporary residence for them in the community. Halfway houses are small (usually about fifteen residents living under supervision in a large, old house), have a familylike living arrangement (the occupants are residents, not patients, and they live in the house as if in a family), are in an open setting (they live openly in a particular neighborhood), and are intended to integrate the individual back into the community by stimulating him or her to function normally in a community setting.

As for community mental health centers, in 1990 there were nearly 700 centers in the United States, compared with about 300 in 1972. Although the goal of 2,000 such centers has obviously not been met, community mental health centers are an integral part of this nation's mental health services. To meet federal funding requirements, community mental health centers are required to provide both inpatient and outpatient services, day-care services, twenty-four-hour emergency service, and educational services for community agencies and professional personnel. Although community mental health programs are now well established in many communities, the funding of these programs through various federal, state, and local resources does limit their services.

Community mental health centers were initially intended to be self-supporting after the federal government had provided money for construction and staffing with qualified personnel. It was believed that enough income could be generated from individual fees, insurance payments, and state and local government revenues. That turned out to be a false assumption because the great majority of people who use community mental health center services are poor (Brown 1985; Issac and Armat 1990). More-affluent people go to private practitioners, private and general hospital outpatient clinics, or free-standing clinics. Thus, the federal government has had to continue to shoulder much of the cost of community mental health centers. Another financial obstacle is that of insurance reimbursements. Neither private nor federal health insurance has provided sufficient coverage. Coverage for mental problems has always been less extensive than that provided for physical disorders.

As for public, government-sponsored health insurance, Medicare and Medicaid, Medicare provides some limited inpatient coverage for the elderly in state mental hospitals and somewhat more extensive coverage for general hospital inpatient status—but little for outpatient services. Medicaid is administered by the states, who define their own benefits, and is intended to help the poor. At least half of the money comes from the federal government, however, and coverage is not provided for mentally disordered people between the ages of twenty-one and sixty-five if they are hospitalized in facilities that are exclusively psychiatric, including halfway houses. It does provide for inpatient care in general hospitals and for some nursing home services. Outpatient care is given very limited coverage. There is also the Supplemental Security Income program, which pays a small amount to support former mental patients if they live in a nonpsychiatrically oriented facility like a boarding house, hotel, or nursing home without psychiatric services. Sometimes the states also contribute funds to this program. On balance, existing coverage is inadequate at best, and public insurance programs in particular force former mental patients away from living arrangements that have psychiatric treatment programs and outpatient services, toward nursing homes and low-income housing.

Mental Health Reform

In the early 1990s, the United States was the only First World country without national health insurance. In 1993, the newly elected Clinton administration formulated an extensive health reform plan intended to change this situation. The rising cost of health care and the significant proportion of the Americans—about 13.5 percent of the total population—without health insurance were the major causes of the public's demand for change. The Clinton plan, which was intended to provide a basic level of benefits to all Americans, included coverage for both physical and mental health problems. Initially, the plan called for comprehensive coverage of mental health needs, but the projected high cost of health reform as a whole resulted in limits being placed on mental health benefits. The final proposal provided for thirty outpatient visits and sixty hospital days per year (Starr 1994). That was an improvement over most private health plans, which typically provide coverage for twenty outpatient days and thirty days of hospitalization annually, but fell far short of providing comprehensive benefits. Wider mental health coverage was put off until 2000. National health insurance was to be financed by having employers bear 80 percent of the costs for their employees, by new taxes on items like cigarettes, by savings from Medicaid, and by spending limits on Medicare.

The Clinton plan was not enacted following congressional inaction in 1994. Numerous interest groups lobbied Congress to adopt provisions favorable to them or to oppose the plan altogether. For example, the small-business lobby strongly opposed measures requiring businesses with few employees to pay a high percentage of health insurance costs, and the American Medical Association, hospitals, drug companies, and insurance companies opposed price controls or global caps on health spending; labor unions and the elderly were against any losses in benefits; and consumer groups were dissatisfied with the powerful position of insurance companies who were to become providers of health care by sponsoring large health maintenance organizations and with the lack of immediate benefits for the uninsured. The failure of the Clinton plan to be approved by Congress and the stunning success of the Republican Party in capturing control of both the U.S. House and the U.S. Senate in the November 1994 elections make future efforts at health reform uncertain. Whether some type of national health insurance program will eventually be enacted and what type of mental health provisions it might contain are unclear as this book is being published.

Deinstitutionalization and Public Policy

The current emphasis upon deinstitutionalization has not been matched by an expanded budget for community mental health programs on either the federal or the state level. Although some economy-minded state legislatures and governors have been willing to save money by closing state mental hospitals, they have been less willing to divert money into community mental health. Some small states, such as Hawaii, have had success in treating seriously disturbed mental patients in the community, but larger states such as New York and California have often had more people and problems than they can handle. Advocates of community mental health programs have argued that dumping patients into unprepared communities does not constitute community treatment, and consequently the unhappy results of this practice should not detract from the community mental health movement. These advocates insist that the community mental health movement has not had an opportunity to become fully operational, and therefore should not be condemned as a failure before it has had a chance to demonstrate its merits.

As originally planned, community mental health programs were intended to deliver a comprehensive range of postpatient services through community mental health centers, halfway houses, family and group homes, therapeutic residential centers, foster-care arrangements, and so forth. The overall coordinator of services was to be the community mental health center. In many communities, this comprehensive system has never evolved. Nevertheless, some state mental hospitals have proceeded to discharge their patient population as if these services did exist. A particular problem is that often there is no link between community mental health programs and state hospitals. The result is that the two systems find themselves working independently of each other. Occasionally, a discharged patient simply becomes lost after release from the hospital because community programs are not aware that the patient is in the community. The lack of coordination, communication, and overall responsibility for the patients compounds the problems they face and heightens criticism of community mental health in general.

Many former patients living in the community have unpleasant encounters. Sometimes they are isolated in low-income areas of the community and thus are prone to become so disorganized, despondent, or perhaps even violent that readmission is required. About one-half of all discharged mental patients are readmitted within a year of their release from mental hospitals. Ineffective measures in providing care for discharged patients also mean a lack of follow-up services. Many patients are shunted into nonpsychiatric facilities, including nursing homes. Ellen Bassuk and Samuel Gerson describe the situation as follows:

> Untherapeutic though many nursing homes are, living conditions in most of them are at least tolerable. Conditions may be worse for discharged patients living on their own, without enough money and usually without any possibility of employment. Many of them drift to substandard inner-city housing that is overcrowded, unsafe, dirty and isolated. Often they come together to form a new kind of ghetto subpopulation, a captive market for unscrupulous landlords. Their appearance and their sometimes bizarre behavior may disturb the neighborhood, and they are usually shunned and frequently feared. Even patients who live in recognized residential centers such as halfway houses have been found to have inadequate medical and psychiatric care or none at all, minimal activities and little interaction with people outside the facility. For the significant proportion of ex-patients who return to live with their own families physical conditions may be relatively good, but severe stresses can be placed both on the family and the patient, particularly in the absence of close follow-up treatment; there may be long-term effects, especially on children in the household. Finally, whatever the living arrangements for a discharged patient may be, he is almost sure to find a shortage of vocational rehabilitation, sheltered employment or job referrals, transportation and recreation.[1]

Such problems indicate the growing concern both within and outside the community mental health movement that chronically disturbed patients often receive worse care in the community than in the hospital. Media accounts of the experiences of former patients in the community have sometimes caused shock and outrage among the general public. Such accounts have intensified public awareness of the problem. It is not unusual for some newspaper stories to imply that mental hospitalization is preferred:

> Look in the crevices and on the fringes of any city. They're in the trailer park along the freeway, the old hotels along the railroad tracks, the sagging gingerbread houses with torn shades. Most live in mini-institutions, hotels converted to shelter and nursing care homes—often short on hominess and care.

---

[1] Ellen L. Bassuk and Samuel Gerson, "Deinstitutionalization and Mental Health Services," *Scientific American* 238 (1978), 50.

At the worst, they browse the streets. They move in a shuffle, the result of heavy medication. They sit on the curbs drinking or holding conversations with their private voices.

They are the bag ladies poking through garbage, the people who rant and implore, the ones who shiver in overcoats in summer and go barefoot in winter.

And always some want to go back to hospitals. A middle-aged woman kept returning like a homing pigeon to New York's Bronx State Hospital. She couldn't cope with a troubled daughter, late welfare checks and the East Bronx where she was robbed five times. She began to hear voices.

Often, she would be found curled up asleep in the lobby of the hospital. Once re-admitted, she improved. "It's a jungle in the East Bronx," she says. "I'm afraid to leave the apartment. That's slow death in itself. The hospital is better for me."[2]

Some media stories of mentally ill ex-patients document claims of being forced into migrant labor or getting caught up in drug use and a life of crime. Young female ex-patients may get dumped into a community and eventually find themselves working as prostitutes, still mentally disturbed and unprepared for life on the outside. Others lead empty and isolated lives sitting around the rooming houses and hotels that serve as their homes, without any semblance of the staff supervision that they might receive in mental hospitals. Particularly jarring are the accounts of former patients involved in sensational crimes that could have been avoided if the patients had remained in state hospitals. Two of the most sensational cases that helped focus early attention on the problems of deinstitutionalization were the 1973 cases of Edmund Kemper and Sheila Broughel. Edmund Kemper III, a six-foot-nine-inch, 280-pound man living in California, had killed his grandparents at the age of fifteen and was held in a state hospital for the criminally insane until he was twenty-one. The psychiatrist in charge of his care believed that he should not be returned to society, but a parole board disagreed, and Kemper was sent to live with his mother. Three years later, he was convicted on eight counts of first-degree murder and sentenced to life in prison. Since his release, he had killed, raped, and mutilated six hitchhiking college coeds and had stabbed to death and dismembered his mother and her friend.

In stark contrast to Kemper, Sheila Broughel was the *victim* of a particularly brutal crime. An intelligent but mentally ill twenty-six-year-old Vassar College graduate, she had worked as a secretary for the *New Yorker* magazine. She had been under psychiatric treatment for some time and had developed a deep distrust of both psychiatrists and mental hospitals. She went to Washington, D.C., to "talk with the nation's leaders about mental health" and found herself living in Washington's Union Station. Usually she could be found, day or night, rain or shine, standing in the entrance to the station. Paul Hodge, a newspaper reporter for the *Washington Post,* took an interest in her:

---

[2]"Community Mental Health: Does It Exist?" *Champaign-Urbana News-Gazette,* November 27, 1977, p. A8.

He was at the station covering another story, discussed her with a station policeman who told him she was "crazy" but that there was nothing he could do since she was not a danger to herself or others. Hodge bought her lunch—she said she was hungry and broke—and persuaded her to go with him to see a psychiatrist he knew at St. Elizabeth's Hospital.

The psychiatrist thought she needed help and advised her to sign herself into the hospital voluntarily. She refused and asked to be taken back home—the "home" being Union Station. The reporter left her there. The next day she disappeared. Writes Hodge, "When her mutilated body, sexually assaulted and stabbed almost 30 times, was found in an abandoned garage a dozen blocks from Union Station, some of her friends and even a relative said they were not surprised and thought it to be a kind of suicide."

Hodge quotes a New Haven lawyer whose firm had twice secured her release from Connecticut mental hospitals a few years earlier: He said lawyers in his office had discussed "how would we feel if something like this happened. Suppose she ends up in an alley we said. . . . Still I think we made the right decision in working to keep her out of hospitals. She was not dangerous and she passionately wanted to be free. That's what it means to have a free society, not to lock people up all the time."[3]

A more recent case is the 1995 escape of a mentally ill man from a New York City psychiatric center who should have been classified as dangerous but—for some reason—was not and who was able to simply walk away from the treatment facility. Despite a twenty-year history of violence and mental problems, the man had been given grounds privileges, which meant he had the freedom to move about the hospital unescorted. He disappeared on the city streets. Hospital officials heard nothing about him until eleven days later, when he was arrested for pushing a woman in front of an oncoming train and killing her.

Reaction to these kinds of reports produces a backlash in some communities where local citizens argue against mental patients being housed in their midst. Some community residents have gone to court to prevent mental health centers and halfway houses from being set up in their neighborhoods. The concern has usually focused on the possible decline of property values and the possible threat to the well-being of the neighborhood posed by having significant numbers of mentally disturbed persons in the area. Resistance ranges from outright threats to changes in zoning laws, city ordinances, bureaucratic delays, and informal pressure. Rejection of this nature, which some argue is actually prejudice, combines with inadequate funding to push former patients into living in slum areas, where their chances of staying out of the hospital are clearly diminished. Severely mentally ill African Americans and males generally are most likely to experience low-quality housing arrangements (Uehara 1994)

However, there have been successes. For example, New York City's Fountain House, which was founded by former mental patients in 1948, serves

---

[3]Jonas Robitscher, "Moving Patients Out of Hospitals—in Whose Interest?" in *State Mental Hospitals*, ed. P. Ahmed and S. Plog (New York: Plenum, 1976), pp. 158–59.

about two thousand persons, mostly schizophrenics. The staff numbers about sixty and works with an annual budget of over $1 million (40 percent of which comes from private sources). Fountain House leases apartments, arranges employment, provides banking services, offers day and night programs, and provides cheap meals. The Cambridge-Somerville Mental Health Center near Boston has forty facilities under its management, which include halfway houses, day-care clinics, and a cooperative housing project. Besides a staff of mental health professionals, paraprofessional workers are employed to maintain contact with former mental patients living in the area. These workers can return the patients to nearby mental hospitals on short notice if an emergency arises.

Success, however, can be measured in different ways. Segal and Aviram (1978) report on a study of sheltered care in California involving about five hundred mental patients placed among families, in boarding houses, or in halfway houses. Most of the patients were on welfare, with the majority receiving Supplemental Security Income from the federal government to pay for their housing. These patients were not particularly difficult to deal with, and their symptoms were not especially severe. Some were very dependent on others for such things as buying groceries and clothing and obtaining transportation. They tended to keep to themselves or interact mostly with other patients or the people they lived with. Those who were successful in bridging the social gap between them and the outside community had been able to do so largely because of the friendly responses of their neighbors. Particularly important was the availability of spending money for the patients so that they could participate in community activities. Segal and Aviram found that these patients had never been fully integrated into the wider society and that the sheltered care program was not likely to reintegrate them on any broad scale. But the program was able to enhance involvement with the outside world and within the facility that supported them. If enhanced social involvement is a goal of community care, it is possible to achieve it. Segal and Aviram conclude:

> The outcome of community care then must not be assessed in terms of the number of people, the head count, returning to independent economic activity but must be assessed in terms of the number of people maintaining an adequate level of functioning who, given our past experience, might deteriorate to a less than adequate level of social functioning if they were confined to large institutional settings.[4]

Another example of success is found in Sarah Rosenfield's (1992b) study of The Club/Habilitation Services founded in 1973 as a unit of the University of Medicine and Dentistry of New Jersey–Community Mental Health Center in Piscataway, New Jersey. Particular services, including psychiatric treatment,

---

[4]Steven P. Segal and Uri Aviram, *The Mentally Ill in Community-Based Sheltered Care* (New York: Wiley-Interscience, 1978), p. 286.

training in daily living and social skills, vocational rehabilitation, social contacts, structured activities, and temporary jobs, provided patients with a sense of empowerment and financial resources. This situation promoted feelings of mastery and control among the patients, which significantly increased their overall quality of life. Rosenfield suggests that her results underscore the importance of interventions in the lives of the chronically mentally ill that can increase life satisfaction.

Deinstitutionalization is a desired process for many—including what may be a majority of mental patients. Mechanic (1979) states that despite allegations of patient "dumping" and the possible adverse living conditions and victimization, most patients prefer community living. We can see that attitude, for example, in a patient quoted in a newspaper interview concerning the problems of community mental health care. The patient, "Eddie," points out that he and the other ex-patients live like "brothers" and "sisters" because it can be "rough out there" (meaning life outside the hotel filled with the former patients). He notes that some people in the town do not like him and his friends and that once or twice he has been refused service in business establishments because he was too loud or rude. But he gets by and much prefers his life as an outpatient to life in the hospital:

> "I've had 10 years of incarceration in hospitals and I've bounced around a bit. I'm an alcoholic and a real kook," Eddie says cheerfully. "I prayed for the day they would let us out and we could live like human beings again."[5]

What has happened, says Mechanic (1979:71), is that "deinstitutionalization has been accompanied by a strong social ethic of personal freedom and independent living, reflected in our social policies." Many patients have come to share this view of freedom and personal autonomy and to regard it as their social right, even though it may have negative consequences for them. Moreover, many courts are moving toward adopting the least restrictive alternative for mental patients and allowing them the greatest degree of personal freedom possible, although that freedom may result in adverse life conditions. Mechanic notes:

> Deinstitutionalization is not simply a matter of cost, or even a matter of what professionals and patients might wish. It is a social process influenced by ideologies, trends in civil liberties, conflicting conceptions of freedom and rehabilitation, and trade-offs between the choices of clients and what the state conceives to be in their interests.[6]

For some mentally disordered people, community care is in their interest and undoubtedly is a more humane and effective mode of treatment and

---

[5] *Champaign-Urbana News-Gazette*, p. A8
[6] Mechanic, *Future Issues in Health Care*, p. 70.

maintenance. Unfortunately, the community mental health movement took on too large an assignment and was never funded to the extent its programs required. As noted by Robin and Wagenfeld (1977), critiques of the community mental health movement have articulated one common theme: The mandate of community mental health programs to treat the mentally ill and to eliminate adverse social conditions spawning mental disorder was too broad. Community mental health centers were expected to provide psychiatric treatment and at the same time try to locate and help people who simply had problems with day-to-day living. Although community mental health centers have failed to remove the causes of mental disorder from community life, they have been successful in helping many people with mental problems to adjust satisfactorily to life outside mental institutions, and they have been able to provide significant psychiatric resources at the community level. H. Warren Dunham presents what is probably the best summary of the situation:

> If one expected the mental health centers to contribute to the solution of such perennial problems as war, racial conflict and/or poverty, why then obviously the centers have not been successful. However, if one expected the centers to provide quick and easy access to psychiatric care and treatment for persons in a community, to break down misconceptions about the nature of mental illness, to develop a followup for the treatment plan developed for each patient and to furnish a type of psychiatric intervention that would keep certain patients from ever entering a mental hospital, then one might argue that by these standards the centers have achieved a modicum of success.[7]

However, the 1980s and 1990s have been witness to an increase in the number of homeless people in America, many of whom are mentally ill. This situation led the American Psychiatric Association as early as 1984 to conclude that deinstitutionalization has been a failure and a major social tragedy. The association stated that the concept of shifting the chronically mentally ill from state and county mental hospitals to community treatment facilities was essentially a good one, but implementation of the policy was flawed. There had been a failure to provide adequate mental health care in the community and to meet such basic needs as shelter and food. A principal problem in large cities was the availability of inexpensive housing. Many mentally ill people found themselves living on the street or in alleys as part of the nation's homeless population (Brown 1985; Issac and Armat 1990; Johnson 1990; LaFond and Durham 1992). Treating the mentally ill as outpatients rather than in institutions was a primary factor in causing the population of homeless mentally ill to increase. After release from a mental hospital, many patients simply had no place to go. Moreover, some of them were incapable of making decisions for themselves or following a consistent program of treatment. In some com-

---

[7]H. Warren Dunham, *Social Realities and Community Psychiatry* (New York: Human Sciences, 1976), p. 196.

munities, the ability to respond to the needs of mentally ill people was inadequate because of a lack of resources (Hollingsworth 1994).

Whereas some patients had benefited from community care, for others the policy meant increased suffering. What was needed was a revamping of the nation's mental health system with markedly increased funding for sheltering the homeless mentally ill and providing them with adequate food, clothing, and medical and mental health care.

Therefore, at present it appears that the policy of deinstitutionalization has not brought the quality of life to the mentally ill that was intended. The 1990s are likely to see increased debate over this issue as local, state, and federal governments attempt to cope with the problem.

DELIVERY OF MENTAL HEALTH SERVICES IN THE UNITED STATES: AN APPRAISAL

If the goals of a society are to be realized, behavior should be predictable. Typically, this is achieved by establishing formal institutions and organizations. By virtue of their existence, such institutions and organizations control human behavior by setting up rules, regulations, and predefined patterns of conduct that channel behavior in a certain direction, as opposed to the many other possible directions. Those individuals and groups responsible for setting policy for such institutions and organizations define the relationships among the various subunits they administer and determine what is necessary to reach the goals of the collective enterprise. In a complex society, institutions and organizations with similar goals are usually blended into a common system so that coordinated effort from all entities can be applied to solving the problem at hand. Thus, we see in this approach the basis of a logical strategy for dealing with threats to the well-being of society because it allows for the rational management of resources to overcome problems and promote a better life for all.

Unfortunately, the system for health care delivery in the United States, in regard to physical *and* mental health, is neither logical nor a system. In reality, it is a *nonsystem*. The existing health care delivery system is a conglomerate of health practitioners, agencies, and institutions, all of which operate more or less independently. There often is little or no effective planning or coordination, with the result that there has been (1) a duplication of services, which increases the cost of care; (2) a maldistribution of services, which translates into a relative abundance of resources in affluent urban areas in contrast to limited resources in urban poverty and rural areas; and (3) a lack of comprehensiveness and continuity of care. Moreover, there is no national system of health insurance, and many people cannot afford by themselves to pay for quality medical care. The United States is the only major industrial country that has no comprehensive program for making health care available to all its citizens. With the failure of the Clinton administration to enact health reform in 1994, modifications in the health care delivery system in the United States—including mental health—received a major setback.

Consequently, the system based on fee-for-service remains in place as this book goes to press. In this system, patients pay for services rendered or pay insurance companies to pay for those services. The poor receive public health insurance at a nominal cost, but the nonpoor are expected to pay, and care is expensive. Private insurance companies, although providing a crucial service, nevertheless operate at a profit and pass their costs on to those they insure. This approach is based upon the concept of free enterprise and the open market, in which the consumers of health care, like the consumers of other products, are supposedly free to choose the health care providers that offer the best services at the best price. The assumed benefit is an improvement in services as a result of competition among the providers. Incompetent physicians and inadequate hospitals will theoretically be driven out of the market by more competent, more reasonably priced, and more efficient physicians and better hospitals. The fee-for-service system is highly attractive to physicians, and it is obviously no coincidence that it is the dominant form of *private* practice. It allows physicians to decide what branch of medicine they should specialize in, where they should practice medicine, how many patients they should have, how many hours they should work, and how much money they should charge for their services. Professional ethics are supposed to block any desire they might have to make as much money as possible.

The delivery of mental health services, however, presents a somewhat different problem from that of services intended to improve physical health. The majority of mental hospital patients are involuntarily committed and thus have no choice of where they go. In addition, county, state, and federal governments have traditionally assumed the responsibility for those persons who are unable to take care of themselves and who pose a threat to either their own safety or that of society. Examples here are institutions for the mentally ill, the mentally retarded, the blind, and the deaf. These persons receive care financed by public funds and are inmates of social agencies designed to prevent them from disrupting the usual patterns of social life or hurting themselves. As a rule, they have chronic, incurable problems, although for many of the mentally ill there is the possibility of returning to a relatively normal life. Many of the blind and the deaf also are returned to society after training. Yet for the mentally ill, it is clear that there is no "system" of public or private care to coordinate and supervise their treatment. There are community mental health centers, freestanding clinics, psychiatric wards in general and Veterans Administration hospitals, state and county mental hospitals, and private practices and private hospitals, but patients can easily become lost or misplaced when referred from one care provider to another. Also, each agency or provider maintains its own records, so that important information about the patient may not be passed on as well. Mental health services, whether public or private, are fragmented and disjointed.

All social organizations and systems have some conflict and structural strain. Such conflict is apparent in the health field—especially psychiatry. Psychiatrists in private practice are oriented toward curing or achieving and maintaining some state of normality. Psychiatrists in mental hospitals are oriented in this direction but also act as custodians for uncurable patients and as police officers for violent patients. Psychiatrists in private practice make the most money and have the greatest prestige and the best surroundings for working at their craft. Psychiatrists in mental hospitals have the lowest prestige, make less money, and in general may not be as well trained. Often, medical doctors in state and county mental hospitals are foreign trained, are not psychiatrists, or both. The fee-for-service system usually draws off the best psychiatrists and the most affluent patients, causing the conditions, the standards, and often the personnel in the public mental hospitals to be substandard. Besides the strain of the maldistribution of services, there is also conflict regarding the most important forms of therapy. Many psychiatrists favor drug therapy; others emphasize psychoanalysis, behavior modification, and so forth. Some use a combination of techniques, but there is no clear consensus.

The United States is clearly struggling to improve both the quality and the availability of mental health services for the majority of its citizens, but it has failed to do so to date. The rudiments for a comprehensive system of mental health services exist. What is needed are ways to coordinate and pay for these services, but there is no agency that can assume the responsibility for managing patients moving between the public and private sectors or between various providers within those sectors. Additionally, as for paying for mental health services in general, as might be provided by national health insurance, such funding is not a prominent concern in current debates. Nonetheless, the country sorely needs adequate funding for the public's mental health needs and coordinating centers where the mentally ill can be received, diagnosed, and then referred to the most appropriate mental health provider in such a way that their patient experience can be monitored. This is the sort of system used in various European countries, such as Sweden, Great Britain, and Germany. In Western European countries, a parallel system of private practice is also available, but the focus is on public services financed by tax revenues, with little or no out-of-pocket cost to the individual. Taxes may be high, but the burden is shared and the cost is much lower than that of any other method for the patient. In addition, the system offers comprehensive care through coordinated management. Americans, however, have traditionally been reluctant to pay high taxes and support government-run health care for the entire population.

SUMMARY

This chapter has reviewed the present American system of delivery of mental health services. In the specialty mental health sector alone, in the past twenty years there has been a significant shift in the form of such services from institutional (inpatient) services to community (outpatient) services. The majority of people with mental problems, often minor in nature, are still treated in primary care settings by physicians who are not psychiatrists.

Much of this chapter has examined community mental health centers, which have been the source of much enthusiasm and promise but also the subject of severe criticism. Community mental health centers have failed to eradicate social conditions that promote mental disorder. But they have had some success in making psychiatric care more accessible to the community. Through programs of outpatient care, crisis intervention, and primary prevention, many people have been helped. Currently, the most important public issue in the community mental health movement is deinstitutionalization. Many mental hospital patients have been literally dumped into communities, where they have been exploited and their mental problems have been exacerbated by having to cope with adverse living conditions. Other patients have done well in the community, and this arrangement is undoubtedly best for them. Often, the mental hospitals and community mental health centers have not been well coordinated, so that sometimes patients became lost after discharge from the hospital, or the community mental health centers were not prepared to cope with the influx of patients thrust upon their services. Frequently, they have had more patients and problems than they could realistically serve adequately. Since their inception, community mental health centers have had serious funding problems, and they have never had the financial resources to realize their potential.

In the final analysis, public policy should be oriented toward what is best for the patient, although federal and state budgets have to be taken into account. In fact, most discussions of mental health reform begin with considerations of financing. The review of policy issues in this chapter suggests that the most pressing needs of the mental health care delivery system in the United States today are (1) to develop a comprehensive system of mental health services, ranging from mental hospitals to transition facilities (such as halfway houses and other forms of supervised living arrangements) to readily available psychiatric services in the community that would include private practice psychiatrists, freestanding outpatient clinics, general hospital outpatient clinics, and community mental health centers with outpatient, crisis intervention, and primary prevention services; (2) to coordinate all these services on state, county, and local levels; (3) to upgrade the quality of state and county mental hospital services and facilities; and (4) to provide greater insurance coverage for both inpatient and outpatient mental health needs.

14

Mental Disorder and the Law

An important part of any discussion of public policy and mental disorder is mental health law, for it is in the law that a society's concepts about abnormal behavior are articulated into formal rules and regulations. Those who fail to follow the law place themselves in jeopardy as nonconformists. Thus, the law is society's vehicle for enforcing conformity. In criminal cases, the intent of the law is to assess blame and to punish in relation to the severity of harm and the extent of guilt. It is presumed that the individual who commits a criminal act is not only responsible but also able to understand the nature of the offense. The law consequently serves as a process by which society acts against those who willingly disrupt the social order and harm the individuals and institutions within it.

Mental disorder, however, is different in that the mentally disturbed individual may not be able to understand or comprehend the consequences of his or her behavior and therefore may not be responsible for it. The issue, then, is ascertaining the extent of a person's mental shortcomings and placing that person into the custody of mental health professionals rather than sentencing that person to prison. The intent is not to punish but to provide psychiatric treatment. But again, as in other fields pertaining to mental disorder, mental health law is ill defined and subject to controversy. The purpose of this chapter, accordingly, will be to review the present status of mental health law. The discussion will center on the following topics: (1) the concept of dangerousness, (2) false commitment, (3) insanity as a defense in a criminal trial, and (4) the right to treatment.

THE CONCEPT OF DANGEROUSNESS

Each year, several thousand people are diagnosed as mentally ill and are committed to mental hospitals without their consent on the grounds that they are likely to be dangerous to self, others, or property. Their commitment is based upon a psychiatric prediction that they are likely to engage in harmful conduct, a prediction that is made *before* they actually have acted as predicted. Under criminal law, a person has to be found guilty of committing a crime before being confined. What we are dealing with here is the situation in which someone is locked up because of an estimate that he or she might cause harm sometime in the future.

This action is justified primarily by the legal doctrine of *parens patriae,* which has been interpreted to allow the state to invoke civil commitment proceedings against the mentally ill to protect both the individuals concerned and society at large from possible harm. The doctrine of *parens patriae* evolved from Anglo-Saxon law and began as a protection for the property interests of the sovereign rather than for the interests of the insane. The idea was that if a noble acted "insanely" and squandered his or her property, from which the sovereign derived revenue in the form of taxation, the king or queen was to have the right to intercede and control the property in the interest of the insane person. Of course, it was also in the sovereign's interest to control the property because it provided him or her with money. But as the power of the English monarchs began to wane, the doctrine of *parens patriae* was used to protect the property of nobles from their insane acts, not because of the sovereign's interest in the property, but for the welfare of the noble who owned it. Although the emphasis shifted from protecting the monarch's interest to protecting the noble's interest, the chief concern was still the property, not the person. Insane nobles were not involuntarily committed to mental hospitals under this doctrine. They could wander about mostly as they pleased, as long as their property was secure and protected.

It was not until the late nineteenth century that the doctrine of *parens patriae* was used to justify the protection of the insane person's property from that person *and* the person's involuntary commitment to a mental hospital. Both are supposed to be in the mentally disturbed person's best interest. Under the modern interpretation of *parens patriae,* the state has the right and the duty to take care of those adjudged unable or unwilling to take care of themselves because of mental disorder. Such people are construed as belonging to a potentially dangerous class of persons because they may harm themselves, others, or property. By linking dangerousness to mental disorder, society is allowed to enact preventive detention against the mentally ill, a practice that otherwise would be unconstitutional because the detention of persons merely presumed to be dangerous is prohibited in the absence of an overt act.

The attractiveness of dangerousness as the paramount criterion for involuntary civil commitment of the mentally ill is that most people readily agree that dangerousness, violence, or harmful conduct is just cause for state intervention whenever such behavior is displayed. The concept of dangerousness is also consistent with the premises of criminal law in that it invokes the power of the state to deal with people who would commit harm. Moreover, dangerousness is a concept compatible with the popular stereotype of a mental patient as someone who is unpredictable and potentially dangerous (Link, Andrews, and Cullen 1992; Link et al. 1987; Szasz 1987). Thomas Scheff (1984) argues, for example, that the meaning of "crazy" is understood even by grade-school children and is part of our culture, as illustrated by phrases like "the boogeyman will get you."

The debate over involuntary civil commitment in the United States centers on the possible denial to mental patients of the legal safeguards of due process under the Fourteenth Amendment to the Constitution (Hiday 1988; Issac and Armat 1990). At issue is whether dangerousness, as a basis for civil commitment, meets the high standard of proof ("beyond a reasonable doubt") required in criminal trials or even the standard of proof ("a preponderance of the evidence") in many civil actions. This question arises from the vague definitions, the exceedingly low predictive accuracy of psychological tests and clinical judgments purporting to assess dangerousness, and the high rates of overprediction of such behavior.

Problems in Defining Dangerousness

Few concepts linking law and psychiatry are as difficult to define as dangerousness. The existing definitions are almost as diverse as the various courts and judges who are called upon to decide the issue. Even though the statutory language of all but fourteen states in the United States explicitly or implicity bases involuntary civil commitment on dangerousness, there are few or no statutory guidelines defining the concept or describing types of dangerous conduct (Brooks 1974; Hiday 1988; LaFond and Durham 1992; Teplin 1984).

Although involuntary civil commitment is usually justified on three grounds—(1) dangerousness to self, (2) dangerousness to others, and (3) need for treatment—it is difficult to make a general statement about the various state statutes regulating involuntary civil commitment. As Paul Keen (1974:773) observes, the statutes are as varied as the legislatures that promulgated them. There remains a considerable difference among the states in regard to definitions and interpretations of dangerousness.

Whether a person is committed involuntarily to a mental hospital on the grounds of being dangerous to self, others, or property is therefore dependent upon the decisions of judges and perhaps jurors and the testimony of psychiatrists or other physicians as expert witnesses. Yet on what basis should the courts find a person likely to injure self or others? When is the likelihood of harm substantial enough to warrant confinement? And how much and what types of "injury" must result? These are questions that state statutes usually do not answer, and the courts often look at how prior cases have determined appropriate action.

Danger to self   As for danger to self, attention is directed to both the threat of direct physical violence and the physical injury that might result from the inability, neglect, or refusal of a person to care for his or her ordinary needs. In cases in which physical injury has been self-inflicted, courts have typically had little difficulty reaching a finding of dangerousness. However, problems sometimes arise when the inability to care properly for one's own personal needs is the sole basis upon which civil commitment is sought. Of the courts that have spoken in this area, some have been willing to include personal neglect in the definition of dangerousness. For instance, a West Virginia court said in *State ex rel. Hawks* v. *Lazaro:* ". . . when it can be demonstrated that an individual . . . is so mentally retarded or mentally ill that by sheer inactivity he will permit himself to die either of starvation or lack of care, then the state is entitled to hospitalize him."[1] The Oregon Court of Appeals, in *Oregon* v. *Johnson,* upheld a homeless woman's civil commitment on the grounds that a mental disorder impaired her ability to meet her food and shelter needs.[2] In Minnesota, in *In re Harvego,* the appeals court found that a lack of income, a job, or a place to stay, along with an inability to care for one's self and extensive drug use, constituted a danger to self,[3] and in *In re Schaefer,* failure on the part of a woman to provide for her basic needs was reaffirmed as grounds for being a danger to self.[4]

When faced with the less extreme situation of physical injury, rather than death, resulting from self-neglect, a federal court in Alabama said in *Lynch* v. *Baxley:*

> In the case of dangerousness to self, both the threat of physical injury and discernible neglect may warrant a finding of dangerousness. Although he does not threaten actual violence to himself, a person may be properly committable under

---

[1] *State ex rel. Hawks* v. *Lazaro,* 202 S.E. 2d 109 (1973).
[2] *Oregon* v. *Johnson,* 843 P. 2d 985 (Or. Ct. App. 1992).
[3] *In re Harvego,* 389 N.W. 2d 266 (Minn. Ct. App. 1987).
[4] *In re Schaefer,* 498 N.W. 2d 298 (Minn. Ct. App. 1993).

the dangerousness standard if it can be shown that he is mentally ill, that his mental illness manifests itself in neglect or refusal to care for himself, that such neglect or refusal poses a real and present threat of substantial harm to his well being, and that he is incompetent to determine for himself whether treatment for his mental illness would be desirable.[5]

Other examples found in case law include alcoholism[6] and even writing bad checks[7] as a danger to one's self. Consequently, it seems that several types of behavior can be construed as causing a person difficulty or harm if that person persists in doing it.

Danger to others   The cases causing the least amount of controversy are those in which direct physical violence has been inflicted upon another person. Two questions must be answered when an injury has occurred: (1) How substantial must the danger be to the other person to warrant civil commitment, and (2) is physical injury necessary or can psychological injury also qualify as danger to other people?

The most extreme provocation is obviously murder. In 1907, a Washington court held in *State ex rel. Thompson* v. *Snell* that murder was conclusive proof of dangerousness.[8] No court has disagreed with this finding. The only contention in murder cases is whether the act was precipitated by mental disorder. For dangers other than murder, the courts have not always agreed on the degree of harm necessary to require civil commitment. The United States Supreme Court spoke most directly to this issue in *Humphrey* v. *Cady* when interpreting a Wisconsin statute on defining requirements for civil commitment and treatment.[9] The Court stated that an individual's potential for doing harm had to be great enough to justify such a massive curtailment of liberty as that represented by commitment to a mental hospital. In *Lynch* v. *Baxley,* the court interpreted this finding to mean that the mental illness must pose a *serious* threat of *substantial* harm to self or others.[10] Other cases have demonstrated that it is necessary to find "significant" or "substantial" danger before the liberty of a person can be taken away. Representative of this trend is the New Jersey case of *State* v. *Knol,* which held:

> Dangerous conduct involves not merely violation of social norms enforced by criminal sanctions, but significant physical or psychological injury to persons or

---

[5]*Lynch* v. *Baxley,* 386 F. Supp. 378, 390 (M.D. Ala. 1975).

[6]*Dudley* v. *Texas,* 730 S.W. 2d 51 (Tex. Ct. App. 1987).

[7]*U.S.* v. *Charnizan,* 232 A. 2d 587 (1967); *Overholser* v. *Russell,* 283 F. 2d 195 (1960).

[8]*State ex rel. Thompson* v. *Snell,* 89 P. 931 (1907).

[9]*Humphrey* v. *Cady,* 405 U.S. 504 (1972).

[10]*Lynch* v. *Baxley,* footnote 5.

substantial destruction of property. Persons are not to be indefinitely incarcer-
ated because they present a risk of future conduct which is merely socially undesirable. Personal liberty and autonomy are of too great value to be sacrificed to
protect society against the possibility of future behavior which some may
find odd, disagreeable or offensive, or even against the possibility of future non-
dangerous acts which would be grounds for criminal prosecution if actually committed.[11]

What is suggested here is that the most important criterion in determining danger to others is the degree of harm, rather than the activity, criminal or
otherwise. Although other cases have held that "any criminal activity" is a form
of dangerousness sufficient to merit civil commitment if mental disorder is
implicated,[12] most courts seem to agree that some notion of substantial harm is
necessary. As previously stated, murder is clearly a circumstance of "significant"
and "substantial" harm. Other violent acts inflicted on others also usually qualify as dangerousness.

State v. *Knol* addressed the time element in determining dangerousness.[13]
This case required that such anticipated conduct occur within the *reasonably
foreseeable* future. Because no specific time limitation was set in this case, it is
presumed that the "reasonably foreseeable future" is to be ascertained by the
facts in each particular case.

Psychological harm also may be claimed. The few courts that have dealt
with this issue have rejected the contention that dangerousness to self and others is confined solely to physical injury. In cases in California (*People* v. *Stoddard*) and the District of Columbia (*Carras* v. *District of Columbia*), the argument
was dismissed that physical injury was the only form of injury to self and others.[14] Both cases concerned persons involved in sex crimes (indecent exposure), and the courts held that the word "injury" includes injury to feelings
and that the word "pain" includes mental suffering. This interpretation was
described as not being limited to sex crimes. However, in the case *State ex rel.
Hawks* v. *Lazaro,* the court held that the degree of psychological injury definitely must be ascertainable.[15]

Danger to property   Several state statutes include danger to property as
inherent in the concept of dangerousness in regard to civil commitment.
Again, the problem of ascertaining the degree of injury is as necessary as it is
in determining possible harm to people. Courts in New Jersey and Maryland

---

[11]*State* v. *Knol,* 344 A. 2d 282, 301–302 (1975).
[12]See *Cross* v. *Harris,* 418 F. 2d 1095 (1969); *Davy* v. *Sullivan,* 354 F. Supp. 1320 (1973).
[13]*State* v. *Knol,* footnote 11.
[14]*People* v. *Stoddard,* 38 Cal. Rptr. 407 (1964); *Carras* v. *District of Columbia,* 183 A. 2d (1962).
[15]*State ex rel. Hawks* v. *Lazaro,* footnote 1.

have ruled that persons dangerous to property are subject to commitment. In New Jersey, the case of *State* v. *Knol* accepted the concept of danger to property but held that substantial injury to property was required.[16] In Maryland, the court in *Director of Patuxent Institution* v. *Daniels* offers a good summary:

> When this mental illness exists, it is no less real because an outward manifestation has been an offense against property rather than an offense against a person. One who is a menace to the property of others easily fits within the definition of a danger to society, and the legislative power is not abused when it concludes that one only violating property rights is potentially a danger to the person of others.[17]

However, as further illustration of the contradictions that can be found in case law, a court decision in Hawaii stipulated that a danger to property did not, in itself, warrant involuntary civil commitment. This court, in the case of *Suzuki* v. *Yuen,* stated that dangerousness to property is not a constitutional basis for commitment in either an emergency or a nonemergency and that only danger to self or others is a sufficient requirement for hospitalization.[18] It was noted that the state's interest could be adequately protected by the use of criminal statutes prohibiting damage to property. The court said that even if not committed to a mental health facility, a person could still be jailed to prevent future property damage if the evidence justified it.

Necessity of an overt act   There is disagreement as to whether an *overt* act of harm is necessary to justify commitment or whether a decision to commit a person without a prior act will afford the defendant the proper safeguards he or she is entitled to. The issue of whether any criminal act will justify civil commitment of the mentally ill as being dangerous has not been answered uniformly by the courts. The cases of *Overholser* v. *Russell* and *U.S.* v. *Charnizan* in the District of Columbia regard any criminal act as creating a sufficient level of dangerousness to justify civil commitment.[19] Conversely, the Illinois case of *People* v. *Bradley,* although primarily concerned with the standard of proof necessary in a civil commitment case, held that criminal charges alone are not sufficient evidence that a person may be reasonably expected to harm self or others.[20]

---

[16]*State* v. *Knol,* footnote 11.

[17]*Director of Patuxent Institution* v. *Daniels,* 243 Md. 2d 16, 49, 221 A. 2d 397, 416 (1966).

[18]*Suzuki, et al.* v. *Yuen, G., et al.* Civil 73-3854, Hawaii (1977).

[19]*Overholser* v. *Russell,* footnote 7; *U.S.* v. *Charnizan,* footnote 7.

[20]*People* v. *Bradley,* 318 N.E. 2d 267 (1974).

In the 1946 Iowa case of *Gahwiller* v. *Gahwiller,* a jury made a finding of dangerousness based on Mr. Gahwiller's repeated threats to kill his brother, after an eighteen-year dispute between them over some property.[21] Before making those threats, Mr. Gahwiller had attempted to choke his brother but in the intervening years had committed no other acts of violence. It was found that the threats alone were sufficient to justify a determination of dangerousness, and no subsequent Iowa court has questioned the finding. Other cases have held that the mere threat of harm, combined with continuing mental disorder, will sustain a finding of dangerousness. For example, in a 1987 Montana case, *In re R.J.W.,* the act of carrying a concealed weapon, in addition to mental illness, was found to be sufficient evidence of dangerousness. In this case, a mentally ill man threatened his landlord and displayed a concealed gun. That action was viewed as an imminent threat of future injury that qualified as proof of dangerousness beyond a reasonable doubt. The court held that it was not required to wait until a person actually uses weapons against other people before deciding the question of dangerousness.[22]

Another case, the 1974 Illinois decision in *People* v. *Sansome,* flatly rejected the claim that a prior overt act was necessary to predict the dangerousness of a patient.[23] Mr. Sansome demonstrated what one psychiatrist defined as "unrealistic thinking" in believing himself to be a senator and in thinking that people were trying to occupy his land illegally. He had been arrested ordering people off his property, but he had never stated he would harm anyone. Sansome's attorney claimed that to find him dangerous on those grounds was to confine him *only* because he was diagnosed as mentally ill. (For involuntary civil commitment in many states, it is necessary to be *both* mentally ill and dangerous; being just "mentally ill" or just "dangerous" is not sufficient justification.) The Illinois court rejected Sansome's contention, stating that a decision to commit a person based upon a medical opinion that the person is reasonably expected to engage in dangerous conduct without out previous harmful acts is acceptable and constitutional.

Still other courts have maintained that an overt act is indeed necessary for a finding of dangerousness to others. *Lessard* v. *Schmidt,* a 1972 federal case interpreting a Wisconsin law, required that the determination of dangerousness be based on a finding of a recent overt act, attempt, or threat to do harm.[24] The 1975 *Lynch* v. *Baxley* case in Alabama used almost the same language in requiring evidence of an overt act before civil commitment can be

---

[21] *Gahwiller* v. *Gahwiller,* 25 N.W. 2d 484 (1946).

[22] *In re R.J.W.,* 736 P. 2d 110 (Mont. Sup. Ct. 1987).

[23] *People* v. *Sansome,* 309 N.E. 2d 733 (App. Ct. Ill. 1974).

[24] *Lessard* v. *Schmidt,* 349 F. Supp. 1078 (E. D. Wis. 1972).

justified—a decision reaffirmed by an Alabama federal court in the 1991 *Wyatt v. King* case.[25]

All courts are apparently willing to justify civil commitment if there has been a serious overt act or threat by a mentally ill person; not all courts are willing to do so in the absence of overt action.

Likelihood of harm   Although rarely articulated, most courts view dangerousness as a product of the magnitude of the harm and the probability that the defendant will cause it to occur.[26] As the New Jersey court stated in *State v. Knol,* evaluation of the possible risk considers both the likelihood of dangerous conduct and the seriousness of the harm that may ensue if the feared conduct takes place.[27] A sliding-scale approach is implied; that is, as the probability of harm increases, the seriousness of the harm required for a finding of dangerousness decreases. Most state statutes use broad language such as "dangerous to others" or "for the welfare of others," thus allowing the courts to draw whatever standards they feel are appropriate. The California Supreme Court in 1915 established a standard in *Ex Parte Harcourt* followed by all courts that have spoken on the subject.[28] The court stated that there must be more than the mere possibility that the person will be a danger if allowed to remain at large. It maintained that the defendant's mental condition must make it *reasonably certain* that he or she will endanger himself or herself or be a menace to society.

Two Illinois decisions provide standards similar to that of *Ex Parte Harcourt.* The first, *People v. Sansome,* states that a "reasonable expectation," not a specific degree of probability, that a person is likely to engage in dangerous conduct is required.[29] In this case, a psychiatrist testified that Sansome's actions "strongly" indicated that he believed people were after him and that patients whom the psychiatrist had known in the past with the same type of delusion had injured or attempted to injure others. The facts, the court stated, clearly led to a finding that the patient could reasonably be expected to injure others, thereby justifying the commitment.

The second case, *People v. Bradley,* was built on the rather ambiguous standard of "reasonable expectations."[30] The state sought to commit Mr. Bradley based on his refusal to leave his wife's hospital bed, his attempt to strike a court bailiff, and his uncooperative attitude when examined by a psychiatrist. The

---

[25]*Lynch v. Baxley,* footnote 5; *Wyatt v. King,* 781 F. Supp. 750 (M.D. Ala. 1991).

[26]See *People v. Stoddard,* footnote 14.

[27]*State v. Knol,* footnote 11.

[28]*Ex Parte Harcourt,* 150 P. 1001 (1915).

[29]*People v. Sansome,* footnote 23.

[30]*People v. Bradley,* footnote 20.

psychiatrist testified that Bradley "could conceivably be dangerous." The Illinois Supreme Court strongly criticized commitment based on those facts, which it indicated was to "disregard the individual's right not to be unjustly or unreasonably confined." The facts in *People* v. *Bradley* did not lead to a finding of dangerousness, and the decision by the lower court to authorize civil commitment was reversed.

The determination of whether dangerousness exists is always based on medical testimony, but as is apparent from this discussion, any civil commitment proceedings can be challenged in the courts. Therefore, the decision is ultimately a legal one, not a medical one.

Burden of proof   In most civil cases, the applicable burden of proof is "preponderance of the evidence." This standard is the least demanding standard available in the law. The preponderance of the evidence standard holds that the evidence that produces the strongest impression has the greatest weight and is the most convincing. Although vague, the standard is frequently used by courts in civil commitment cases with the state normally charged with providing the alleged facts of dangerousness.

However, some courts have found the preponderance-of-the-evidence standard unconstitutional because it is not strict enough to protect what they feel are the fundamental liberties of the patient. In turning to a stricter standard, many of these courts have adopted the standard of "clear and convincing evidence." This standard has not been well defined but is generally said to require more than "preponderance of the evidence" and less than "beyond a reasonable doubt." The Supreme Court of New Mexico, when considering the issue for the first time in the 1975 case of *Matter of Valdez*, justified its requirement of clear and convincing evidence by stating that civil commitment is a hybrid procedure, involving elements of both criminal and civil law.[31] The court went on to say that the very nature of civil commitment rules out the stricter standard of "beyond a reasonable doubt" because psychiatry is not an exact science and therefore is unable to make exact predictions. As a result, such a stringent standard was argued as being unworkable in this area. Examples of what the courts have found to be "clear and convincing evidence" of dangerousness of civil commitment cases are shooting a police officer,[32] a paranoid belief that people were after one's property and that one would have to protect it,[33] the crime of breaking and entering,[34] and exhibitionism.[35]

The most stringent standard of proof required of the state is the one required in àll criminal cases—proof "beyond a reasonable doubt." Some

---

[31] *Matter of Valdez*, 540 P. 2d 818 (1975).

[32] *State* v. *Carter*, 316 A. 2d 449 (1974).

[33] *People* v. Sansome, footnote 23.

[34] *In re Levias*, 517 P. 2d 588 (1973).

[35] *People* v. *Stoddard*, footnote 14.

courts have adopted this standard because they feel that the same standard that applies to criminal cases should also apply to civil commitment cases. The significance of the distinction between the different standards of proof can be seen in cases in which commitment would be justified under one standard, but not under the more stringent requirements of another standard. An example is the case of *In re Balley*.[36] Mr. Balley was more of a nuisance than anything else. He had appeared at the White House three times asking to see the president while posing as an Illinois senator. The jury was instructed to follow the preponderance-of-the-evidence standard and found Balley to be dangerous according to that criterion. A higher court, however, declared that applying this standard deprived the defendant of due process and ordered that the standard of beyond a reasonable doubt be followed. Balley was released because it could not be shown that he was dangerous beyond a reasonable doubt.

Along those same lines, a district court of appeals in Florida found that a twenty-nine-year-old woman, showing no signs of mental illness other than periodic absences from home and one instance of embezzlement of $960 (no criminal charges were filed), could not be committed, because the evidence did not prove beyond a reasonable doubt that she would be dangerous in the future.[37] In New Jersey, a patient was found to be disoriented as to time and place and was diagnosed as paranoid but found not to be dangerous if allowed to remain at liberty.[38] The court instructed the jury that any reasonable doubt in their minds about the potential dangerousness of the patient had to be resolved in the patient's favor.

Conclusion The mere designation of mental illness is not sufficient grounds in many states for the civil commitment of an individual. There must also be a finding that the insanity is of such a degree that if the person remained at large he or she would be a danger to self, others, or property. Unfortunately, there are few applicable standards. Decisions are usually made on a case-by-case basis, aided by medical testimony. But in the end it is a legal decision. In case law, actions ranging from murder to writing bad checks to neglect of one's own physical needs have been found to constitute dangerousness. But there is little agreement about what constitutes dangerous conduct, except for the most obvious of behaviors: *overt physical violence or harm*. In fact, some courts have required proof of an overt act as a constitutional necessity. Other courts have rejected the claim that a previous overt act is necessary to predict dangerousness. As Allen Fagin (1976:491) states: "It is clear, therefore, that the exercise of the power to commit is a form of predictive decision-making under conditions of uncertainty." There is no

---

[36] *In re Balley*, 482 F. 2d 648 (1973).

[37] *In re Pickles Petition*, 170 S. 2d 603 (Fla. 1965).

[38] *In re Heukenikian*, 94 A. 2d 501 (N.J. 1953).

judicial consensus on any but the most obvious acts of dangerousness—that is, murder and direct physical assault—and the issue remains one of the most unsettled areas of the law.

The Problem of Predicting Dangerousness

The controversial definition of dangerousness is compounded by the difficulty in predicting it accurately. Psychiatrists are called upon to testify in this regard as expert witnesses, and it is their testimony that is the usual basis for commitment. However, no psychological tests have yet been developed that predict dangerousness precisely (Megargee 1970; Monahan 1981). Reliance upon psychiatrists' clinical judgments are matters of professional opinion and not scientific fact. Indeed, it has been argued that clinical judgments based on insight, intuition, and experience as a mode of predicting dangerousness are perhaps no better than lay judgments (Cocozza and Steadman 1976; Laves 1975). Stone (1975) suggests that although there may be relatively unusual clinical symptoms that can be best diagnosed by psychiatrists or other mental health practitioners, psychiatric intuition and clinical experience may not be especially valuable in predicting whether patients will be dangerous. There are some patients for whom anyone could predict potentially dangerous acts because of their obvious behavior or past history of violence. For those patients, a psychiatric prediction would do little more than confirm what was obvious to all. Psychiatric predictions of dangerousness, for example, have a relatively high degree of short-term validity for persons brought to hospital emergency rooms for acting violently (McNiel and Binder 1987).

Studies of discharged mental patients   Before the mid-1960s, most studies of discharged mental patients found them to be not particularly dangerous, because they had lower arrest rates as a group than the general population did (Brill and Malzberg 1962; Cohen and Freeman 1945). But later studies have modified this conclusion. In studies of ex–mental patients in Maryland in the 1960s, it was found that when compared with the general population, male ex-patients had higher arrest rates for rape and robbery (Rappaport and Lassen 1965), and female ex-patients had higher arrest rates for aggravated assault (Rappaport and Lassen 1966). Other research on the experiences of 1,142 former Veterans Administration mental patients found higher arrest rates for robbery but not for sex crimes (Giovannoni and Gurel 1967). Although alcoholism was not their primary diagnosis (95 percent were diagnosed as schizophrenic), almost half of these patients had serious drinking problems. Additional research in New York State has also found that arrest rates for rape, aggravated assault, and robbery were higher for a group of discharged mental patients than for "normal" citizens (Zitrin et al. 1976) and that the proportion of male mental patients with police records is steadily increasing (Melick, Steadman, and Cocozza 1979). Other research in New York City found that mental patients have elevated rates of violent and illegal behavior compared with nonpatients in the community, but differences were modest and largely due to patients with psychotic symptoms (Link, Andrews, and Cullen 1992).

Studies such as these do not mean that mentally disordered people are all exceptionally dangerous and unpredictable. What they do mean is that such people are not less dangerous than the general population (as was previously thought) and may be slightly more dangerous in regard to certain crimes, primarily crimes against persons, such as robbery and assault (Issac and Armat 1990).

Psychiatrists are criticized most for their predictions of dangerousness when their assessments have been demonstrated to be wrong. Besides the occasional media reports of mentally disturbed persons who harm themselves or other people after being classified as not dangerous, there have been studies of patients defined as dangerous who have subsequently shown themselves to be relatively harmless. One of the best-known of these studies is of the Baxstrom patients, conducted by Henry Steadman and Joseph Cocozza (1974). The United States Supreme Court in 1966 ruled in *Baxstrom* v. *Herold* that Johnnie K. Baxstrom, who was sent to prison for second-degree assault, found to be insane, then transferred to a state hospital for the criminally insane, could not be held in the hospital longer than his prison sentence without a judicial review of his case.[39] This decision eventually resulted in the transfer of 967 patients from New York's two maximum-security hospitals for the criminally insane to regular state mental hospitals. As Steadman and Cocozza note, these patients were considered to be among the most dangerous in the state and were expected to display their dangerousness in the hospitals to which they were being sent or in the communities if they were released. After four years, only 26 of the 967 patients had been so troublesome that they had to be returned to a maximum-security hospital. Seven years later, it was found that only 2.7 percent of all the original Baxstrom patients had been returned to hospitals for the criminally insane at any time after their transfer in 1966. If the Baxstrom patients had not been transferred, most of them would have spent several more years, without being especially dangerous, in a hospital for the criminally insane.

To place this discussion in perspective, it is relevant to note that the mentally ill do not constitute the most dangerous group in society when compared with criminals, ex-felons, or even persons convicted of drunk driving (Shah 1975). However, as Steadfast (1981) observes, ex–mental patients, as a group, are arrested more often than the general population. And the perception that the mentally ill can be dangerous influences the extent to

---

[39]*Baxstrom* v. *Herold*, 383 U.S. 107 (1966).

which individuals want to interact with them (Link and Cullen 1986; Link et al. 1992).

The tendency to overpredict   Psychiatrists often overpredict dangerousness on the basis that it is better to commit a person (commitment by itself is not thought likely to be harmful) than to allow that person to remain at large and possibly harm someone (Hiday 1977, 1988; Scheff 1984; Shah 1975; Stone 1975). According to Scheff (1984), this "medical decision rule" is based upon an important norm for dealing with uncertainty in medical diagnosis. This norm holds that it is better to judge a well person sick than to judge a sick person well. Scheff (1984) summarizes the logic of this approach with respect to mental health by pointing out that there is an element of danger to self or others in most cases of mental disorder; therefore, it may be better to risk unnecessary hospitalization than the harm that the patient might do to himself or herself or others.

In discussing the bias among physicians toward finding illness, Eliot Freidson states that because the work of the physician is supposed to be for the good of the patient,

> the health professional typically assumes that it is better to impute disease than to deny it and risk overlooking or missing it. This posture is in contrast with the legal sector, in which it is assumed that it is better to allow a guilty man to go free than to mistakenly convict an innocent man. In short, the decision-rule guiding the medical activity of practitioners to be safe by diagnosing illness rather than health.[40]

Psychiatrists, then, in line with their medical training, seem generally to follow the "safe" approach and to commit individuals who might be harmless, rather than to fail to commit persons who might attempt to kill or harm themselves or other people. Too often, psychiatrists have been taken to task by people in their community for failing to commit someone who later proved dangerous. As Allen Fagin (1976:519) explains, psychiatrists almost never find out about patients for whom they have been wrong in predicting violence. But they almost always learn about their errors in predicting nonviolence, and often it is from newspapers telling of the crime. "The fact that errors of underestimating the possibilities of violence are more visible than errors of overestimating," states Fagin (1976:519), "inclines the psychiatrist—whether consciously or unconsciously—to err on the side of confining rather than releasing. His modus operandi becomes: When in doubt, don't let them out." We can see an example of that attitude in Scheff's study of the screening process for civil commitment in a midwestern state. One medical examiner employed by the court was reported as saying:

---

[40]Eliot Freidson, *Profession of Medicine* (New York: Dodd, Mead, 1970), pp. 255–56.

We always take the conservative side. [Commitment or observation] Suppose a patient should commit suicide. We always make the conservative decision. I had rather play it safe. There's no harm in doing it that way.[41]

The result is that the great majority of mental patients involuntarily committed on the grounds of being dangerous to self, others, or property may not really be dangerous and can be categorized as "false positives." A false positive is a person who is predicted to act in a certain manner and who does not do so. In contrast, a "true positive" is someone who does act as predicted.

The most important influence on a psychiatrist's decision to commit an individual is that person's alleged offense. The more violent the offense, the more likely it is that psychiatrists (and courts) will reach a finding of dangerousness (Cocozza and Steadman 1976; Hiday 1977, 1988; Levinson and Ramsay 1979).

Although the decision to commit is a judicial one, Cocozza and Steadman note that the courts tend to acquiesce in favor of what psychiatrists recommend as expert witnesses. In their study, they found that recommendations by psychiatrists in regard to the probability of dangerous behavior were accepted by the court in 87 percent of the cases. Other research in Milwaukee found that the average length of time for a civil commitment hearing was thirteen minutes, during which the judges routinely accepted the psychiatrists' conclusions (Zander 1976). Usually, the psychiatrists would make rather sweeping statements to the effect that the patient suffered from a major psychiatric disorder and would be dangerous to others, without going into any details. Nor would they be asked to explain the basis for their opinion or what they meant by saying that a patient was "dangerous." One attorney, representing a patient, approached a judge after a hearing decided in favor of commitment, and remarked that he really did not think full-time inpatient hospitalization was necessary for his client. The judge replied, "My feelings are the same as yours, but I can't disregard the expert testimony" (Zander 1976:526).

There is research showing that judges seem more willing and in need of less certainty to commit people than psychiatrists (Simon and Cockerham 1977). If psychiatrists tend to be predisposed toward commitment (as Scheff, 1984, and others report) on the grounds that commitment in itself is not harmful and may be beneficial and that it is better to protect society by recommending commitment than to gamble on possible harmful conduct, judges may subscribe to this tendency even more than psychiatrists. The implications of this for defendants in civil commitment cases is that both judges and psychiatrists tend to lean toward commitment but that judges may be more likely to do so because they have greater responsibility for protecting society from harm.

---

[41]Thomas J. Scheff, "The Societal Reaction to Deviance: Ascriptive Elements in the Psychiatric Screening of Mental Patients in a Midwestern State," *Social Problems* 11 (1964), 410.

In sum, the concept of dangerousness remains highly controversial and no doubt misrepresents the mental state of many patients who are involuntarily committed under its auspices. Yet the potential for dangerousness continues to be the primary basis for civil commitment.

FALSE COMMITMENT

When the first state mental hospitals were established in the United States during the early part of the nineteenth century, commitment laws were nonexistent or extremely lax. In some states, a person could be committed just on the word of someone else, supposedly responsible and of sound mind, that he or she needed hospitalization. This was particularly true in regard to husbands committing their wives on very little evidence. This deficiency was aided by the tendency to believe, as Richard Fox (1978:130) observed, the "common assumption that women possessed a weak nervous constitution and were particularly susceptible to breakdowns." This was changed in 1860 by the famous Illinois case of Mrs. E.P.W. Packard, who was committed to a state mental hospital on the word of her husband, the Reverend Packard, and required to stay there for three years. Mrs. Packard (who may actually have been mildly schizophrenic) claimed that her husband had simply wanted "to get rid of her." Her commitment had been legal under a state statute that read:

> *Married women* and *infants* who, in the judgment of the medical superintendent of the state asylum at Jacksonville are evidently insane or distracted, may be entered or detained in the hospital at the request of the *husband of the woman* or the guardian of the infant, *without evidence of insanity required in* other cases.[42]

The case of Mrs. Packard, who complained in two books and on a nationwide tour that her husband had "railroaded" her into a mental hospital, had a direct effect on several states by instituting trials by jury in civil commitment cases and otherwise tightening up their requirements for involuntary hospitalization. Even though there were occasional warnings during the remainder of the nineteenth century that the nation's commitment system threatened individual liberties and could result in a sane person being committed or "railroaded" into an insane asylum, by the early twentieth century false commitment had become less of a public concern.

This is not to say that all people sent to mental hospitals are insane. Fox (1978:136) explains that in San Francisco between 1906 and 1929, court records disclosed that "the insane comprised a motley assortment of deviants, some of whom were doubtless 'mentally ill' and incapable of caring for themselves, but others of whom appear from the record not to have been men-

---

[42]Thomas S. Szasz, *Law, Liberty, and Psychiatry* (New York: Collier, 1968), p. 58.

tally ill even when that elastic category is stretched to the limit." The people in this latter group were largely those who were "undesirables" for reasons of morals, personality, age, and so forth. Often they were a financial burden to their relatives or to the community, and civil commitment was a way of getting rid of the problem. The legal criterion for commitment was that a person was "so far disordered in mind" as to be a danger to self or others, but Fox found few examples of dangerous behavior in court records. Most people had simply shown inappropriate or peculiar behavior (for example, "wouldn't wear shoes and masturbated openly," or "acted silly and lost interest in things that should interest women," or "calls strangers 'brothers' and speaks exclusively on religious subjects"). "Commitment proceedings," states Fox (1978:137), "were initiated in most cases not because the behavior of the accused revealed either grave disability or destructiveness, but because relatives, doctors, police, or neighbors decided they could no longer tolerate his or her behavior."

Today, a person who is the subject of a hearing for civil commitment has, in many states, the right to an attorney (who is appointed by the court if the defendant cannot pay for legal services), the right to a hearing, and the right to a trial by jury. The person may also have the right to an independent psychiatric evaluation, the right to confront witnesses, and the right to bail, and the state may even be required to demonstrate that the person is dangerous "beyond a reasonable doubt." And if falsely committed, in some states the person has the right to sue for damages. Assuming one lives in a state that has all or most of these rights accorded by statute and has a capable attorney and perhaps the testimony of a psychiatrist to support one's claims to freedom, one can avoid false commitment.

Once committed involuntarily and not as a result of a criminal action, a person has only two ways to secure release from a mental hospital. One is to cooperate with the hospital staff and become certified by them as "cured" or no longer disturbed to the point that it is necessary to have one's freedom restricted. Of course, this means that the person has to accept the hospital's idea of what is wrong with the individual, conform to the staff's notion of the "ideal" or "good" patient, and impress the staff sufficiently that one is normal enough to be released. The second way to gain release from a mental hospital is to hire a lawyer and file a writ of habeas corpus on the grounds that one's freedom has been abridged. That action will result in a legal hearing for release. A problem with that, however, which is common to most proceedings in which a person attempts to avoid civil commitment, is that it requires having a psychiatrist testify on one's behalf that another psychiatrist is wrong. Professionals are sometimes reluctant to make such statements in court against their colleagues.

An example of the use of habeas corpus to secure release from a mental hospital is a highly publicized 1960 case in Louisiana. This involved the governor of Louisiana, Earl Long. Governor Long had reportedly "gone off his rocker" during the May session of the state legislature in attempting to push through civil rights legislation that revoked a law that had stood since Reconstruction and gave parish (county) registrars the authority to disqualify black voters. The law was strongly supported by a white racist element in the legislature. Tired, overworked, on a diet (which probably did not help his disposition), and having problems with his wife and the legislature, Long became exhausted and incoherent. His wife had him flown to Texas to be committed for psychiatric treatment.

Once in Texas, Long managed to persuade a judge in Houston to release him on the basis of a promise to readmit himself to a mental hospital in Louisiana. Long, after all, was a resident of Louisiana and not Texas. Long returned to Louisiana, checked himself into a private mental hospital in New Orleans, and promptly checked himself out again. He then headed for Baton Rouge, the state capital, to assume power as governor, but he was stopped by sheriff's deputies. They arrested him at the request of his wife, who had him committed to the state hospital at Mandeville. Long telephoned his lawyer, who drove to Mandeville and found him sitting naked in a locked room. Long had the attorney obtain a writ of habeas corpus, which allowed him to regain his liberty temporarily, pending a final hearing. Long returned to the capital, assumed power as governor, and promptly *fired* the state director of the Department of Hospitals and the superintendent of the mental hospital at Mandeville, who, in the usual course of events, would have testified in court that he was mentally disturbed. He also fired any other staff members who might have testified against him. And then he took a vacation in the West with a favorite New Orleans showgirl.

A. J. Liebling (1961), a writer for the *New Yorker* magazine, went to Louisiana to investigate the story. Liebling found few people, even among Long's enemies, who believed he was really insane. Although some people saw his frantic betting at horse races, his impulsive purchases of such items as nearly fifty cases of cantaloupes and several hundred dollars' worth of cowboy boots at roadside stands, his endless long distance telephone calls throughout the night, arguments with friends, and his romance with a stripper as evidence that he was mentally ill—other people saw this conduct during Long's vacation to be evidence that Long was indeed his usual self. People who knew him pointed out that he had always been like that. He was obviously a colorful character, and found a writ of habeas corpus to be a useful measure in avoiding incarceration for his noncriminal behavior.

INSANITY AS A DEFENSE IN A CRIMINAL TRIAL

A traditional defense against prosecution in Anglo-American law has been to admit one's guilt but to claim insanity as the cause in order to escape punishment (Finkel 1988; Goldstein 1967; La Fond and Durham 1992). Typically, then, the defense of insanity is raised only in those criminal cases in which the defendant takes the position that "I committed the crime, but I am not responsible for my actions because I did not know what I was doing by reason of insanity." By introducing this defense, the defendant is in effect conceding that he or she cannot demonstrate innocence in the conventional manner. Thus, the defendant attempts to shift responsibility away from himself or herself to the presence of mental disorder. The culprit then becomes the "mental disorder" in that *it* kept the person from doing whatever a normal person would have done in those circumstances. At that point, says Abraham Goldstein (1967:19), "the search becomes one for information regarding what the accused was *really* thinking when he committed the crime, how he was *really* functioning, rather than for inferences drawn from his acts at the time of the crime."

Usually, the insanity defense is raised only in the case of an individual who is competent to stand trial. Insanity in some cases precludes an individual from standing trial because of being unable to understand the charges against him or her or to assist the lawyer in preparing a defense. If found mentally ill, the defendant will be committed in all likelihood to a hospital for the criminally insane. He or she might remain there even longer than if sentenced to prison. Yet defendants can be severely mentally ill and still be legally competent to stand trial, as determined in *Adams v. United States*,[43] because, as Ennis and Emery (1978) explain, the real issues in competency evaluations are essentially legal issues. The most relevant issue is the defendant's ability to understand the nature and consequences of a guilty plea. If the defendant can do this, a trial can be held. Whether a defendant can help in his or her defense, is willing or able to testify, or can stand the strain of a prolonged court hearing is decided by the lawyer and the client. The burden of the defense falls not on the defendant but on the attorney.

The use of mental disorder as an excuse for criminal action can be traced to the reign of Edward I (1272–1307) of England. The landmark case in Anglo-American law that established the modern-day approach to the insanity defense is the 1843 *M'Nagthen* case.[44] While operating under the paranoid delusion that he was being persecuted by certain people, M'Nagthen mistakenly killed the secretary of a man he really intended to kill. He was found not guilty by reason of insanity and sent to a mental hospital. The M'Nagthen rule that came out of this trial and became so influential in subsequent, similar hearings was the following:

> . . . that to establish a defence on the grounds of insanity, it must be clearly proved that, at the time of the committing of the act, the party accused was labouring under such a defect of reason, from disease of the mind, as not to

---

[43] *Adams v. United States*, 297 F. Suppl. 596 (S.D.N.Y. 1969).
[44] *M'Nagthen's Case*, 10 Clark & Fin. 200 (1843).

know the nature and quality of the act he was doing; or if he did know it, that he did not know he was doing what was wrong.[45]

A major problem with the M'Nagthen rule is that some critics took the view that it referred to intellectual awareness alone and did not take emotional feelings into account (Goldstein 1967). Consequently, a supplement to the M'Nagthen rule evolved, which was the *irresistible impulse test*. This test holds that there are certain situations in which people are irresistibly driven to act in certain ways. In other words, they lose control of themselves through an over-stimulation of emotions—such as when a man discovers his wife in bed with another man and commits murder. This kind of action would be placed under the category of "accident" because it is not planned or purposefully executed. The irresistible impulse test was very popular during the 1930s because it played to the strengths of psychoanalytic theory and emphasized the motivating influences behind emotions. However, in what Goldstein (1967:68) calls "a remarkable reversal of opinion," the test has been rejected in most states because it adds little to the M'Nagthen rule, is impossible to apply with any scientific accuracy, and expands the insanity-as-a-defense concept too far for many courts. Indiana, for example, excludes the irresistible impulse as a separate and independent excuse for the commission of a criminal act.[46] However, the irresistible impulse test persists in some states. In a highly publicized 1994 case in a county court in Manassas, Virginia, a woman, Lorena Bobbitt, was acquitted of criminal charges in cutting off her husband's penis on the grounds of temporary insanity. A jury concluded that she had yielded to an irresistible impulse after being raped by her husband. Before that event, Mrs. Bobbitt had allegedly suffered continued physical and psychological abuse from her spouse.

In 1954, the M'Nagthen rule was superseded by the *Durham rule*.[47] The greatest criticism of the M'Nagthen rule was that if it were to be applied strictly, it would be applicable only to people with psychotic symptoms. It did not address the whole range of mental disorders and thus was not a comprehensive measure of insanity. The Durham rule was hailed as a great advance at the time because it offered a "broader test." The basic premise of the Durham rule was that an accused person cannot be held criminally responsible if his or her unlawful act is the "product of mental disease or mental defect." This approach suggested that there are two modes of social existence for the court to consider in a trial in which insanity is a defense: the sane and the insane. If a person is insane (as broadly defined), he or she is therefore not blameworthy of the criminal act in question. The question of insanity was to be a "matter of fact" to be determined by a jury as it interpreted the evidence.

---

[45] *M'Nagthen's Case*, footnote 44.

[46] *Benefiel* v. *Indiana*, 578 N.E. 2d 338 (Ind. Sup. Ct. 1991).

[47] *Durham* v. *United States*, 94 U.S. App. D.C. 228, 214 F.2d 862 (1954).

The Durham rule had its problems, too. In practice it was vague and led to the undue dominance of court proceedings by psychiatrists as expert witnesses. There was no generally accepted understanding by juries or by most laypeople of what was meant by "product of mental disease." It was necessary to rely on experts testifying on the nature of the "product." Here, "product" referred to the outcome of a disorder rather than the disorder itself. As a result, psychiatrists, in defining "product," were defining a concept that is legal and ethical instead of medical. In essence, psychiatrists found themselves making legal conclusions rather than stating medical opinions.

In 1955, the year after the Durham rule, the American Law Institute (ALI) rejected the advice of its own psychiatric committee and did not endorse the Durham rule. Instead, it drafted its own recommendations on mental disorder for its Model Penal Code and came up with a different formulation: the ALI rule, which states:

> (1) A person is not responsible for criminal conduct if at the time of such conduct as a result of mental disease or defect he lacks substantial capacity either to appreciate the criminality of his conduct or to conform his conduct to the requirements of law.
> (2) As used in this Article, the terms "mental disease or defect" do not include an abnormality manifested only by repeated criminal or otherwise antisocial conduct.[48]

According to Goldstein (1967:87), the ALI rule "is a modernized and much improved rendition of *M'Nagthen* and the 'control tests.' " The key words in the first paragraph of the rule are "appreciate," which implies awareness, and "conform," which gets away from the notions of "control," and "irresistible impulse." The word "appreciate" is intended to describe an impairment of feeling or judgment rather than cognition. It describes a state of mind that is insufficiently aware of, or sensitive to, the consequences of one's behavior, because of mental disorder. Also, the ALI rule requires only "substantial incapacity" rather than a total loss of mental reality and normal functioning. The result is that the ALI rule is midway between the M'Nagthen rule (criticized as too limited) and the Durham rule (criticized as too broad). Moreover, the language of the ALI rule requires psychiatrists to judge medical matters (that is, the extent of the "mental disease or defect") and not the outcome ("product") of a disorder. By 1995, twenty states had adopted the ALI rule, twenty-eight states followed the M'Nagthen rule, one state (New Hampshire) had the Durham rule, and one state (Idaho) had abolished the insanity defense.

In 1984, however, a dramatic change took place in insanity laws with the passage of the Insanity Defense Reform Act. This law was passed by Congress as

---

[48]American Law Institute, *Model Penal Code* (1962), par. 4.01.

a result of adverse public reaction to the acquittal of John Hinckley, Jr., in the attempted assassination of President Ronald Reagan in 1981. Hinckley was found innocent by reason of insanity, even though he shot and wounded the president and three others.[49] Because Hinckley, tried in a federal court in the District of Columbia, had claimed insanity as his defense, the government could convict him only if it could prove that he was sane at the time of the shooting. The jury in the case had some doubt that he was completely sane and therefore was required to find him not guilty. Hinckley did not have to serve a prison sentence but was committed to a mental hospital until such time that a judge (on the recommendation of a psychiatrist) decides that he can go free.

The Insanity Defense Reform Act has two principal provisions: (1) It provides that whether a defendant is insane is to be determined by deciding if, at the time of the act, the defendant was unable to appreciate the nature and quality or wrongfulness of his or her act; and (2) it shifts to the defendant the burden of proving by clear and convincing evidence the defense of insanity. Consequently, in criminal cases involving insanity currently tried in all federal courts and many state jurisdictions, the *defendant* must now prove that he or she was insane at the time the crime was committed—instead of the government having to prove that the defendant was sane. Thus, the burden of proof is clearly shifted to the defense instead of the prosecution. As of 1995, thirty-eight states place the burden of proof in insanity as a defense on the defendant, and twelve states still require the state to prove sanity if the insanity defense is raised in criminal trials.[50]

Usually, being found insane and therefore not responsible for one's criminal act does not lead to freedom. It leads to confinement, often long-term, in a mental hospital and to psychiatric treatment. This is seen in a 1993 federal court decision in Kansas where it was held that a person found not guilty by reason of insanity cannot be released from treatment because of the potential for dangerousness.[51] Once one's mental condition has been improved or restored, that person may be returned for a hearing to determine whether further criminal prosecution and perhaps prison are in order. Or the person may be set free. In 1992, the United States Supreme Court overturned a Louisiana law under which people found not guilty of a crime by reason of insanity must remain in a mental institution, even if no longer insane, until they can prove they are no longer dangerous.[52] The court held that once an

---

[49] *United States* v. *Hinckley*, Crim. 81–306 (D.D.C. 1982).

[50] The twelve states leaving the burden of proof on the state are Colorado, Florida, Kansas, Massachusetts, Michigan, Mississippi, New Mexico, North Dakota, Oklahoma, South Dakota, Tennessee, and Utah.

[51] *United States* v. *Burns*, 812 F. Suppl. 190 (D. Kan. 1993).

[52] *Foucha* v. *Louisiana*, 112 U.S. 1780 (1992).

inmate is no longer mentally ill, dangerousness alone is not a constitutionally adequate reason for continued confinement.

Few defendants claim insanity as a defense because it is difficult to prove and is expensive; fewer still are acquitted by reason of insanity (LaFond and Durham 1992; Simon and Aaronson 1988). Typically, the defense is used only in very serious crimes in which lengthy confinement in a hospital for the criminally insane is preferred to the likely consequences of a criminal conviction (that is, death or a life sentence) and evidence of possible insanity exists.

THE RIGHT TO TREATMENT

Another significant legal issue with implications for social policy is the mental patient's right to treatment. In the past, mental patients have often had no rights at all, and mental hospitals were nothing more than warehouses for society's undesirables. In contemporary society, the role of the mental hospital is not just custodial but also therapeutic (or at least is intended to be). A landmark legal decision in this regard is the 1966 *Rouse* v. *Cameron* case in the District of Columbia.[53] Rouse was confined for psychiatric treatment, and he demanded that it be provided when it was allegedly not forthcoming. The court held simply that the hospital should try to provide such treatment and that failure to do so could not be justified by a lack of resources. This decision implied that there might be a constitutional right to treatment.

Then in 1971 came the *Wyatt* v. *Stickney* case in Alabama. Alabama had three mental institutions at that time, one for whites, one for blacks, and one for the mentally retarded. A federal court in 1965 had ordered that the three institutions be integrated. Each of the institutions was overcrowded, understaffed, and seriously underfinanced. Conditions in these institutions were reportedly very bad. The state delayed in honoring the court order for integration and consequently lost several million dollars in federal subsidies for the hospitals. A fiscal crisis followed, which made hospital conditions even worse than before. Over a hundred employees, including psychologists, social workers, and occupational therapists, were laid off. Finally, several employees and a patient, Ricky Wyatt, brought suit in federal court to halt the firing of employees on the grounds that it would prohibit treatment for many of the patients. The court held in the case of *Wyatt* v. *Stickney* that although the hospital had the right to fire its employees, it also had the duty to provide treatment. The court stated:

---

[53] *Rouse* v. *Cameron*, 373 F. 2d 451 (D.C. Cir. 1966).

To deprive any citizen of his or her liberty upon the altruistic theory that confinement is for humane and therapeutic reasons and then fail to provide adequate treatment violates the very fundamentals of due process.[54]

The court in *Wyatt* v. *Stickney* also defined the minimum standards of care and stated that if the hospital could not provide such care, it could not hold a patient there against that patient's will. The Alabama state legislature refused to appropriate additional money to support the hospitals, and subsequently, many patients were released. Nevertheless, *Wyatt* v. *Stickney* gives patients the right to treatment or release.

As Arlene Kanter (1989:115) points out, the legal theory in *Wyatt* v. *Stickney* is straightforward: When the state deprives a person of liberty in order to provide treatment, it has an obligation to provide treatment. If treatment cannot be provided, the patient should be released. A subsequent U.S. Supreme Court decision expanded this view in 1975 in *O'Connor* v. *Donaldson* where the Court held that patients who are not dangerous to themselves and others, are receiving only custodial care, and are able to live in the community by themselves or with the help of family or friends cannot be institutionalized against their will.[55]

If mental patients have a right to treatment, the question logically arises as to whether they have the right to refuse treatment. The right to refuse treatment poses several problems, for it would require that patients be mentally competent to decide for themselves whether the treatment prescribed for them was appropriate. Yet how do you obtain "informed consent" from a mentally disturbed and legally incompetent person, and what are the implications of withholding psychiatric treatment from a patient involuntarily committed and in need of that treatment? A federal court in Boston in 1979 ruled that mental patients have the right to refuse the drugs and seclusion ordered by their physicians on the grounds that patients have a constitutional right to decide what happens to them in reference to psychiatric treatment.[56] Attorneys in the suit brought against Boston State Hospital argued that their clients had the right to reject medication, such as Thorazine and Haldol, used to control manic and violent behavior, because of the potential side effects of the drugs. It was shown that force had been used to administer the drugs to some of the defendants. It was the court's position that even though hospitalized mental patients do suffer at least some impairment of their ability to relate to reality, most are able to appreciate

---

[54]*Wyatt* v. *Stickney*, 325 F. Suppl. 781 (M.D. Ala. 1971); 334 F. Suppl. 1341 (M.D. Ala. 1971); enforced by 344 F. Suppl. 373, 344 F. Suppl. 387.

[55]*O'Connor* v. *Donaldson*, 422 U.S. 563 (1975).

[56]*Rogers* v. *Department of Mental Health*, 478 F. Suppl. 1342 (1979).

the benefits, risks, and discomfort that may be expected to result from receiving psychoactive drugs. However, the hospital staff was accorded the right to use force in rendering medication or seclusion if there was a substantial likelihood that the patient was a danger to self or others because of the high probability of suicide, violent behavior against others, or personal injury.

In *Washington* v. *Harper,* a 1990 U.S. Supreme Court decision, the Court ruled that inmates of prisons have only a limited constitutional right to refuse psychiatric medication.[57] It was held that, regardless of a prisoner's competency to make decisions about psychiatric medications, such drugs can be administered involuntarily, following an independent administrative hearing in which a majority of the panel agree that the prisoner is mentally ill and dangerous to self or others, and that the medication is in the prisoner's medical interest. In such situations, the state's concerns will outweigh those of the prisoner. Although it is not clear to what extent the *Washington* v. *Harper* ruling will apply in nonprison settings, this decision is likely to provide an important basis for court intervention in treatment refusal cases generally.

The current trend in court decisions is that forced medication is to be permitted in emergencies, at least in institutions; but in nonemergencies and outside of institutions, the right to refuse treatment receives much stronger support (Kanter 1989). In *Rennie* v. *Klein,* for example, a federal appeals court held that an individual not committed to a mental institution has a right to refuse medication administered against his or her will.[58] And when civil authorities in New York City in a highly publicized act took a homeless woman off a sidewalk where she had been living for a year and a half, a state appeals court in the case of *Boggs* v. *New York City Health and Hospitals Corp.* determined that the woman could not be forcibly medicated in a nonemergency under New York law.[59] Finally, in *Riggins* v. *Nevada,* the United States Supreme Court ruled that a state cannot force a mentally ill defendant to take antipsychotic medications during a trial in which the person has claimed insanity as a defense without overriding justification.[60] An earlier safeguard provided by the Supreme Court in *Ake* v. *Oklahoma* was to require a state to give a defendant access to competent psychiatric assistance when (1) insanity is likely to be an issue at a trial and (2) the issue of future dangerousness has been raised by the prosecution.[61]

---

[57]*Washington* v. *Harper,* 494 U.S. 210 (1990).
[58]*Rennie* v. *Klein,* 653 F.2d 836, 843 (3d Cir. 1981).
[59]*Boggs* v. *New York City Health and Hospitals Corp.,* 523 N.Y.S. 2d 71 (N.Y. App. Div. 1987).
[60]*Riggins* v. *Nevada,* 112 U.S. 1810 (1992).
[61]*Ake* v. *Oklahoma,* 470 U.S. 68 (1985).

MENTAL HEALTH LAW AND SOCIAL CONTROL

Definitions of dangerousness, false commitment, insanity as a defense, and the right to treatment are bound up in a society's interest in maintaining social order, yet at the same time providing mentally disturbed patients with legal rights that will protect them as individuals from being unduly punished and being allowed no choice of what happens to them. Sociologists have tradition-ally focused on the concept of social control as harmonizing personal and group behavior with the general goals of society. The alternative to such control is, of course, chaos and a breakdown of social constraints that enable an orderly and less threatening life to exist. Mental health law, accordingly, is an expres-sion of a society's determination to remove mentally disturbed deviants from its midst and to place them in controlled settings, where they can receive treat-ment for their condition and, one hopes, be returned to normal functioning. For incurable patients, removal from society tends to be permanent, however.

Social control of the mentally disturbed is dependent upon subjective judgments of the behavior in question, because of the inexact nature of psy-chiatric practice. In most physical disorders, physicians can locate and treat identifiable diseases; in criminal law, cases do not come to trial unless it is clear that a crime has been committed. So in both medicine and criminal law, prac-titioners generally work with concrete cases in which there is clear, tangible evidence of either a health or a legal problem. Unfortunately, mental prob-lems are not subject to the same degree of consensus that is found elsewhere in medicine and law (although there can be disagreement and uncertainty in those areas), nor is there the tangible "proof" of a disorder, except in the most obvious cases. People are therefore committed to psychiatric facilities on the basis of how others view their behavior based on what they think is normal for the circumstances.

In attempting to formulate guidelines that allow a civilized society to incarcerate its citizens in the absence of an illegal act, the concept of danger-ousness was formulated as the capstone of the civil commitment process. This concept is consistent with the legal philosophy of criminal law in that it equates mental disorder with harm to self, others, or property. Because harmful con-duct cannot be tolerated in the interest of social order, the mentally disturbed, like criminals, thus become liable to removal from the mainstream of society. The justifications for this removal are, of course, that such people are *likely* to be harmful and that it can be shown they are also mentally ill—according to the professional judgment of psychiatrists who act as society's agents in such matters. Even though most mental patients committed on grounds of potential dangerousness are false positives, the dangerousness concept does provide a legal vehicle for getting the mentally ill out of the community and into a psy-chiatric hospital. This is the primary reason why the concept of dangerousness persists in mental health law and why it is likely to continue to persist, despite its inexactness. Currently, there is nothing better to replace it.

As for false commitment, we see it as a social problem when other mechanisms of social control (for example, the family, religion) fail and people turn to the state through the process of civil commitment to remove those they consider unpleasant, deviant, embarrassing, or obnoxious. Conversely, the persecuted in this situation can use the law through a writ of habeas corpus as a social control mechanism to restore them to their usual place in society, in the absence of acceptable evidence that their behavior is also mentally ill. Hence, when we see social control failing, we see the use of the law as a remedy to restore control, both on the part of those who would commit others and on the part of those committed who want their freedom. We also see an appeal to the law in the use of insanity as a defense in criminal trials. In this instance, social control has clearly failed, and the guilty individual attempts to avoid punishment by blaming a pathological mental condition. The law thereby becomes a way for them to obtain psychiatric treatment instead of life imprisonment or a death sentence. In sum, use of law seems to increase when the influence of other social controls decreases.

Once a person is committed, the norms of a humane society demand that the person receive therapeutic care to alleviate the condition. This was not always so in the past, with the result that there have been increasing demands for the right to treatment, with patients having some control over the type of treatment they receive. Again, this result is essentially one of social control in that it promotes cooperation between patient and practitioner, supposedly leading to better conditions for the insane. This is in accordance with society's desire to restore mental patients, if possible, to a normal life. It restrains an institution's attempts to do what is best for the institution rather than what is best for the individual patient and ultimately society. This assumes, however, that mental patients demanding the right of treatment are able to make decisions regarding their own welfare. After all, in the final analysis, mental health law does pertain to the welfare of society and the individual. For society, mental health is intended to control deviant behavior; for the individual, mental health law is intended to protect a person's interests and allow him or her to obtain treatment. In both instances, problems are theoretically solved and social order is maintained.

SUMMARY

The purpose of this chapter has been to review the current state of mental health law as an expression of public policy. Mental health law is an unsettled field, continuing to change and develop as it moves toward more definitive concepts, legal safeguards, and the establishment of rights for mental patients for whom in the past there were none. Most of this chapter was devoted to examining the various issues in the concept of "dangerousness" as grounds for civil commitment to a mental hospital. This concept is the most controversial in mental health law today and is still unresolved. It requires that mentally ill patients be committed involuntarily because they are likely to be a danger to self, others, or property. The likelihood of such action depends upon the assessment of psychiatrists, who have a demonstrated tendency to overpredict dangerousness and to commit many people who are, in fact, harmless. Other issues discussed in this chapter include the problems of establishing a legal standard reflecting society's and the individual's needs in determining the parameters of false commitment, insanity as a defense, and the right to treatment.

15

Mental Disorder and Public Policy in Selected Countries

This chapter discusses mental health policy in Great Britain, Italy, Germany, and China, four countries that have opted for an emphasis on community care of the mentally ill. Mental health policy in Japan and Poland is also reviewed for comparative purposes. An examination of the experiences of other nations in dealing with mental disorder helps to place the American situation in an international perspective. All countries formulate policies to cope with mental illness and can learn from one another in determining the best approach in dealing with the problem.

GREAT BRITAIN

Mental health services in Great Britain have undergone significant changes since the 1960s (Goldberg and Huxley 1980; Jones 1988; Miles 1981; Pilgrim and Rogers 1993; Ramon 1994). The strategy used to implement change was the Mental Health Act of 1959, which formally recommended an "open-door" policy for mental patients. The idea was that patients would be as free to seek help for mental disorders as they were for physical illnesses. Mental patients were also to be treated in the least restrictive environment compatible with their safety and the safety of the general public. That meant that the majority of patients would be given treatment in community settings and in most cases continue to live at home. Hospitalization, if necessary, would take place largely on a voluntary basis, and most patients would be kept on unlocked wards. For those patients who were a threat to themselves or other people, the National Health Service Act of 1977 set aside four special mental hospitals to house the criminally insane and others considered violent or dangerous. Since 1960, admissions to mental hospitals in England alone have declined over 50 percent from 135,000 patients in 1960 to about 50,000 in 1990 (Pilgrim and Rogers 1993).

However, implementing a community mental health program was not as easy as planning it. As Kathleen Jones (1988) explains, funding was limited, rising admissions to mental hospitals caused significant overcrowding and poor living conditions, and a series of allegations about the mistreatment of mental hospital patients by male nurses received extensive media attention in the 1970s. Gradually, funding was somewhat improved, overcrowding reduced, and reports of cruelty to patients investigated and dealt with. A few nurses were sentenced to prison.

Although the overall care of mental patients improved during the 1980s, significant problems remain with respect to the funding of health care delivery in general and for mental health in particular. Great Britain is not a wealthy country, and its spending on health lags behind that of many other advanced nations. Britain spends about 6 percent of its gross domestic product on health care, which exceeds that of Greece and is about the same as Spain and Denmark but ranks behind the other Western European countries, Canada, and the United States. There are political issues as well. One major dispute is over whether community care for the mentally ill should be controlled by local authorities or the National Health Service. The 1988 Griffiths Report recommended local control over community care, but this measure was strongly opposed by the central government, since it involved authority over large amounts of funding (Jones 1988).

Great Britain's National Health Service was formed in 1948 when the government took responsibility for health care delivery. The government assumed the ownership of hospitals and became the employer of physicians and the other health care workers. Health services were financed out of tax revenues, and care was provided free to patients. The first line of medical care remained the general practitioner, who screens all patients and decides whether to provide treatment or refer the patient to a specialist (called a "consultant") or to a hospital. Although some patients receive care on a private basis and are responsible for paying for the services rendered, the great majority are treated free of charge by the National Health Service.

Great Britain, like the United States, emphasizes community care for mental illness. The first level of care for mental problems is the general practitioner, who treats directly about 95 percent of all patients with psychiatric complaints (Goldberg and Huxley 1980). Normally, a patient is not referred to a psychiatrist unless he or she does not respond to initial treatment. Most mentally disturbed people continue to live in their usual environment and to be seen by their local doctor. Or they may be placed in group homes. While the general practitioners provide medical care (typically psychoactive drugs), social workers deal with the patient's social problems. Consequently, mentally disturbed people in Great Britain do not usually go directly to a psychiatrist for treatment, but must first be seen by a general practitioner, who decides whether to refer the patient to a specialist. Admissions to mental hospitals, however, are usually made through psychiatrists. Nearly 90 percent of all mental hospital admissions are voluntary (Goldberg and Huxley 1980), with schizophrenia and depressive disorders the two leading diagnoses (Ramon 1994).

To meet community needs, the number of psychiatric units in general hospitals has been increased, community mental health centers have been established (fifty-four such centers existed in 1987), the use of community psychiatric nurses has increased, and greater emphasis has been placed on voluntary services and informal care by family and friends (Pilgrim and Rogers 1993).

To prevent former mental patients from being lost and neglected in the community, the 1990 National Health Service and Community Care Act stipulates that patients cannot be discharged from mental hospitals without a plan for care in the community; however, implementation of the plan is not mandatory—only planning is obligatory (Ramon 1994). In reality, adequate housing and services in many British communities for mental patients are lacking, and government funding for such services remains low. As in the United States, deinstitutionalization in Britain has not been a great success (Hollingsworth and Hollingsworth 1994; Ramon 1994).

ITALY

Italy has taken an extreme approach to community care of the mentally ill by essentially abolishing mental hospitals (Bollini, Reich, and Muscettola 1988; Donnelly 1992; Isaac and Armat 1990; Jones 1988). Public Law 180, passed in 1978, completely rearranged the organization of Italian psychiatric services. This law stipulated that no new patients could be admitted to mental hospitals, that small (fifteen-bed) psychiatric units were to be established in general hospitals, that patients could stay only forty-eight hours in these units (or seven days with a court order), and that alternative structures were to be set up in the community. The law also decreed that no new mental hospitals could be constructed, so that ultimately Italy's system of mental hospitals would disappear as the inpatient population declined with the end of new admissions or readmissions after discharge. Regional governments were given the responsibility to carry out the legislation in a manner consistent with local needs.

This action, as Paola Bollini and his colleagues (1988) explain, came during a period of general reform of Italy's health care system and was the primary goal of *Psichiatria Democratica* (Democratic Psychiatry) reform movement. This movement had developed under the leadership of Franco Basaglia, a hospital psychiatrist in northwest Italy who had tried to develop a program of community services for the mentally ill in his hometown but was prevented from doing so by the local government. In 1971, however, Basaglia became director of mental health services in Trieste, near the former Yugoslav border. According to Jones (1988), Basaglia was a gifted clinician and able to inspire both patients and hospital staffs to try new approaches. He had worked in a community mental health center in New York City and was familiar with the antipsychiatric views of Michel Foucault (1965), R. D. Laing (1967, 1969), and Thomas Szasz (1968, 1970, 1974).

Receiving considerable support from left-wing groups, Basaglia made the treatment of the mentally ill a major political issue by arguing that mental patients were discriminated against and forced to live on the margin of society. In Trieste, for example, mental patients were held involuntarily in a mental hospital on the edge of town. What could be more marginal than that? reasoned Basaglia. He proceeded to discharge patients and establish psychosocial centers that patients could visit as they wished. Group homes were established where small numbers of patients could be assisted by psychiatric aides, social workers, nurses, and psychiatrists. Basaglia, who died in 1980, believed that confinement in a mental hospital was inhumane and essentially political, a measure to remove undesirables from the mainstream of society. His ideas gained in popularity, aided by media accounts of poor conditions in many mental hospitals, and they formed the basis for Italy's psychiatric reform.

Just how effective these reforms have been is contained in an account by Jones (1988). Jones visited Trieste first and visited the city's psychosocial centers. She reports:

> . . . the centres in the city . . . are cheerful, casual and informal. There are no appointments—patients come when they wish, for as long as they wish, and are on first-name terms with staff. The only formal event is the daily meeting, at which staff and patients who wish to attend can discuss anything of the moment—the running of the centre, the problems of individuals, the nature of mental illness, or their daily experiences, in the Italian manner, there is much hugging and exclaiming and hand-holding, and there are many cigarettes and cups of coffee. A good lunch is provided in a nearby cafe, or in the centre itself. The contrast between this cheerful, happy and spontaneous interaction, and the strained atmosphere of the average outpatient clinic is marked.
>
> Patients are housed in the surrounding area—some in their own accommodation, some in group flats. Community nurses (usually unqualified but with mental hospital experience) call regularly, helping patients with cooking, cleaning, and shopping. One chops garlic in a spotless little kitchen. Another breezes in with bags of shopping, exclaiming at the prices. They are mostly young, and wear jeans and T-shirts. Though they also check medication and call in the psychiatrist when required, these professional duties are subordinated to a simple friendliness and companionability.[1]

---

[1]Kathleen Jones, *Experience in Mental Health* (London: Sage, 1988), pp. 56–57.

Jones found some of these patients to be severely disturbed, most likely schizophrenic, but they were aware of their problems, and received a great deal of social support from other patients and the staff, and doctors were on call to help them. The mental hospital in Trieste was an entirely different situation, however. Some patients, referred to as "guests," were still living there, and those with highly severe forms of mental disorder were locked up. Other patients were elderly and suffering from afflictions associated with old age; the mental health service did not provide care to patients over the age of sixty-five, and their wards were poorly maintained and locked. Besides the elderly, the mental health service does not treat adolescents (who are the responsibility of their families), the mentally retarded, drug abusers, and inpatients choosing to remain in the mental hospitals. Consequently, many groups are excluded from community care.

The question thus arises as to how far the reforms have spread. In traveling throughout Italy, Jones found that the Trieste area was the best; it has an international character, ample housing, and a supportive local government. Other urban centers, however, have an acute housing shortage, and many former mental hospital patients have joined the population of the homeless. The small psychiatric units in general hospitals were usually the worst accommodations in those facilities, and some patients stayed there for months—not the forty-eight hours required by law. And despite efforts by the staffs in some mental hospitals to improve conditions for the inmates, many hospitals were run-down and understaffed, with unattractive living conditions. In some hospitals, maintenance work had virtually ceased, and there was no new construction. Few hospitals had any organized activities for their patients. And some patients continued to be locked up (having agreed to restraint to remain there), although technically they were "guests." "Guests" were found locked on wards, placed in straitjackets, and strapped to their beds. Mental hospitals in the south of Italy were especially bad; Jones (1988:67) states, for example, that the "conditions in some hospitals in the south must be among the most inadequate to be found anywhere in Western Europe."

Italy's psychiatric reforms are uneven. In areas like Trieste and elsewhere in the north, the reforms have seen some success. In the south, the poorest and most underdeveloped area of the country, expectations have not been met. As Jones (1988) and Bollini and his associates (1988) observe, important regional differences in the implementation of Italy's psychiatric reforms persist. Both Jones and Bollini and associates found a much larger mental hospital population in the south, and considerably fewer facilities and staff personnel for community care. In addition, the south had significantly higher rates of severely disabling disorders like schizophrenia and dementia than the north. Bollini and associates state:

> Many factors probably contribute to this difference: a true higher prevalence of severe mental disorders in Southern Italy due to low socioeconomic status; cul-

tural differences in family attitudes, with Southern Italy's extended families being able to cope with most mentally ill members but not with the most disturbed; an inadequate provision and quality of mental health facilities in the South, limiting access for milder cases but providing services for the most severe and disabled cases.[2]

At the present, the Italian government is reviewing the effects of psychiatric reform and considering major revisions of the law. Deinstitutionalization in Italy has produced many of the same problems as found in Britain and the United States (Donnelly 1992).

GERMANY

Germany has an unfortunate history in psychiatry. During the 1933–45 Nazi period, large numbers of mentally ill and mentally retarded people were put to death by lethal injections, by overdoses of sedatives, and later by gassing (Lifton 1986). These activities were carried out as part of a "life unworthy of life" eugenics program that reflected the Nazi obsession with racial superiority and later became a prototype for the Holocaust. Families were informed that the patients had died of pneumonia or other natural causes, since the program was kept hidden from the general public. Arthur Kleinman (1988) describes this period as psychiatry's darkest hour.

The situation in modern Germany, however, is far different. German mental patients today are treated within an extensive system of mental hospitals, psychiatric wards in general hospitals, psychiatric clinics, group homes, and the offices of private practitioners. As in the United States, most German patients receive care in community settings, and large networks of outpatient psychiatric services exist in major urban areas; rural patients are generally treated by local doctors, usually general practitioners, with more serious cases sent to regional psychiatric hospitals (Dilling and Weyerer 1984; Häfner 1987).

Germany has a system of government-sponsored national health insurance that covers the cost of mental health services for approximately 94 percent of the German population. Those persons excluded from the national health insurance programs are the most wealthy whose income exceeds the limits for government coverage; they can purchase national health insurance coverage or private health insurance. Otherwise, participation in the national program is mandatory, and Germans are required to be insured by one of Germany's public health insurance organizations. There are several different health insurance groups, and membership in a particular plan is usually determined by one's occupation or place of employment. About 12.6 percent of a

---

[2]Paola Bollini, Michael Reich, and Giovanni Muscettola, "Revision of the Italian Psychiatric Reform: North/South Differences and Future Strategies," *Social Science and Medicine* 26 (1988), 1333.

worker's monthly gross earnings goes to pay for health insurance, with half paid by the employee and half by the employer. Special provisions are made for the unemployed and the self-employed. Health care is free to the individual, and the costs of care are paid by the public health insurance companies based upon a set schedule of fees established through negotiation between the insurance companies and organizations representing doctors and hospitals. The government monitors and regulates the system.

Although insurance coverage for mental health services is widely available, and an extensive network of psychiatric facilities and practitioners is in place, this does not mean that the German system lacks problems. Most countries, including Germany, still do not have enough well-equipped and well-staffed psychiatric units in general hospitals and a well-functioning network of complementary services in the community to discharge the majority of patients requiring long-term hospital care (Häfner 1987). Some mental hospitals have inadequate facilities to house large numbers of patients, and mental health is not among the highest priorities in the financing of health care services (Thielen 1986).

In many ways, the Germans face the same obstacles as Americans in providing psychiatric care to the general population. However, there are some important differences between Germany and the United States as well. First, mental health may not be perceived as a serious social problem in Germany to the degree it is in the United States (Müller 1985). Second, some beliefs of Germans and Americans about mental disorders are fundamentally different. Germans tend to think that mental problems either are emotional disturbances caused by stress and are transitory, or are genetic in origin, long-term, and relatively incurable; Americans, on the other hand, tend to believe that mental disorders can generally be overcome through professional care, personal effort, and willpower (Townsend 1978). Thus, Germans tend to show greater pessimism about outcomes for severely disabled mental patients. And third, Germany has a highly developed system of spas in which patients suffering from anxiety and affective disorders, tension, stress, and other problems can be treated through rehabilitation medicine (the *Kur*)—involving therapeutic baths and drinking water from local mineral springs, special diets, walks through gardens, hiking, and rest and relaxation in a pleasant environment (Maretzki 1987). These treatments are covered by national health insurance and are widely used.

The extent of mental disorder in the general German population is not known, because few studies of psychiatric epidemiology have been conducted. Sociological research in the area of mental health is practically nonexistent, and the field of social psychiatry is highly underdeveloped (Angermeyer 1986; Müller 1985; Siedow 1985). The reason for this seems to be that psychiatry is not a focal point of public interest, nor generally considered an attractive area of research (Müller 1985). Epidemiological studies in psychiatry have been generally limited to the Mannheim area (Häfner 1986, 1987) and some field studies in Northrhine-Westphalia (Cockerham et al. 1988) and rural Bavaria (Dilling and Weyerer 1984; Fichter and Weyerer 1985; Weyerer and Dilling 1984). Germans appear to have relatively low rates of anxiety in comparison with other Europeans (O'Brien 1984); in comparison with Americans, Germans may have somewhat higher rates of depression but otherwise are not essentially different when it comes to anxiety tendencies or overall psychological distress (Cockerham et al. 1988).

CHINA

China has focused on community care as the only way it can realistically cope with mental disorder in a large, underdeveloped nation of over one billion people and relatively limited resources. Furthermore, the Chinese claim that there is much less mental illness in their country than in Western society (Butterfield 1989; Cockerham 1984; Kleinman and Mechanic 1979; Livingston and Lowinger 1983; Mechanic and Kleinman 1980). Whether that is actually the case is not known, because of a lack of data and official statistics, and assertions of an ideological nature espousing the virtues of Chinese-style communism for mental health that cannot be independently verified (Cockerham 1984; Kleinman and Mechanic 1979; Jones 1988).

Arthur Kleinman and David Mechanic (1979) point out other difficulties in ascertaining the extent of mental disorder in China. They note that mentally disordered people in China have historically been subject to stigma, and there may still be a reluctance to label someone mentally ill. It also appears that there is a tendency to diagnose many mental problems as physical problems. Furthermore, "barefoot" doctors (paramedics who are neither barefoot nor doctors) and medical doctors may not be trained to recognize anything but the most obvious psychiatric symptoms. Jones (1988) found that Chinese medical students receive little training in psychiatry. Consequently, Chinese psychiatrists may typically see patients whose symptoms are severe and untreatable by other practitioners.

Also, China is a vast rural nation characterized by strong family ties and cohesive work organizations that Victor and Ruth Sidel (1982) describe as a total community support system. This social network can more easily control the expression of bizarre behavior and provide effective social support in the interest of the larger society than is possible in the West. Sidel and Sidel describe the small study groups of fellow workers and neighbors who meet regularly to discuss both personal and public matters on an intimate basis with one another. They suggest that the availability of these groups serves to minimize the number of psychological problems that require medical treatment because such problems are topics of group discussion and efforts at resolution.

Kleinman and Mechanic (1979) conclude that cases of sexual deviance, alcoholism, drug abuse, and suicide are uncommon in China and hypothesize that the extent of mental disorder is about the same as in the Chinese populations in Hong Kong, Taiwan, Singapore, and the United States. If that hypothesis is correct, China may indeed have a relatively low rate of mental disorder. Studies in the United States of Chinese Americans show increasing but still low rates of psychiatric problems and alcoholism in comparison with other Americans (Gallagher 1987; Kitano 1969, 1985). Rates of schizophrenia in China are estimated to be 0.6 percent of the total population, which is somewhat less than the 1.0 percent estimated for the United States; the Chinese maintain that anxiety is their biggest mental health problem but that depression is not widespread (Cockerham 1984). A low prevalence of depression may be due more to the tendencies of Chinese doctors to diagnose symptoms of depression as physical illnesses, such as kidney deficiency (Kleinman and Mechanic 1979). There may be more depression than the Chinese admit (Butterfield 1989).

Chinese mental patients are treated with a combination of traditional Chinese and Western medicine, along with an extensive use of family and neighborhood and work-study groups in providing social support, counseling, and management of therapy. Drugs and psychotherapy are both employed to help patients, but the psychotherapy seems to consist largely of counseling (Cockerham 1984). Most patients remain at home unless they are violent and likely to hurt themselves or other people. In rural areas, people with mental disorders visit clinics on agricultural communes; urban residents are usually treated at hospital outpatient clinics. Medical personnel also visit patients in their homes to give them and their families information on how to take care of themselves.

Work or neighborhood groups are usually placed in charge of monitoring a patient's progress and treatment schedule, especially when the individual's symptoms have been stabilized. Patients will also perform manual labor consistent with their capabilities when recovering and be paid a small amount of money for their effort. The group will supervise the taking of medications prescribed by the doctor, participate in therapy, and provide ideological instruction. The groups also monitor the patient's behavior and make reports to the medical personnel in charge of the case. In addition, they help solve whatever social and psychological difficulties exist at home or elsewhere that might cause the patient stress.

With only about sixty thousand beds available in mental hospitals and fewer than four thousand psychiatrists for such a large population, the treatment of mental disorder does not appear to be a high priority in Chinese society. However, detailed information on the Chinese system of mental health care delivery is clearly lacking. To what extent China's approach to mental health can contribute to mental health programs of other nations is uncertain because of China's unique social and political system. There seem to be unusually high levels of community and group involvement in dealing with mental problems, but the effectiveness of this approach and other aspects of mental health care in China await clarification by future research. For the present, the Chinese believe that mental disorder is not a significant health problem and that their needs are being met.

JAPAN

Japan, in distinct contrast to the other nations discussed in this chapter, strongly supports the management of mental disorders through a custodial system of psychiatric care (Munakata 1986). This approach is reflected in the statistics presented in Table 15–1, which shows the number of beds, inpatients, and patients committed involuntarily, along with the percent of involuntary patients, in Japanese mental hospitals between 1970 and 1990. As Table 15–1 indicates, the number of beds for mental patients increased nationwide from 242,022 in 1970 to 358,128 in 1990 and the number of inpatients increased from 253,433 to 348,859 over the same period. These figures are dramatically different from those in the United States, Great Britain, and Italy, where the numbers of beds and patients in mental hospitals steeply declined over the same period. The trend in Japan, however, does not signify that Japanese mental patients are being hospitalized in large numbers without their consent; on the contrary, as shown in Table 15–1, the number of involuntarily committed patients declined from 76,597 in 1970 to 12,572 in 1990 and the percentage of such patients dropped from 30.2 to 3.6. The overwhelming majority of Japanese mental patients are hospitalized voluntarily.

According to Tsunetsugu Munakata (1986, 1989), factors such as health insurance coverage, the aging of the population, and the rise of national income explain the increase in the number of admissions and beds in psychiatric hospitals. Japan has a national health insurance system that covers the cost of health services for all people age seventy and older. Patients under the age of seventy pay 30 percent of their health care expenses under the national

Table 15–1 Number of beds, resident patients, and involuntarily admitted patients in Japanese mental hospitals, 1970–1990.

YEAR	BEDS	RESIDENT PATIENTS	INVOLUNTARY ADMISSIONS	PERCENT OF INVOLUNTARY ADMISSIONS
1970	242,022	253,433	76,597	30.2
1975	275,468	281,127	65,571	23.3
1980	304,469	311,584	47,400	15.2
1985	333,570	339,989	30,543	9.0
1990	358,128	348,859	12,572	3.6

Source: Ministry of Health and Welfare, Japan, 1993.

health insurance plan, but they are reimbursed for any expenses exceeding 60,000 yen (about $580) during any given month. Low-income patients are reimbursed for amounts spent over 33,600 yen (about $325) monthly. Not all Japanese are covered by the national health insurance program. Many business firms and public institutions provide health insurance for their employees, and some large business corporations even employ doctors and own hospitals. Japanese are thus assured of medical care and hospitalization. Also, the Japanese government sets fees for both doctors and hospitals; this means that costs tend to be low because the government refuses to pay high rates and providers are prevented by law from charging more than the government fee schedule allows (Cockerham 1995).

Extensive health insurance coverage, the relatively low cost of hospitalization, and the national rise in personal income in Japan, resulting from its major role in the world economy in the latter part of the twentieth century, have established a financial environment conducive to hospitalization. This situation, combined with the rapid aging of Japan's population, explains why increasingly large numbers of Japanese enter mental hospitals. The Japanese are growing older at a faster rate than the population of any other country. About 12 percent of Japan's population was age sixty-five or older in 1990; however, the proportion of elderly is estimated to reach 23 percent by 2014, which represents a pace of aging unexceeded elsewhere in the world. As Munakata (1986) points out, there is a significant relationship between the number of beds in psychiatric hospitals and the ratio of persons age sixty-five and older. "As the population increases," states Munakata (1986:353), "beds of psychiatric hospitals tend to increase in number." Part of this development is undoubtedly due to increases in dementia in Japan because of the growth of the elderly population. Japan's Ministry of Health and Welfare estimated in 1992 that 6.7 percent of Japan's elderly population suffered from dementia, with the percentage expected to rise to 7 percent in 2000.

Additionally, psychiatric hospitals in Japan appear to provide many of the functions that nursing homes provide in the United States. In Japan, it is common for elderly people to be cared for by their family at home; it is when the family is unable to cope with the tasks associated with home care, especially abnormal behavior on the part of the aged family member, that the person is likely to be admitted to a psychiatric hospital. It may, in fact, be several years before a family gives up caring for the mentally ill family member at home (Munakata 1989). The Japanese thus appear similar to the Chinese in stressing care within the family, but once that care falters, they are more likely to seek custodial care for the mentally disordered family member in Japan's extensive system of mental hospitals. The notion of care of the mentally ill in the community (deinstitutionalization) beyond that provided by the family, as found in the United States and Western Europe, is not strong in Japan. Ultimately, it falls to the family to be responsible for its sick and dependent members. According to Munakata:

A Japanese mental hospital takes the place of the family in assuming the responsibility for care of the precious sick member at a time when the family has reached the point of exhaustion of material and/or psychological resources. As a rule, the family and the patient expect that the mental hospital will function as a surrogate family. This expectation of a family style mental hospital in Japan usually goes both ways: the hospital administrator or medical director acts like the head of a family and often lives within the premises of the hospital while attempting to create a family-like warm atmosphere in the hospital. The small size of most mental hospitals (the national average is 250 beds) is well suited for maintaining a family-like atmosphere.[3]

The family-like environment expected in mental hospitals is consistent with the cultural tendency of the Japanese to find psychological security within the context of group life. Japanese psychiatrist Takeo Doi (1981, 1985) notes the extreme importance of close family and friendship ties in Japan by explaining the concept of *amae*. *Amae* has no equivalent meaning in any Western language or culture and therefore cannot be easily translated. It refers to an emotional need common to the Japanese to feel united with other people. In adult life, that need is satisfied primarily by close relations with friends and coworkers. Although conforming to group norms and values means that the Japanese surrender some of their individuality, Doi (1981:174) states that "by becoming one with the group the Japanese are able to display a strength beyond the scope of the individual." Doi suggests that this typically Japanese characteristic is not necessarily bad, despite its negative evaluation by Westerners, because it promotes a feeling of belonging and being cared for. Doi points out that this situation provides a sense of strong social support for psychologically distressed people in Japan, whereas in the West such people are often isolated and left on their own to deal with their problems.

Unfortunately, this does not mean that care in Japanese mental hospitals is always a positive experience. Despite its supportive environment, Japanese psychiatric facilities typically pay low wages to workers, lack adequate training programs, and have low status as a place to be employed. Consequently, they tend to have a high turnover rate in personnel, low staff morale in comparison with general hospitals, and difficulty keeping competent workers (Munakata 1986).

Most mental hospitals (86 percent) in Japan are privately owned. Mental hospital admissions are highest among those who are aged, have low incomes, and live in rural areas. Length of mental hospitalization is among the longest in the world—close to six hundred days on the average, compared with about fifteen days in the United States. Weakened family ties as a result of mental illness, the custodial function for elderly patients, extensive health insurance

---

[3]Tsunetsugu Munakata, "The Socio-Cultural Significance of the Diagnostic Label 'Neurasthenia' in Japan's Mental Health Care System," *Culture, Medicine and Psychiatry* 13 (1989), 207.

Table 15–2   Percentage distribution by diagnosis of Japanese mental patients, 1987.

DIAGNOSIS	INPATIENTS	OUTPATIENTS
Schizophrenia	61.0	18.2
Mood disorders	4.6	12.7
Anxiety disorders	6.2	33.1
Alcohol-related	6.0	1.8
Mental retardation	4.4	1.8
Dementia	9.3	3.5
Epilepsy	3.5	17.1
Other	5.0	11.8
TOTALS	100.0%	100.0%

Source: Ministry of Health and Welfare, Japan, 1991.

coverage, low costs, and the hospital's desire to increase earnings all promote long hospital stays for Japanese mental patients (Munakata 1986).

As in the United States, the majority of inpatients in Japanese mental hospitals have a primary diagnosis of schizophrenia. Table 15–2 shows the percentage distribution by primary diagnosis of Japanese mental patients in 1987, the most recent year data were available as this book was being published. Table 15–2 shows that schizophrenia was the leading diagnosis for inpatients (61 percent), followed by dementia or senile disorders (9.3 percent). For outpatients, anxiety disorders were the leading diagnosis (33.1 percent), followed by schizophrenia (18.2 percent). Most outpatients in Japan are treated in doctors' offices, since psychiatric clinics with outpatient facilities are rare. In 1989, 344,378 persons were inpatients and 10.3 million were outpatients. The future direction of mental health care in Japan may be toward greater outpatient care, since the Japanese government directed in 1994 that the number of beds in mental hospitals be reduced.

POLAND

Poland is included in this chapter as an example of the manner in which widespread societal change has an impact on the mental health of a nation. Along with the other formerly socialist countries of Eastern Europe and the former Soviet Union, Poland experienced massive social, economic, and political change with the collapse of communism in the region during 1989–1990. Change brought a free-market economy and multi-party political system, while ending the power of the Communist Party and overturning a social system that had been in place since 1947. Despite the fact that Poland's standard of living was low in comparison to the West's and political freedom was curtailed, job security and lower prices for goods and services existed under communism's controlled economy. Consequently, positive values like democracy and freedom were counterbalanced by negative effects like increased poverty, higher unemployment, and decreased feelings of security (Brodniak and Ostrowska 1993). For Poles, the new conditions were a radical change from the past.

Prior to communism's fall, the level of physical health in Poland, as well as in Eastern Europe generally and in the former Soviet Union, was in a state of decline. Beginning in the mid-1960s, health care delivery on the basis of welfare capitalism in the West and socialism in the East had produced increasingly different outcomes for Europe's population. The formerly socialist countries, like Poland, witnessed a downturn in life expectancy and rise in mortality—especially for men. The transition to capitalism in the early 1990s did not immediately reverse the trend, and the nations in Eastern Europe still reflect an adverse health situation in comparison to the West.

The existing Polish health care delivery system, including mental health services, is a continuation of the old Soviet-style system in which care is provided by personnel and facilities organized and financed by the state. Cooperative clinics, established by industrial and agricultural workers, also provide outpatient care, and some private clinics exist. But most of the former communist health care delivery system, consisting of state-owned clinics and hospitals, is still in place. The long-term goal of Polish health policy, however, is a complete conversion from a state-supported socialist system to a private system supported by an obligatory national health insurance program financed largely by contributions from employers and workers.

When it comes to mental health, Poland has 653 psychiatric outpatient clincs distributed throughout the country, but only 49 mental hospitals. Psychiatric wards also exist in some general hospitals, and there are centers for the treatment of alcohol and drug dependence. Additionally, there are few sources of intermediate care between outpatient clinics and hospitals. As a result, most mental patients lack access to care beyond the local level unless they have a particularly severe condition that requires hospitalization.

It is estimated that between the late 1980s and the early 1990s, some 700,000 Poles, or about 2 percent of the total population, were treated annually in the nation's mental health facilities (Brodniak and Ostrowska 1993). For 1990–1993, the period immediately following the end of communism, there were no major increases in the incidence of mental disorder, except for alcohol psychoses (a 15-percent increase) and drug dependence (a 48-percent increase). Poland's Ministry of Health and Social Welfare estimated the consumption levels of alcohol had increased from 35 to 40 percent during this period, while the use of illicit drugs also increased substantially. Inpatient admissions to mental hospitals for schizophrenia and mood disorders also rose somewhat, but the overall incidence of such problems in the general population remains relatively stable over the last two decades (Brodniak and Ostrowska 1993).

The rise in substance-related disorders appears linked to Poland's current economic crisis, which has lowered the quality of life for many people and impeded the nation's transition to capitalism. Studies of the general population show a significant increase in feelings of fatigue, nervousness, irritability, apathy, discouragement, headaches, and sleeplessness—thereby suggesting a deterioration of mental well-being (Brodniak and Ostrowska 1993). It therefore appears that the greatest impact of changed societal conditions for Poland is a rise in alcohol and drug abuse and feelings of lessened well-being, but not significantly higher rates of schizophrenia and major mental problems such as anxiety and mood disorders.

SUMMARY

Like the United States, four of the countries discussed in this chapter have formulated mental health policies emphasizing community care of the mentally ill. Great Britain relies heavily upon general practitioners to treat the majority of mentally disturbed people in their usual home environment. Psychiatrists are called in to deal with the most severe problems generally, and they typically decide whether admission to a mental hospital is warranted. Italy has taken the extreme measure of attempting to abolish mental hospitals and treat all patients in a community setting. However, the mental hospitals have not disappeared, and considerable regional disparity exists between the services available for mental patients in northern Italy and those available in the more disadvantaged southern part of the country. Germany emphasizes community care in an extensive system of hospitals and outpatient facilities, but mental health is not regarded as a major social problem and little research on its true prevalence is conducted. China attempts to contain and treat mental disorder within a group context as much as possible in a social system that places intense group pressure on individuals, which may minimize all but the most bizarre symptoms.

Japan, the fifth country discussed, takes a different approach to the delivery of mental health care. First, care is emphasized in the family, with primary care practitioners treating patients on an outpatient basis. If that is ineffective, the mentally ill person is likely to be admitted to a mental hospital, where a lengthy stay is common. Care in the community is practically unknown, although some halfway houses exist. Nevertheless, the future of mental health care in Japan may be in increased outpatient services, since the government has directed a reduction in the number of beds in psychiatric hospitals. Poland, faced with massive social and economic change, has not seen a significant rise in mental disorders, except for substance abuse.

The general trend in the Western world today appears to be toward increasing emphasis on community care, with other nations leaving mentally disturbed people to be treated on the local level, especially by the family and local medical practitioners. Admissions to mental hospitals are declining in the West, with schizophrenics remaining the largest group needing long-term residential care (Häfner 1987). On balance, however, it cannot be claimed that the provision of mental health services ranks as a top priority in either health care delivery or public policy, or receives ample funding in any one particular health care system. In the British and Italian systems, as well as in the United States, mental health services are important but do not receive extensive funding. The Chinese appear to ignore the problem of mental illness as much as possible. Mental disorder thus remains a major social problem demanding solutions.

References

ABEL, THEODORA, RHODA METRAUX, AND SAMUEL ROLL. 1987. *Psychotherapy and culture.* Albuquerque: University of New Mexico.

AGRAS, W. STEWART. 1989. "Learning theory." Pp. 262–70 in H. Kaplan and B. Sadock (eds.), *Comprehensive textbook of psychiatry,* Vol. 1, 5th ed. Baltimore: Williams & Wilkins.

AKERS, RONALD L. 1967. "Problems in the sociology of deviance: Social definitions and behavior." *Social Forces* 46:455–65.

———. 1977. *Deviant behavior: A social learning approach.* 2nd ed. Belmont, CA: Wadsworth.

AKERS, RONALD L., AND RICHARD HAWKINS (eds.). 1975. *Law and control in society.* Englewood Cliffs, NJ: Prentice Hall.

ALEXANDER, FRANZ G., AND SHELDON T. SELESNICK. 1966. *The history of psychiatry.* New York: Mentor Books.

ALLEN, GILLIAN, AND ROY WALLIS. 1976. "Pentecostalists as a medical minority." Pp. 110–37 in R. Wallis and P. Morley (eds.), *Marginal medicine.* New York: Free Press.

ANESHENSEL, CAROL S., RALPH R. FRERICHS, AND VIRGINIA A. CLARK. 1981. "Family roles and sex differences in depression." *Journal of Health and Social Behavior* 22:379–93.

ANESHENSEL, CAROL S., CAROLYN M. RUTTER, AND PETER A. LACHENBRUCH. 1991. "Social structure, stress, and mental health: Competing conceptual and analytic models." *American Sociological Review* 56:166–78.

ANGERMEYER, MATTHIS C. 1986. "Im Dickicht der Journals auf der Suche nach der Psychiatrischen Soziologie." *Mensch Medizin Gesellschaft* 11:127–33.

ANTONOVSKY, AARON. 1974. "Conceptual and methodological problems in the study of resistance resources and stressful life events." Pp. 245–55 in B. S. Dohrenwend and B. P. Dohrenwend (eds.), *Stressful life events: Their nature and effects.* New York: Wiley.

———. 1979. *Health, stress, and coping.* San Francisco: Jossey-Bass.

ANTUNES, GEORGE, CHAD GORDON, CHARLES GAITZ, AND JUDITH SCOTT. 1974. "Ethnicity, socioeconomic status, and the etiology of psychological distress." *Sociology and Social Research* 58:361–68.

ARMSTRONG, BARBARA. 1976. "Preparing the community for the patient's return." *Hospital and Community Psychiatry* 27:349–56.

ASELTINE, ROBERT H., AND RONALD C. KESSLER. 1993. "Marital disruption and depression in a community sample." *Journal of Health and Social Behavior* 34:237–51.

ASKENASY, ALEXANDER R., BRUCE P. DOHRENWEND, AND BARBARA S. DOHRENWEND. 1977. "Some effects of social class and ethnic group membership on judgments of the magnitude of stressful life events: A research note." *Journal of Health and Social Behavior* 18:432–39.

ASTRUP, C., AND O. ÖDEGAARD. 1960. "Internal migration and mental disease in Norway." *Psychiatry Quarterly Supplement* 34:116–30.

AUSUBEL, D. P. 1961. "Personality disorder is a disease." *American Psychologist* 16:69–74.

AVIRAM, U., AND S. SEGAL. 1973. "Exclusion of the mentally ill." *Archives of General Psychiatry* 29:126–31.

AVISON, WILLIAM R., AND DONNA D. MCALPINE. 1992. "Gender differences in symptoms of depression among adolescents." *Journal of Health and Social Behavior* 33:77–96.

BACHMAN, JERALD D., LLOYD D. JOHNSTON, AND PATRICK O'MALLEY. 1990. "Explaining the recent decline in cocaine use among young adults: Further evidence that perceived risks and disapproval lead to reduced drug use." *Journal of Health and Social Behavior* 31:173–84.

BACHMAN, JERALD G., AND PATRICK M. O'MALLEY. 1984. "Black–white differences in self-esteem: Are they affected by response styles?" *American Journal of Sociology* 90:624–39.

BAKER, DONALD, JOHN BEDELL, AND LORRAINE PRINSKY. 1982. "Children's perceptions of mental illness: A partial test of Scheff's hypothesis." *Symbolic Interaction* 5:343–56.

BALDASSARE, MARK. 1978. *Residential crowding in urban America*. Berkeley and Los Angeles: University of California Press.

———. 1981. "The effects of household density on subgroups." *American Sociological Review* 46:110–18.

BANDURA, ALBERT. 1969. *Principles of behavior modification*. New York: Holt, Rinehart & Winston.

BARRY, ANNE. 1971. *Bellevue is a state of mind*. New York: Harcourt Brace Jovanovich.

BART, PAULINE B. 1974. "The sociology of depression." Pp. 139–57 in P. Roman and H. Trice (eds.), *Explorations in psychiatric sociology*. Philadelphia: Davis.

BASSUK, ELLEN L., AND SAMUEL GERSON. 1978. "Deinstitutionalization and mental health services." *Scientific American* 238:46–53.

BASTIDE, ROGER. 1972. *The sociology of mental disorder*. Trans. J. McNeil. New York: McKay.

BATESON, G., D. JACKSON, J. HALEY, AND J. WEAKLAND. 1956. "Towards a theory of schizophrenia." *Behavioral Science* 1:251–64.

BAUGHMAN, E. E. 1971. *Black Americans: A psychological analysis*. New York: Academia.

BECKER, HOWARD S. 1973. *Outsiders: Studies in the sociology of deviance*. New York: Free Press.

BELLACK, ALAN S., MICHEL HERSEN, AND ALAN E. KAZDIN (eds.). 1990. *International handbook of behavior modification and therapy*. 2nd ed. New York: Plenum.

BEM, S. L. 1974. "The measurement of psychological androgyny." *Journal of Consulting and Clinical Psychology* 42:155–62.

BENTZ, W. K., J. W. EDGERTON, AND M. KHERLOPIAN. 1969. "Perceptions of mental illness among people in a rural area." *Mental Hygiene* 53:459–65.

BENTZ, W. K., J. W. EDGERTON, AND F. T. MILLER. 1969. "Perceptions of mental illness among public school teachers." *Sociology of Education* 42:400–406.

BERGER, PETER L., AND THOMAS LUCKMANN. 1967. *The social construction of reality*. Garden City, NY: Doubleday, Anchor Books.

BERGER, PHILIP B., BEATRIX HAMBURG, AND DAVID HAMBURG. 1977. "Mental health: Progress and problems. Pp. 261–76 in J. Knowles (ed.), *Doing better and feeling worse: Health in the United States*. New York: Norton.

BERK, BERNARD B., AND VICTOR GOERTZEL. 1975. "Selection versus role occupancy as determinants of role-related attitudes among psychiatric aides." *Journal of Health and Social Behavior* 16:183–91.

BITTNER, EGON. 1967. "Police discretion in emergency apprehension of mentally ill persons." *Social Problems* 14:278–92.

BLUMER, HERBERT. 1969. *Symbolic interactionism*. Englewood Cliffs, NJ: Prentice Hall.

BOCOCK, ROBERT. 1981. *Freud and modern society*. Walton-on-Thames, England: Nelson.

BOLLINI, PAOLA, MICHAEL REICH, AND GIOVANNI MUSCETTOLA. 1988. "Revision of the Italian psychiatric reform: North/south differences and future strategies." *Social Science and Medicine* 27:1327–35.

BOOCOCK, SARANE S. 1972. *An introduction to the sociology of learning*. New York: Houghton Mifflin.

BOOTH, ALAN. 1976. *Urban crowding and its consequences.* New York: Praeger.

BOOTH, ALAN, AND JOHN COWELL. 1976. "Crowding and health." *Journal of Health and Social Behavior* 17:204–20.

BOOTH, ALAN, AND JOHN N. EDWARDS. 1976. "Crowding and family relations." *American Sociological Review* 41:308–21.

BOURNE, PETER G. 1970. *Men, stress, and Vietnam.* Boston: Little, Brown.

BRADY, JOHN P. 1975. "Behavior therapy." Pp. 1824–31 in A. Freedman, H. Kaplan and B. Sadock (eds.), *Comprehensive textbook of psychiatry,* Vol. 2, 2nd ed. Baltimore: Williams & Wilkins.

BRAGINSKY, BENJAMIN M., DOROTHEA D. BRAGINSKY, AND KENNETH RING. 1969. *Methods of madness: The mental hospital as a last resort.* New York: Holt, Rinehart & Winston.

BRANDT, ANTHONY. 1975. *Reality police: The experience of insanity in America.* New York: Morrow.

BRENNER, M. HARVEY. 1973. *Mental illness and the economy.* Cambridge, MA: Harvard University Press.

BRILL, H., AND B. MALZBERG. 1962. "Statistical report on the arrest record of male expatients, age 16 or over, released from New York State mental hospitals during the period 1946–48." Mental Hospital Service Supplemental Report 153. Washington, DC: American Psychiatric Association.

BRINES, JULIE. 1994. "Economic dependency, gender, and the division of labor at home." *American Journal of Sociology* 100:652–88.

BRODNIAK, WLODZIMIERZ A. 1994. "The mental health promotion in Poland: Concepts, risks to mental health, current state and strategies." Paper presented to the European Society for Medical Sociology meetings, Vienna, Austria.

BRODNIAK, WLODZIMIERZ, AND ANTONINA OSTROWSKA. 1993. "Systemic transformation in the mental health of Polish society." *Polish Demographic Review* 3:139–51.

BROMAN, CLIFFORD C. 1987. "Race differences in professional help-seeking." *American Journal of Community Psychology* 15:473–87.

BROMBERG, WALTER. 1975. *From shaman to psychotherapist.* Chicago: Henry Regnery.

BROOKS, ALEXANDER D. 1974. *Law, psychiatry and the mental health system.* Boston: Little, Brown.

BROVERMAN, I. K., D. M. BROVERMAN, F. E. CLARKSON, P. S. ROSENKRANTZ, AND S. R. VOGEL. 1970. "Sex-role stereotypes and clinical judgments of mental health." *Journal of Consulting and Clinical Psychology* 34:1–7.

BROWN, DIANE R., LAWRENCE E. GARY, ANGELA D. GREENE, AND NORWEETA G. MILBURN. 1992. "Patterns of social affiliation as predictors of depressive symptoms among urban blacks." *Journal of Health and Social Behavior* 33:242–53.

BROWN, GEORGE W. 1974. "Meaning, measurement, and stress of life events." Pp. 217–43 in B. S. Dohrenwend and B. P. Dohrenwend (eds.), *Stressful life events: Their nature and effects.* New York: Wiley.

BROWN, GEORGE W., AND J. L. T. BIRLEY. 1968. "Crises and life changes and the onset of schizophrenia." *Journal of Health and Social Behavior* 9:203–14.

BROWN, G. W., J. L. T. BIRLEY, AND J. K. WING. 1972. "Influence of family life on the course of schizophrenic disorders." *British Journal of Psychiatry* 121:241–58.

BROWN, G. W., MARGARET BONE, BRIDGIT DALISON, AND J. K. WING. 1966. *Schizophrenia and social care: A comparative follow-up study of 339 schizophrenia patients.* New York: Oxford University Press.

BROWN, GEORGE W., AND TIRRIL HARRIS. 1978. *Social origins of depression: A study of psychiatric disorder in women.* New York: Free Press.

BROWN, PHIL. 1985. *The transfer of care.* London: Routledge.

BURGESS, ROBERT L., AND RONALD L. AKERS. 1966. "A differential association-reinforcement theory of criminal behavior." *Social Problems* 14:128–47.

BURNAM, M. AUDREY, RICHARD L. HOUGH, MARVIN KARNO, JAVIER I. ESCOBAR, AND CYNTHIA A. TELLES. 1987. "Acculturation and lifetime prevalence of psychiatric disorders among Mexican Americans in Los Angeles." *Journal of Health and Social Behavior* 28:89–102.

BURNAM, M. AUDREY, DIANNE M. TIMBERS, AND RICHARD L. HOUGH. 1984. "Two measures of psychological distress among Mexican Americans, Mexicans and Anglos." *Journal of Health and Social Behavior* 25:24–33.

BUTTERFIELD, FOX. 1989. *China: Alive in the bitter sea.* Rev. ed. New York: Bantam.

CANTOR, NORMAN F. 1969. *Medieval history.* 2nd ed. New York: Macmillan.

CARNAHAN, D. L., W. GOVE, AND O. GALLE. 1974. "Urbanization, population density and overcrowding: The quality of life in urban America." *Social Forces* 53:62–72.

CARR, LESLIE G., AND NEAL KRAUSE. 1978. "Social status, psychiatric symptomatology, and response bias." *Journal of Health and Social Behavior* 19:86–91.

CATALANO, RALPH, AND C. DAVID DOOLEY. 1977. "Economic predictors of depressed mood and stressful life events in a metropolitan community." *Journal of Health and Social Behavior* 18:292–307.

CENTER FOR MENTAL HEALTH SERVICES. 1992. *Mental health, United States, 1992.* Washington, DC: U.S. Government Printing Office.

———. 1994a. *Mental health, United States, 1994.* Washington, DC: U.S. Government Printing Office.

———. 1994b. "Additions and resident patients at end of year, state and county mental hospitals, by age and diagnosis, by state, United States, 1992. Rockville, MD: Center for Mental Health Services.

———. 1994c. "Male–female admission differentials in state mental hospitals, 1880–1990. Mental Health Statistical Note 211. Rockville, MD: Center for Mental Health Services.

CIBA FOUNDATION SYMPOSIUM. 1965. *Transcultural psychiatry.* Boston: Little, Brown.

CLANCY, KEVIN, AND WALTER GOVE. 1974. "Sex differences in mental illness: An analysis of response bias in self-reports." *American Journal of Sociology* 80:205–16.

CLAUSEN, JOHN A. 1983. "Sex roles, marital roles, and response to mental disorder." *Research in Community and Mental Health* 3:165–208.

CLAUSEN, JOHN A., AND CAROL L. HUFFINE. 1975. "Sociocultural and social/psychological factors affecting social responses to mental disorder." *Journal of Health and Social Behavior* 16:405–20.

CLEARY, PAUL D., AND DAVID MECHANIC. 1983. "Sex differences in psychological distress among married people." *Journal of Health and Social Behavior* 24:111–21.

COCKERHAM, WILLIAM C. 1978. "Interactional considerations in studying American Indians: The case of adolescent self-esteem." *Symbolic Interaction* 2:43–58.

———. 1979. "Labeling theory and mental disorder: A synthesis of psychiatric and social perspectives." Pp. 257–80 in N. Denzin (ed.), *Studies in symbolic interaction,* Vol. 2. Greenwich, CT: JAI Press.

———. 1984. "Mental disorder in the People's Republic of China." *Journal of International and Comparative Social Welfare* 1:40–51.

———. 1985. "Sociology and Psychiatry" Pp. 265–73 in H. Kaplan and B. Sadock (eds.), *Comprehensive textbook of psychiatry,* Vol. 1, 4th ed. Baltimore: Williams & Wilkins.

———. 1990a. "Becoming mentally ill: A symbolic interactionist model." Pp. 339–50 in N. Denzin (ed.), *Studies in symbolic interaction.* Greenwich, CT: JAI Press.

———. 1990b. "A Test of the relationship between race, socioeconomic status, and psychological distress." *Social Science and Medicine* 31:1321–26.

———. 1991. *This aging society.* Englewood Cliffs, NJ: PrenticeHall.

———. 1995. *Medical Sociology,* 6th Edition. Englewood Cliffs, NJ: PrenticeHall.

COCKERHAM, WILLIAM C., AND AUDIE L. BLEVINS, JR. 1976. "Open school vs. traditional school: Self-identification among Native American and white adolescents." *Sociology of Education* 49:164–69.

COCKERHAM, WILLIAM C., GERHARD KUNZ, AND GUENTHER LUESCHEN. 1988. "Psychological distress, perceived health status, and physician utilization in West Germany." *Social Science and Medicine* 26:829–38.

COCOZZA, JOSEPH J., AND HENRY J. STEADMAN. 1976. "The failure of psychiatric predictions of dangerousness: Clear and convincing evidence." *Rutgers Law Review* 29:1084–1101.

———. 1978. "Prediction in psychiatry: An example of misplaced confidence in experts." *Social Problems* 25:265–76.

COHEN, L. H., AND H. FREEMAN. 1945. "How dangerous to the community are state hospital patients?" *Connecticut State Medical Journal* 9:697–99.

COHEN, ROSALIE. 1974. "Neglected legal dilemmas in community psychiatry." Pp. 69–82 in P. Roman and H. Trice (eds.), *Sociological perspectives on community mental health.* Philadelphia: Davis.

CONGER, RAND D., FREDERICK O. LORENZ, GLEN H. ELDER, JR., RONALD L. SIMONS, AND XIAOJIA GE. 1993. "Husband and wife differences in response to undesirable life events." *Journal of Health and Social Behavior* 34:71–88.

COOPER, BRIAN. 1961. "Social class and prognosis in schizophrenia." *British Journal of Preventive and Social Medicine* 15:17–27.

COOPER, BRIAN, AND BIRGITT LACKUS. 1984. "The social-class background of mentally retarded children: A study in Mannheim." *Social Psychiatry* 19:3–12.

COSER, ROSE LAUB. 1976. "Suicide and the relational system: A case study in a mental hospital." *Journal of Health and Social Behavior* 17:318–27.

CROCETTI, G., AND P. LEMKAU. 1963. "Public opinion of psychiatric home care in an urban area." *American Journal of Public Health* 53:409–17.

CROCETTI, G. M., H. R. SPIRO, AND I. SIASSI. 1974. *Contemporary attitudes toward mental illness.* Pittsburgh: University of Pittsburgh Press.

CUMMING, E., AND J. CUMMING. 1957. *Closed ranks: An experiment in mental health education.* Cambridge, MA: Harvard University Press.

———. 1965. "On the stigma of mental illness." *Community Mental Health* 1:135–43.

D'ARCY, CARL, AND JOAN BROCKMAN. 1976. "Changing public recognition of psychiatric symptoms? Blackfoot revisited." *Journal of Health and Social Behavior* 17:302–10.

DAVIS, JOHN M. 1985. "Antipsychotic drugs." Pp. 1481–1513 in H. Kaplan and B. Sadock (eds.), *Comprehensive textbook of psychiatry,* Vol. 2, 4th ed. Baltimore: Williams & Wilkins.

DEAN, ALFRED, BOHDAN KOLODY, AND PATRICIA WOOD. 1990. "Effects of social support from various sources on depression in elderly persons." *Journal of Health and Social Behavior* 31:148–61.

DEAUX, KAY. 1976. *The behavior of women and men.* Monterey, CA: Brooks/Cole.

DEFOE, DANIEL, SIR JOHN FORTESQUE-ALAND, AND JOHN CONOLLY. 1973. "Observations on psychiatric confinement, 1728–1830." Pp. 7–11 in T. Szasz (ed.), *The age of madness.* Garden City, NY: Doubleday, Anchor Books.

DENZIN, NORMAN K. 1968. "The self-fulfilling prophecy and patient-therapist interaction." Pp. 349–58 in S. Spitzer and N. Denzin (eds.), *The mental patient: Studies in the sociology of deviance,* New York: McGraw-Hill.

———. 1970a. "The methodologies of symbolic interaction: A critical review of research techniques." Pp. 447–65 in G. Stone and H. Farberman (eds.), *Social psychology through symbolic interaction.* Waltham, MA: Ginn-Blaisdell.

———. 1970b. "Rules of conduct and the study of deviant behavior." Pp. 120–59 in J. Douglas (ed.), *Deviance and respectability.* New York: Basic Books.

———. 1977. *Childhood socialization.* San Francisco: Jossey-Bass.

———. 1984. *On understanding emotion.* San Francisco: Jossey-Bass.

DERSHOWITZ, ALAN. 1973. "Preventive confinement: A suggested framework for constitutional analysis." *Texas Law Review* 51:1277–1324.

Diagnostic and statistical manual of mental disorders, 4th Edition (DSM-IV). Washington, DC: American Psychiatric Association.

DILLING, H., AND S. WEYERER. 1984. "Prevalence of mental disorders in the small-town–rural region of Traunstein (Upper Bavaria)." *Acta Psychiatrica Scandinavia* 69:60–79.

DINITZ, SIMON, AND NANCY BERAN. 1971. "Community mental health as a boundaryless and boundary-busting system." *Journal of Health and Social Behavior.* 12:99–107.

DOHERTY, EDMUND G. 1978. "Are differential discharge criteria used for men and women psychiatric inpatients?" *Journal of Health and Social Behavior* 19:107–16.

DOHRENWEND, BARBARA S. 1973. "Life events as stressors: A methodological inquiry." *Journal of Health and Social Behavior* 14:167–75.

DOHRENWEND, BARBARA S., AND BRUCE P. DOHRENWEND. 1969. *Social status and psychological disorder.* New York: Wiley.

DOHRENWEND, BARBARA S., AND BRUCE P. DOHRENWEND (eds). 1974. *Stressful life events: Their nature and effects.* New York: Wiley.

DOHRENWEND, BARBARA S., LARRY KRASNOFF, ALEXANDER R. ASKENASY, AND BRUCE P. DOHRENWEND. 1978. "Examplification of a method for scaling life events: The PERI life events scale." *Journal of Health and Social Behavior* 19:205–29.

DOHRENWEND, BRUCE P. 1966. "Social status and psychological disorder: An issue of substance and an issue of method." *American Sociological Review* 31:14–34.

———. 1974. "Problems in defining and sampling the relevant population of stressful life events." Pp. 275–310 in B. S. Dohrenwend and B. P. Dohrenwend (eds.), *Stressful life events: Their nature and effects.* New York: Wiley.

———. 1975. "Sociocultural and social-psychological factors in the genesis of mental disorders." *Journal of Health and Social Behavior* 16:365–92.

DOHRENWEND, BRUCE P., V. W. BERNARD, AND L. C. KOLB. 1962. "The orientations of leaders in the urban area toward problems of mental illness." *American Journal of Psychiatry* 118:683–91.

DOHRENWEND, BRUCE P., AND E. CHIN-SONG. 1967. "Social status and attitudes toward psychological disorder: The problem of tolerance of deviance." *American Sociological Review* 32:417–33.

DOHRENWEND, BRUCE P., AND BARBARA S. DOHRENWEND. 1976. "Sex differences and psychiatric disorders." *American Journal of Sociology* 81:1447–54.

DOI, TAKEO. 1981. *The anatomy of dependence.* Trans. J. Bester. Tokyo: Kodansha International.

———. 1985. *The anatomy of self.* Trans. M. Harbison. Tokyo: Kodansha International.

DONNELLY, JOHN 1985. "Psychosurgery." Pp. 1563–69 in H. Kaplan and B. Sadock (eds.), *Comprehensive textbook of psychiatry,* Vol. 2, 4th ed. Baltimore: Williams & Wilkins.

DONNELLY, MICHAEL. 1992. *The politics of mental health in Italy.* London: Routledge.

DOOLEY, DAVID, AND RALPH CATALANO. 1984. "Why the economy predicts help-seeking: A test of competing explanations." *Journal of Health and Social Behavior* 25:160–76.

DUBOS, RENÉ. 1959. *Mirage of health.* New York: Harper.

DUNHAM, H. WARREN. 1976. *Social realities and community psychiatry.* New York: Human Sciences.

———. 1977. "Schizophrenia: The impact of sociocultural factors." *Hospital Practice* 12:61–68.

DURKHEIM, EMILE. 1950. *The rules of sociological method.* New York: Free Press.

———. 1951. *Suicide.* New York: Free Press.

DUVALL, DONNA, AND ALAN BOOTH. 1978. "The housing environment and women's health." *Journal of Health and Social Behavior* 19:410–17.

EATON, JOSEPH W., AND ROBERT J. WEIL. 1955. *Culture and mental disorders.* Glencoe, IL: Free Press.

EATON, WILLIAM W., JR. 1974a. "Medical hospitalization as a reinforcement process." *American Sociological Review* 39:252–60.

———. 1974b. "Residence, social class, and schizophrenia." *Journal of Health and Social Behavior* 15:289–99.

———. 1978. *Life events, social supports, and psychiatric symptoms: A reanalysis of the New Haven data.* Journal of Health and Social Behavior 19:230–34.

———. 1980a. "A formal theory of selection for schizophrenia." *American Journal of Sociology* 86:149–58.

———. 1980b. *The sociology of mental disorder.* New York: Praeger.

EATON, WILLIAM W., AND LARRY G. KESSLER. 1985. *Epidemiologic field methods in psychiatry.* Orlando, FL: Academic Press.

EDGERTON, W. J., AND W. K. BENTZ. 1969. "Attitudes and opinions of rural people about mental illness and program services." *American Journal of Public Health* 59:470–77.

EDWARDS, JOHN N., ALAN BOOTH, AND PATRICIA KLOBUS EDWARDS. 1982. "Housing type, stress, and family relations." *Social Forces* 61:241–57.

EHRENREICH, JOHN 1978. "Introduction: The cultural crisis of modern medicine." Pp. 1–35 in J. Ehrenreich (ed.), *The cultural crisis of modern medicine.* New York: Monthly Review Press.

EITINGER, L. 1964. *Concentration camp survivors in Norway and Israel.* London: Allen & Unwin.

———. 1973. "A followup of the Norwegian concentration camp survivors." *Israel Annals of Psychiatry and Related Disciplines* 11:199–209.

ELLIOT, RODNEY D., AND BERNARD N. MELTZER. 1981. "Symbolic interactionism and psychoanalysis: Some convergences, divergences, and complementaries." *Symbolic Interaction* 4:225–44.

EMERICK, ROBERT E. 1991. "The politics of psychiatric self-help: Political factions, interactional support, and group longevity in a social movement." *Social Science and Medicine* 32:1121–28.

ENNIS, BRUCE J., AND RICHARD D. EMERY. 1978. *The rights of mental patients.* Rev. ed. New York: Avon Books.

ERIKSON, ERIK H. 1968. *Identity, youth and crisis.* New York: Norton.

ERIKSON, KAI T. 1976. *Everything in its path.* New York: Simon & Schuster.

ESTERSON, AARON. 1972. *The leaves of spring: A study in the dialectics of madness.* Harmondsworth, England: Pelican Books.

EYSENCK, HANS J. 1961. "The effects of psychotherapy." Pp. 697–725 in H. Eysenck (ed.), *Handbook of abnormal psychology.* New York: Basic Books.

FADIMAN, JAMES, AND DONALD KEWMAN (eds.). 1973. *Exploring madness: Experience, theory, and research.* Monterey, CA: Brooks/Cole.

FAGIN, ALLEN. 1976. "The policy implications of predictive decision: 'Likelihood' and 'dangerousness" in civil commitment proceedings." *Public Policy* 24:491–528.

FARINA, A., R. D. FELNER, AND L. A. BOUDREAU. 1973. "Reactions of workers to male and female mental patient job applicants." *Journal of Consulting and Clinical Psychology* 41:363–72.

FARIS, ROBERT E., AND H. WARREN DUNHAM. 1939. *Mental disorders in urban areas.* Chicago: University of Chicago Press.

FENWICK, RUDY, AND MARK TAUSIG. 1994. "The macroeconomic context of job stress." *Journal of Health and Social Behavior* 35:266–82.

FICHTER, M. M. AND S. WEYERER. 1985. *Die Oberbayerische Follow-Up FeldStudie.* Munich: University of Munich.

FINK, MAX. 1978. "Electroshock therapy: Myths and realities." *Hospital Practice* 13:77–82.

FINKEL, NORMAN J. 1988. *Insanity on trial.* New York: Plenum.

FISCHER, CLAUDE S. 1973. "Urban malaise." *Social Forces* 52:221–35.

———. 1976. *The urban experience.* New York: Harcourt Brace Jovanovich.

FISHER, SEYMOUR, AND ROGER P. GREENBERG (eds.). 1989. *A critical appraisal of biological treatments for psychological distress.* Hillsdale, NJ: Erlbaum.

FLAHERTY, JOSEPH, AND JUDITH RICHMAN. 1989. "Gender differences in the perception and utilization of social support: Theoretical perspectives and an empirical test." *Social Science and Medicine* 28:1221–28.

FLAX, JAMES W., MORTON O. WAGENFIELD, RUBY E. IVENS, AND ROBERT J. WEISS. 1979. *Mental health and rural America: An overview and annotated bibliography.* Rockville, MD: National Institute of Mental Health.

FOUCAULT, MICHEL. 1965. *Madness and civilization: A history of insanity in the Age of Reason.* New York: Pantheon.

———. 1987. *Mental illness and psychology.* Berkeley and Los Angeles: University of California Press.

FOX, JOHN W. 1980. "Gove's specific sex-role theory of mental illness: A research note." *Journal of Health and Social Behavior* 21:260–67.

———. 1990. "Social class, mental illness, and social mobility: The social selection-drift hypothesis for serious mental illness." *Journal of Health and Social Behavior* 31:344–53.

FOX, RICHARD W. 1978. *So far disordered in mind: Insanity in California 1870–1930.* Berkeley and Los Angeles: University of California Press.

FRACCHIA, J., D. CANALE, E. CAMBRIA, E. RUEST, C. SHEPPARD, AND S. MERLIS. 1975. "The effects of increased information upon community perceptions of ex-mental patients." *Journal of Psychology* 92:271–75.

FRACCHIA, J., C. SHEPPARD, D. CANALE, E. RUEST, E. CAMBRIA, AND S. MERLIS. 1976. "Community perceptions of severity of illness levels of former mental patients: A failure to discriminate." *Comprehensive Psychiatry* 17:775–78.

FREEMAN, ARTHUR M. III, ROBERT L. SACK, AND PHILLIP A. BERGER. 1979. *Psychiatry for the primary care physician.* Baltimore: Williams & Wilkins.

FREEMAN, HOWARD E., AND OZZIE G. SIMMONS. 1961. "Feelings of stigma among relatives of former mental patients." *Social Problems* 8:312–21.

———. 1963. *The mental patient comes home.* New York: Wiley.

FREEMAN, HUGH (ed.). 1984. *Mental health and the environment.* London: Churchill Livingstone.

FREIDSON, ELIOT. 1970. *Profession of medicine.* New York: Wiley.

FRERICHS, ROBERT, CAROL ANESHENSEL, AND VIRGINIA A. CLARK. 1981. "Prevalence of depression in Los Angeles County." *American Journal of Epidemiology* 113:691–99.

FREUD, SIGMUND. 1953–1966. *Standard edition of the complete psychological works of Sigmund Freud.* London: Hogarth Press.

———. 1964. *Moses and Monotheism.* New York: Vintage.

FRIEDRICH, OTTO. 1975. *Going crazy: An inquiry into madness in our time.* New York: Simon & Schuster.

FRITZ, C. E., AND E. S. MARKS. 1954. "The NORC studies of human behavior in disaster." *Journal of Social Issues* 10:26–41.

FUCHS, ESTELLE, AND ROBERT HAVIGHURST. 1973. *To live on this earth: American Indian education.* Garden City, NY: Doubleday, Anchor Books.

FULLER, THEODORE D., JOHN N. EDWARDS, SANTHAT SERMSRI, AND SAIRUDEE VORAKITPHOKATORN. 1993. "Gender and health: Some Asian evidence." *Journal of Health and Social Behavior* 34:252–71.

GALLAGHER, BERNARD J. III. 1987. *The sociology of mental illness.* 2nd ed. Englewood Cliffs, NJ: Prentice Hall.

GALLE, OMER, AND WALTER GOVE. 1978. "Overcrowding, isolation and human behavior: Exploring the extremes in population distribution." Pp. 95–132 in K. Tauber and J. Sweet (eds.), *Social demography.* New York: Academic Press.

GELFAND, MICHAEL. 1964. "Psychiatric disorders as recognized by the Shona." Pp. 156–73 in A. Kiev (ed.), *Magic, faith, and healing: Studies in primitive psychiatry today.* New York: Free Press.

GERSTEN, JOANNE C., THOMAS S. LANGNER, JEANNE G. EISENBERG, AND L. ORZECK. 1974. "Child behavior and life events: Undesirable change or change per se." Pp. 159–70 in B. S. Dohrenwend and B. P. Dohrenwend (eds.), *Stressful life events: Their nature and effects.* New York: Wiley.

GERSTEN, JOANNE C., THOMAS S. LANGNER, JEANNE G. EISENBERG, AND ORA SIMCHA-FAGAN. 1977. "An evaluation of the etiologic role of stressful life events in psychological disorders." *Journal of Health and Social Behavior* 18:228–44.

GIBBS, JACK P. 1971. "A critique of the labeling perspective." Pp. 193–205 in E. Rubington and M. Weinberg (eds.), *The study of social problems.* New York: Oxford University Press.

GILLIS, A. R. 1977. "High-rise housing and psychological strain." *Journal of Health and Social Behavior* 18:418–31.

GIOVANNONI, J. M., AND L. GUREL. 1967. "Socially disruptive behavior of ex-mental patients." *Archives of General Psychiatry* 17:146–53.

GLASS, JENNIFER, AND TETUSHI FUJIMOTO. 1994. "Housework, paid work, and depression among husbands and wives." *Journal of Health and Social Behavior* 35:179–91.

GOFFMAN, ERVING. 1961. *Asylums.* Garden City, NY: Doubleday, Anchor Books.

———. 1963. *Stigma.* Englewood Cliffs, NJ: Prentice Hall.

———. 1971. *Relations in public.* New York: Basic Books.

GOLDBERG, DAVID, AND PETER HUXLEY. 1980. *Mental illness in the community.* London: Tavistock.

GOLDBERG, E. M., AND S. L. MORRISSON. 1963. "Schizophrenia and social class." *British Journal of Psychiatry* 109:785–802.

GOLDENBERG, HERBERT. 1977. *Abnormal psychology: A social/community approach.* Monterey, CA: Brooks/Cole.

GOLDSTEIN, ABRAHAM S. 1967. *The insanity defense.* New Haven, CT: Yale University Press.

GORE, SUSAN. 1978. "The effect of social support in moderating the health consequences of unemployment." *Journal of Health and Social Behavior* 19:157–65.

———. 1981. "Stress-buffering functions of social supports: An appraisal and clarification of research models." Pp. 202–22 in B. Dohrenwend and B. Dohrenwend (eds.), *Stressful life events and their contexts.* New York: Prodist.

———. 1989. "Social networks and social supports in health care." Pp. 306–31 in H. Freeman and S. Levine (eds.), *Handbook of medical sociology,* 4th ed. Englewood Cliffs, NJ: Prentice Hall.

GORE, SUSAN, ROBERT H. ASELTINE, JR., AND MARY ELLEN COLTON. 1992. "Social structure, life stress and depressive symptoms in a high school-aged population." *Journal of Health and Social Behavior* 33:97–113.

GORE, SUSAN, AND THOMAS W. MANGIONE. 1983. "Social roles, sex roles and psychological distress: Additive and interactive models of stress." *Journal of Health and Social Behavior* 24:300–12.

GOVE, WALTER R. 1970a. "Societal reaction as an explanation of mental illness: An evaluation." *American Sociological Review* 35:873–84.

———. 1970b. "Who is hospitalized: A critical review of some sociological studies of mental illness." *Journal of Health and Social Behavior* 11:294–304.

———. 1972. "Sex roles, marital roles, and mental illness." *Social Forces* 51:34–44.

———. 1975a. "Labelling and mental illness." Pp. 35–81 in W. Gove (ed.), *The labelling of deviance: Evaluating a perspective.* New York: Halsted.

———. 1975b. "The labelling theory of mental illness: A reply to Scheff." *American Sociological Review* 40:242–48.

———. 1976. "Deviant behavior, social intervention and labelling theory." Pp. 219–27 in L. Coser and O. Larsen (eds.), *The uses of controversy in sociology.* New York: Free Press.

———. 1978. "Sex differences in mental illness among adult men and women: An examination of four questions raised regarding whether or not women actually have higher rates." *Social Science and Medicine* 12B:187–98.

———. 1979. "Sex, marital status, and psychiatric treatment: A research note." *Social Forces* 58:89–93.

GOVE, WALTER R., AND TERRY FAIN. 1973. "The stigma of mental hospitalization: An attempt to evaluate its consequences." *Archives of General Psychiatry* 28:494–500.

GOVE, WALTER R., AND TERRY R. HERB. 1974. "Stress and mental illness among the young: A comparison of the sexes." *Social Forces* 53:256–65.

GOVE, WALTER R., AND PATRICK HOWELL. 1974. "Individual resources and mental hospitalization: A comparison and evaluation of the societal reaction and psychiatric perspectives." *American Sociological Review* 39:86–100.

GOVE, WALTER R., MICHAEL HUGHES, AND OMER R. GALLE. 1979. "Overcrowding in the home: An empirical investigation of its possible pathological consequences." *American Sociological Review* 44:59–80.

GOVE, WALTER R., MICHAEL HUGHES, AND CAROLYN BRIGGS STYLE. 1983. "Does marriage have positive effects on the psychological well-being of the individual?" *Journal of Health and Social Behavior* 24:122–31.

GOVE, WALTER R., AND JENNIFER TUDOR. 1973. "Adult sex roles and mental illness." *American Journal of Sociology* 77:812–35.

GRANT, VERNON W. 1963. *This is mental illness*. Boston: Beacon Press.

GREBB, JACK A., AND ROBERT CANCRO. 1989. "Schizophrenia: Classic features." Pp. 757–77 in H. Kaplan and B. Sadock (eds.), *Comprehensive textbook of psychiatry*, Vol. 1, 5th ed. Baltimore: Williams & Wilkins.

GREEN, HANNAH. 1964. *I never promised you a rose garden*. New York: Holt, Rinehart & Winston.

GREENLEY, JAMES R. 1979. "Familial expectations, posthospital adjustment, and the societal reaction perspective on mental illness." *Journal of Health and Social Behavior* 20:217–27.

GREENLEY, JAMES R., AND DAVID MECHANIC. 1976a. "Patterns of seeking care for psychological problems." Pp. 177–96 in D. Mechanic (ed.), *The growth of bureaucratic medicine*. New York: Wiley.

———. 1976b. "Social selection in seeking help for psychological problems." *Journal of Health and Social Behavior* 17:249–62.

GRIER, WILLIAM H., AND PRICE M. COBBS. 1992. *Black rage*. New York: Basic Books.

GROB, GERALD N. 1966. *The state and the mentally ill: A history of Worcester State Hospital in Massachusetts, 1830–1920*. Chapel Hill: University of North Carolina Press.

GRÜNBAUM, ADOLF. 1993. *Validation in the clinical theory of psychoanalysis*. Madison, CT: International Universities Press.

GRUSKY, OSCAR, AND MELVIN POLLNER (eds.). 1981. *The sociology of mental illness: Basic studies*. New York: Holt, Rinehart & Winston.

GRUSKY, OSCAR, KATHLEEN TIERNEY, RONALD W. MANDERSCHEID, AND DAVID B. GRUSKY. 1985. "Social bonding and community adjustment of chronically mentally ill patients." *Journal of Health and Social Behavior* 26:49–63.

GUPTA, GIRI RAJ. 1993. *Sociology of mental health*. Boston: Allyn & Bacon.

HÄFNER, HEINZ. 1984. "Psychische Gesundheit im Alter." *Munchener Medizinische Wochenschrift* 24:752–57.

———. 1986. *Psychische Gesundheit im Alter*. Stuttgart: Fischer.

———. 1987. "Do we still need beds for psychiatric patients?" *Acta Psychiatrica Scandinavica* 75:113–26.

HALPERT, H. P. 1969. "Public acceptance of the mentally ill: An experimental study." *Public Health Report* 84:59–64.

HAMILTON, V. LEE, CLIFFORD L. BROMAN, AND WILLIAM S. HOFFMAN. 1990. "Hard times and vulnerable people: Initial effects of plant closing on autoworkers' mental health." *Journal of Health and Social Behavior* 31:123–40.

HARKEY, JOHN, DAVID L. MILES, AND WILLIAM A. RUSHING. 1976. "The relation between social class and functional status: A new look at the drift hypothesis." *Journal of Health and Social Behavior* 17:194–204.

HASSINGER, E. W. 1976. "Pathways of rural people to health services." Pp. 164–87 in E. Hassinger and L. Whiting (eds.), *Rural health services: Organization, delivery and use*. Ames: Iowa State University Press.

HESTON, LEONARD L. 1977. "Schizophrenia: Genetic factors." *Hospital Practice* 12:43–49.

HIDAY, VIRGINIA A. 1977. "Reformed commitment procedures: An empirical study in the courtroom." *Law and Society Review* 11:651–66.

———. 1988. "Civil commitment: A review of empirical research." *Behavioral Sciences & the Law* 11:651–66.

HIRSCH, JERRY. 1970. "Behavior-genetic analysis and its biosocial consequences." *Seminars in Psychiatry* 2:89–105.

HOCHSCHILD, ARLIE RUSSELL. 1973. "A review of sex role research." *American Journal of Sociology* 78:1011–29.

HOLLINGSHEAD, AUGUST B., AND FREDERICK C. REDLICH. 1953. "Social stratification and psychiatric disorders." *American Sociological Review* 18:163–69.

———. 1958. *Social class and mental illness: A community study.* New York: Wiley.

HOLLINGSWORTH, ELLEN JANE. 1994. "Falling through the cracks: Care of the chronically mentally ill in the United States." Pp. 145–72 in J. Hollingsworth and E. Hollingsworth (eds.), *Care of the chronically and severely ill: Comparative social policies.* New York: Aldine de Gruyter.

HOLLINGSWORTH, J. ROGERS, AND ELLEN JANE HOLLINGSWORTH (eds.). 1994. *Care of the chronically and severely ill: Comparative social policies.* New York: Aldine de Gruyter.

HOLMES, T. H., AND M. MASUDA. 1974. "Life change and illness susceptibility." Pp. 45–72 in B. S. Dohrenwend and B. P. Dohrenwend (eds.), *Stressful life events: Their nature and effects.* New York: Wiley.

HOLMES, T. H., AND R. H. RAHE. 1967. "The social readjustment rating scale." *Journal of Psychosomatic Research* 11:213–25.

HOMANS, GEORGE C. 1961. *Social behavior: Its elementary forms.* New York: Harcourt.

HOOK, ERNEST. 1973. "Behavioral implications of the human XXY genotype." *Science* 179:139–50.

HORWITZ, ALLAN. 1977. "The pathways into psychiatric treatment: Some differences between men and women." *Journal of Health and Social Behavior* 18:169–78.

HOUGH, RICHARD L., DIANNE TIMBERS FAIRBANK, AND ALMA M. GARCIA. 1976. "Problems in the ratio measurement of life stress." *Journal of Health and Social Behavior* 17:70–82.

HUFFINE, CAROL L., AND JOHN A. CLAUSEN. 1979. "Madness and work: Short- and long-term effects of mental illness on occupational careers." *Social Forces* 57:1049–62.

HUGHES, MICHAEL, AND WALTER R. GOVE. 1981. "Living alone, social integration, and mental health." *American Journal of Sociology* 87:48–74.

ISSAC, RAEL JEAN, AND VIRGINIA C. ARMAT. 1990. *Madness in the streets: How psychiatry and the law abandoned the mentally ill.* New York: Free Press.

JACKMAN, MARY R., AND ROBERT W. JACKMAN. 1983. *Class awareness in the United States.* Berkeley and Los Angeles: University of California Press.

JACOBSON, DAVID E. 1986. "Types and timing of social support." *Journal of Health and Social Behavior* 27:250–64.

JANIS, IRVING L. 1958. *Psychological stress.* New York: Wiley.

JOHNSON, ANNE BRADEN. 1990. *Out of bedlam: The truth about deinstitutionalization.* New York: Basic Books.

JONES, FRANKLIN DEL, AND ARNOLD W. JOHNSON. 1975. "Medical and psychiatric treatment policy and practice in Vietnam." *Journal of Social Issues* 31:49–65.

JONES, KATHLEEN. 1988. *Experience in mental health.* London: Sage.

KADUSHIN, CHARLES. 1969. *Why people go to psychiatrists.* New York: Atherton.

KALINOWSKY, LOTHAR B. 1975. "The convulsive therapies." Pp. 1969–76 in A. Freedman, H. Kaplan, and B. Sadock (eds.), *Comprehensive textbook of psychiatry,* Vol. 2, 2nd ed. Baltimore: Williams & Wilkins.

KANDEL, DENISE B., MARK DAVIES, AND VICTORIA H. RAVEIS. 1985. "The stressfulness of daily social roles for women: Marital, occupational, and household roles." *Journal of Health and Social Behavior* 26:64–78.

KANTER, ARLENE S. 1989. "Current issues in mental health law." Pp. 113–33 in C. Bonjean, M. Coleman, and I. Iscoe (eds.), *Community care of the chronically mentally ill, Proceedings of the Sixth Robert Lee Sutherland Seminar in Mental Health.* Austin, TX: Hogg Foundation for Mental Health.

KAPLAN, BERT (ed.). 1964. *The inner world of mental illness.* New York: Harper.

KAPLAN, HAROLD L. 1985. "History of psychophysiological medicine." Pp. 1106–13 in A. Freedman, H. Kaplan, and B. Sadock (eds.), *Comprehensive textbook of psychiatry,* Vol. 2, 4th ed. Baltimore: Williams & Wilkins.

KAPLAN, HAROLD L., AND BENJAMIN J. SADOCK. 1989. "Typical signs and symptoms of psychiatric illness." Pp. 460–74 in H. Kaplan and B. Sadock (eds.), *Comprehensive textbook of psychiatry,* Vol. 1, 5th ed. Baltimore: Williams & Wilkins.

KAPLAN, HOWARD B., CYNTHIA ROBBINS, AND STEVEN S. MARTIN. 1983. "Antecedents of psychological distress in young adults: Self-rejection, deprivation of social support, and life events." *Journal of Health and Social Behavior* 24:230–44.

KARP, DAVID A. 1994. "The dialectics of depression." *Symbolic Interaction* 17:341–66.

KASL, STANISLAV V., AND ERNEST HARBURG. 1975. "Mental health and the urban environment: Some doubts and second thoughts." *Journal of Health and Social Behavior* 16:268–82.

KEEGAN, JOHN. 1976. *The face of battle.* New York: Viking.

KEEN, PAUL R. 1974. "Civil commitment of the mentally ill in Kentucky." *Kentucky Law Journal* 62:769–93.

KELLETT, ANTHONY. 1982. *Combat motivation.* Boston: Kulwer.

KENDELL, R. E. 1975. *The role of diagnosis in psychiatry.* Oxford: Blackwell Scientific Publications.

KENDELL, R. E., J. COOPER, A. GOURLEY, AND J. COPELAND. 1971. "Diagnostic criteria of American and British psychiatrists." *Archives of General Psychiatry* 25:123–30.

KESSLER, RONALD C. 1979. "Stress, social status, and psychological distress." *Journal of Health and Social Behavior* 20:259–72.

———. 1982. "A disaggregation of the relationship between socioeconomic status and psychological distress." *American Sociological Review* 47:752–64.

KESSLER, RONALD C., ROGER L. BROWN, AND CLIFFORD L. BROMAN. 1981. "Sex differences in psychiatric help-seeking: Evidence from four large-scale surveys." *Journal of Health and Social Behavior* 22:49–64.

KESSLER, RONALD C., AND PAUL D. CLEARY. 1980. "Social class and psychological distress." *American Sociological Review* 45:463–78.

KESSLER, RONALD C., AND MARILYN ESSEX. 1982. "Martial status and depression: The importance of coping resources." *Social Forces* 61:484–507.

KESSLER, RONALD C., JAMES S. HOUSE, AND J. BLAKE TURNER. 1987. "Unemployment and health in a community sample." *Journal of Health and Social Behavior* 18:51–59.

KESSLER, RONALD C., AND WILLIAM J. MAGEE. 1994. "Childhood family violence and adult recurrent depression." *Journal of Health and Social Behavior* 35:13–27.

KESSLER, RONALD C., KATHERINE A. McGONAGLE, SHANYANG ZHAO, CHRISTOPHER B. NELSON, MICHAEL HUGHES, SUZANN ESHLEMAN, HANS-ULRICH WITTCHEN, AND KENNETH S. KENDLER. 1994. "Lifetime and 12-month prevalence of DSM-III-R psychiatric disorders in the United States: Results from the national comorbidity survey." *Archives of General Psychiatry* 51:8–19.

KESSLER, RONALD C., AND JANE D. McLEOD. 1984. "Sex differences in vulnerability to undesirable life events." *American Sociological Review* 49:620–31.

KESSLER, RONALD C., AND JAMES A. McRAE, JR. 1981. "Trends in the relationship between sex and psychological distress: 1957–1976." *American Sociological Review* 46:443–52.

———. 1982. "The effect of wives' employment on the mental health of married men and women." *American Sociological Review* 47:217–27.

KESSLER, RONALD C., AND HAROLD W. NEIGHBORS. 1986. "A new perspective on the relationships between race, social class, and psychological distress." *Journal of Health and Social Behavior* 27:107–15.

KESSLER, RONALD C., JAMES A. REUTER, AND JAMES R. GREENLEY. 1979. "Sex differences in the use of psychiatric outpatient facilities." *Social Forces* 58:557–71.

KESSLER, RONALD C., J. BLAKE TURNER, AND JAMES S. HOUSE. 1989. "Unemployment, reemployment, and emotional functioning in a community sample." *American Sociological Review* 54:648–57.

KIEV, ARI (ed.). 1964. *Magic, faith, and healing: Studies in primitive psychiatry today.* New York: Free Press.

KIEV, ARI 1968. *Curanderismo: Mexican-American folk psychiatry.* New York: Free Press.

———. 1972. *Transcultural psychiatry.* New York: Free Press.

KILLIAN, L. M., AND S. BLOOMBERG. 1975. "Rebirth in a therapeutic community: A case study." *Psychiatry* 38:39–54.

KIRK, STUART A., AND HERB KUTCHINS. 1992. *The selling of DSM: The rhetoric of science in psychiatry.* New York: Aldine de Gruyter.

KITANO, HARRY H. L. 1969. "Japanese-American mental illness." Pp. 256–84 in S. Plof and R. Edgerton (eds.), *Changing perspectives in mental illness.* New York: Holt, Rinehart & Winston.

———. 1985. *Race relations.* 3rd ed. Englewood Cliffs, NJ: Prentice Hall.

KLEINMAN, ARTHUR. 1988. *Rethinking psychiatry.* New York: Free Press.

KLEINMAN, ARTHUR, AND DAVID MECHANIC. 1979. "Some observations of mental illness and its treatment in the People's Republic of China." *Journal of Nervous and Mental Disease* 167:267–74.

KLERMAN, GERALD L. 1989. "Psychiatric diagnostic categories: Issues of validity and measurement." *Journal of Health and Social Behavior* 30:26–32.

KOHN, MELVIN L. 1969. *Class and conformity: A study in values.* Homewood, IL: Dorsey.
———. 1972. "Class, family, and schizophrenia: A reformulation," *Social Forces* 50:295–304.
———. 1974. "Social class and schizophrenia: A critical review and reformulation." Pp. 113–37 in P. Roman and H. Trice (eds.), *Explorations in psychiatric sociology.* Philadelphia: Davis.
———. 1976. "The interaction of social class and other factors in the etiology of schizophrenia." *American Journal of Psychiatry* 133:177–80.
KRAUSE, ELLIOTT A. 1977. *Power & illness: The political sociology of health and medical care.* New York: Elsevier.
KRAUSE, NEAL, AND KYRIAKOS S. MARKIDES. 1985. "Employment and psychological well-being in Mexican American women." *Journal of Health and Social Behavior* 26:15–26.
KREISMAN, DOLORES E., AND VIRGINIA D. JOY. 1974. "Family response to the mental illness of a relative: A review of the literature." *Schizophrenia Bulletin* 10:34–57.
KROHN, MARVIN D., AND RONALD L. AKERS. 1977. "An alternative view of the labeling versus psychiatric perspectives on societal reaction to mental illness." *Social Forces* 56:341–61.
KULKA, RICHARD A., JOSEPH VEROFF, AND ELIZABETH DOUVAN. 1979. "Social class and the use of professional help for personal problems: 1957 and 1976." *Journal of Health and Social Behavior* 20:2–17.
KUO, WEN H., AND YUNG-MEI TSAI. 1986. "Social networks, hardiness, and immigrants' mental health." *Journal of Health and Social Behavior* 27:133–49.
LAFOND, JOHN Q., AND MARY L. DURHAM. 1992. *Back to the asylum: The future of mental health law and policy in the United States.* New York: Oxford University Press.
LA GORY, MARK, FERRIS J. RITCHEY, AND JEFF MULLIS. 1990. "Depression among the homeless." *Journal of Health and Social Behavior* 31:87–102.
LAGUERRE, MICHAEL. 1987. *Afro-Caribbean folk medicine.* South Hadley, MA: Bergin & Garvey.
LAING, R. D. 1967. *The politics of experience.* New York: Ballantine.
———. 1969. *The divided self.* New York: Pantheon.
LANGNER, T., AND S. MICHAEL. 1963. *Life stress and mental health: The Midtown Manhattan study.* London: Free Press of Glencoe.
LAUER, ROBERT. 1974. "Rate of change and stress." *Social Forces* 52:510–16.
LAVES, RONA G. 1975. "The prediction of 'dangerousness' as a criterion for involuntary civil commitment: Constitutional considerations." *Journal of Psychiatry & Law* 3:291–325.
LEBAR, FRANK M. 1973. *Segregative care in an institutional setting: The ethnography of a psychiatric hospital.* New Haven, CT: Human Relations Area Files.
LEHMANN, S., V. JOY, D. KREISMAN, AND S. SIMMENS. 1976. "Responses to viewing symptomatic behavior and labeling of prior mental illness." *Journal of Community Psychology* 4:327–34.
LEIGHTON, D. C., J. S. HARDING, D. B. MACKLIN, A. M. MACMILLAN, AND A. H. LEIGHTON. 1963. *The character of danger: Psychiatric symptoms in selected communities.* New York: Basic Books.
LEMERT, EDWIN M. 1951. *Social pathology.* New York: McGraw-Hill.
———. 1962. "Paranoia and the dynamics of exclusion." *Sociometry* 25:2–20.
———. 1972. *Human deviance, social problems, and social control.* 2nd ed. Englewood Cliffs, NJ: Prentice Hall.
LEMKAU, P. V., AND G. M. CROCETTI. 1962. "An urban population's opinions and knowledge about mental illness." *American Journal of Psychiatry* 118:692–700.
LENNON, MARY CLARE. 1982. "The psychological consequences of menopause: The importance of timing of a life stage event." *Journal of Health and Social Behavior* 23:353–66.
———. 1987. "Sex differences in distress: The impact of gender and roles." *Journal of Health and Social Behavior* 28:290–305.
———. 1994. "Women, work, and well-being: The importance of work conditions." *Journal of Health and Social Behavior* 35:235–47.
LENNON, MARY CLARE, AND SARAH ROSENFIELD. 1992. "Women and mental health: The interaction of job and family conditions." *Journal of Health and Social Behavior* 33:316–27.
LETORRE, RONALD. 1975. "Gender and age as factors in the attitudes toward those stigmatized as mentally ill." *Journal of Consulting and Clinical Psychology* 43:97–98.
LEVER, JANET. 1978. "Sex differences in the complexity of children's play and games." *American Sociological Review* 43:471–83.
LEVINSON, RICHARD M., AND GEORGEANN RAMSAY. 1979. "Dangerousness, stress, and mental health evaluations." *Journal of Health and Social Behavior* 20:178–87.
LEVINSON, RICHARD M., AND M. ZAN YORK. 1974. "The attribution of 'dangerousness' in mental health evaluations." *Journal of Health and Social Behavior* 15:328–35.

LEVY, LEO, AND LOUIS ROWITZ. 1973. *The ecology of mental disorder.* New York: Behavioral Publications.

LEVY, RENÉ. 1976. "Psychosomatic symptoms and women's protest: Two types of reaction to structural strain in the family." *Journal of Health and Social Behavior* 17:122–34.

LICHTMAN, RICHARD. 1982. *The production of desire: The integration of psychoanalysis into Marxist theory.* New York: Free Press.

LICKEY, MARVIN E., AND BARBARA GORDON. 1991. *Medicine and mental illness.* New York: W. H. Freeman.

LIEBLING, A. J. 1961. *The earl of Louisiana.* New York: Simon & Schuster.

LIEM, RAMSAY, AND JOAN LIEM. 1978. "Social class and mental illness reconsidered: The role of economic stress and social support." *Journal of Health and Social Behavior* 19:139–56.

LIFTON, ROBERT JAY. 1986. *The Nazi doctors.* New York: Basic Books.

LIN, NAN, AND WALTER M. ENSEL. 1989. "Life stress and health: Stressors and resources." *American Sociological Review* 54:382–99.

LIN, NAN, RONALD S. SIMEONE, WALTER M. ENSEL, AND WEN KUO. 1979. "Social support, stressful life events and illness: A model and an empirical test." *Journal of Health and Social Behavior* 20:108–19.

LIN, NAN, MARY W. WOELFUL, AND STEPHEN C. LIGHT. 1985. "The buffering effect of social support subsequent to an important life event." *Journal of Health and Social Behavior* 24:61–69.

LIN, TSUNG-YI. 1953. "A study of the incidence of mental disorder in Chinese and other cultures." *Psychiatry* 16:313–36.

LINDESMITH, ALFRED R. 1968. *Addiction and opiates.* Chicago: Aldine.

LINDESMITH, ALFRED, ANSELM STRAUSS, AND NORMAN DENZIN. 1975. *Social psychology.* 5th ed. Hinsdale, IL: Dryden Press.

LINK, BRUCE G. 1982. "Mental patient status, work, and income: An examination of the effects of a psychiatric label." *American Sociological Review* 47:202–15.

———. 1983. "Reward system of psychotherapy: Implications for inequities in service delivery." *Journal of Health and Social Behavior* 24:61–69.

———. 1987. "Understanding labeling effects in the area of mental disorders: An assessment of the effects of expectations of rejection." *American Sociological Review* 52:96–112.

LINK, BRUCE G., HOWARD ANDREWS, AND FRANCIS T. CULLEN. 1992. "The violent and illegal behavior of mental patients reconsidered." *American Sociological Review* 57:275–92.

LINK, BRUCE G., AND FRANCIS T. CULLEN. 1986. "Contact with the mentally ill and perceptions of how dangerous they are." *Journal of Health and Social Behavior* 27:289–303.

LINK, BRUCE G., FRANCIS T. CULLEN, JAMES FRANK, AND JOHN F. WOZNIAK. 1987. "The social rejection of former mental patients: Understanding why labels matter." *American Journal of Sociology* 92:1461–1500.

LINK, BRUCE G., BRUCE P. DOHRENWEND, AND ANDREW E. SKODOL. 1986. "Socioeconomic status and schizophrenia: Noisome occupational characteristics as a risk factor." *American Sociological Review* 51:242–58.

LINK, BRUCE G., MARY CLARE LENNON, AND BRUCE P. DOHRENWEND. 1993. "Socioeconomic status and depression: The role of occupations involving direction, control, and planning." *American Journal of Sociology* 98:1351–87.

LINK, BRUCE, AND BARRY MILCAREK. 1980. "Selection factors in the dispensation of therapy: The Matthew effect in the allocation of mental health resources." *Journal of Health and Social Behavior* 21:279–90.

LINSKY, ARNOLD S. 1970a. "Community homogeneity and exclusion of the mentally ill: Rejection vs. consensus about deviance." *Journal of Health and Social Behavior* 11:304–11.

———. 1970b. "Who shall be excluded: The influence of personal attributes in community reaction to the mentally ill." *Social Psychiatry* 6:166–71.

LIVINGSTON, MARTHA, AND PAUL LOWINGER. 1983. *The minds of the Chinese people.* Englewood Cliffs, NJ: Prentice Hall.

LORING, MARTI, AND BRIAN POWELL. 1988. "Gender, race, and DSM-III: A study of the objectivity of psychiatric diagnostic behavior." *Journal of Health and Social Behavior* 29:1–22.

LOSCOCCO, KARYN A., AND GLENNA SPITZE. 1990. "Working conditions, social support, and the well-being of female and male factory workers." *Journal of Health and Social Behavior* 31:313–27.

MAAS, JAMES W. 1979. "Biochemistry of the affective disorders." *Hospital Practice* 14:13–20.

MACCOBY, ELEANOR (ed.). 1966. *The development of sex differences.* Stanford, CA: Stanford University Press.

MADSEN, WILLIAM. 1973. *The Mexican-Americans of south Texas.* 2nd ed. New York: Holt, Rinehart & Winston.

MARETZKI, THOMAS W. 1987. "The Kur in West Germany as an interface between naturopathic and allopathic ideologies." *Social Science and Medicine* 24:1061–68.

MARKS, ISAAC. 1979. "Exposure therapy for phobias and obsessive-compulsive disorders." *Hospital Practice* 14:101–8.

MARSHALL, JAMES R., AND GEORGE W. DOWDALL. 1982. "Employment and mental hospitalization: The case of Buffalo, New York, 1914–55." *Social Forces* 60:843–53.

MARSHALL, JAMES R., AND DONNA P. FUNCH. 1979. "Mental illness and the economy: A critique and partial replication." *Journal of Health and Social Behavior* 20:282–89.

MARTIN, BARCLAY. 1971. *Anxiety and neurotic disorders.* New York: Wiley.

MARTIN, WALTER T. 1976. "Status integration, social stress, and mental illness: Accounting for marital status variations in mental hospitalization rates." *Journal of Health and Social Behavior* 17:280–94.

MATT, GEORG E., AND ALFRED DEAN. 1993. "Social support from friends and psychological distress among elderly persons: Moderator effects of age." *Journal of Health and Social Behavior* 34:187–200.

MATZA, DAVID. 1969. *Becoming deviant.* Englewood Cliffs, NJ: Prentice Hall.

MAZUR, ALLAN, AND LEON S. ROBINSON. 1972. *Biology and social behavior.* New York: Free Press.

McLANAHAN, SARA S., AND JENNIFER L. GLASS. 1985. "A note on the trend in sex differences in psychological distress." *Journal of Health and Social Behavior* 26:328–36.

McNEIL, ELTON B. 1967. *The quiet furies.* Englewood Cliffs, NJ: Prentice Hall.

McNIEL, DALE E., AND RENEE L. BINDER. 1987. "Predictive validity of judgments of dangerousness in emergency civil commitment." *American Journal of Psychiatry* 144:197–200.

MEAD, GEORGE H. 1934. *Mind, self, and society.* Chicago: University of Chicago Press.

MECHANIC, DAVID. 1975. "Sociocultural and psychological factors affecting personal responses to psychological disorder." *Journal of Health and Social Behavior* 16:393–404.

———. 1979. *Future issues in health care.* New York: Free Press.

———. 1989. *Mental health and social policy.* 3rd ed. Englewood Cliffs, NJ: Prentice Hall.

MECHANIC, DAVID, AND ARTHUR KLEINMAN. 1980. "Ambulatory medical care in the People's Republic of China: An exploratory study." *American Journal of Public Health* 70:65–72.

MEGARGEE, EDWIN I. 1970. "The prediction of violence with psychological tests." Pp. 97–156 in C. Spielberger (ed.), *Current topics in clinical and community psychology,* Vol. 2. New York: Academic Press.

MEISSNER, WILLIAM W. 1985. "Theories of personality and psychopathology: Classical psychoanalysis." Pp. 337–418 in H. Kaplan and B. Sadock (eds.), *Comprehensive textbook of psychiatry,* Vol. 1, 4th ed. Baltimore: Williams & Wilkins.

MELICK, MARY EVANS, HENRY J. STEADMAN, AND JOSEPH J. COCOZZA. 1979. "The medicalization of criminal behavior among mental patients." *Journal of Health and Social Behavior* 20:228–37.

MENDEL, WERNER M., AND SAMUEL RAPPORT. 1969. "Determinants of the decision for psychiatric hospitalization." *Archives of General Psychiatry* 20:321–28.

MENDELS, JOSEPH. 1970. *Concepts of depression.* New York: Wiley.

MERTON, ROBERT K. 1938. "Social structure and anomie." *American Sociological Review* 3:672–82.

METTLIN, CURT, AND JOSEPH WOELFEL. 1974. "Interpersonal influence and symptoms of stress." *Journal of Health and Social Behavior* 15:311–19.

MILES, AGNES. 1981. *The mentally ill in contemporary society.* Oxford: Robertson.

MILLER, DOROTHY H. 1971. "Worlds that fail." Pp. 102–14 in S. Wallace (ed.), *Total institutions.* Chicago: Aldine.

MILLER, DOROTHY, AND WILLIAM H. DAWSON. 1965. "Effects of stigma on re-employment of ex-mental patients." *Mental Hygiene* 49:281–87.

MIROWSKY, JOHN. 1985. "Depression and marital power: An equity model." *American Journal of Sociology* 91:557–92.

MIROWSKY, JOHN, AND CATHERINE E. ROSS. 1980. "Minority status, ethnic culture, and distress: A comparison of blacks, whites, Mexicans, and Mexican Americans." *American Journal of Sociology* 86:479–511.

———. 1983. "Paranoia and the structure of powerlessness." *American Sociological Review* 48:228–39.

———. 1984. "Mexican culture and its emotional contradictions." *Journal of Health and Social Behavior* 25:2–13.

——. 1989a. "Psychiatric diagnosis as reified measurement." *Journal of Health and Social Behavior* 30:11–25.

——. 1989b. *Social causes of psychological distress.* New York: Aldine de Gruyter.

——. 1990. "Control or defense? Depression and the sense of control over good and bad outcomes." *Journal of Health and Social Behavior* 31:71–86.

——. 1992. "Age and depression." *Journal of Health and Social Behavior* 33:187–205.

MISHLER, ELLIOT G., AND NANCY E. WAXLER. 1963. "Decision processes in psychiatric hospitalization." *American Sociological Review* 29:576–87.

MITCHELL, ROGER E., AND RUDOLF H. MOOS. 1984. "Deficiencies in social support among depressed patients: Antecedents or consequences of stress?" *Journal of Health and Social Behavior* 25:438–52.

MONAHAN, JOHN. 1981. *The clinical prediction of violent behavior.* Beverly Hills, CA: Sage.

MORA, GEORGE. 1985. "History of psychiatry." Pp. 2034–54 in H. Kaplan and B. Sadock (eds.). *Comprehensive text of psychiatry,* Vol. 2, 4th ed. Baltimore: Williams & Wilkins.

MOSKOS, CHARLES C., JR. 1970. *The American enlisted man.* New York: Russell Sage.

MOSS, GORDON E. 1973. *Illness, immunity, and social interaction.* New York: Wiley.

MUELLER, DANIEL P., DANIEL W. EDWARDS, AND RICHARD M. YARVIS. 1977. "Stressful life events and psychiatric symptomatology: Change or undesirability." *Journal of Health and Social Behavior* 18:307–17.

MULFORD, C. L. 1968. "Ethnocentrism and attitudes toward the mentally ill." *Sociological Quarterly* 9:107–11.

MULLAN, HUGH, AND MAX ROSENBAUM. 1978. *Group psychotherapy: Theory and practice.* 2nd ed. New York: Free Press.

MÜLLER, ULRICH. 1985. "Tendezwenden' in der Gesellschaft Paradigmenwandlungen in Soziologie und Psychiatrie?" *Mensch Medizin Gesellschaft* 10:264–72.

MUNAKATA, TSUNETSUGU. 1986. "Sociocultural background of the mental health system in Japan." *Culture, Medicine and Psychiatry* 10:351–65.

——. 1989. "The socio-cultural significance of the diagnostic label 'neurasthenia' in Japan's mental health care system." *Culture, Medicine and Psychiatry* 13:203–13.

MURPHY, H. B. M. 1961. "Social change and mental health." Pp. 280–329 in *Causes of mental disorders: A review of epidemiological knowledge.* New York: Milbank Memorial Fund.

——. 1969. "Migration and the major mental disorders: A reappraisal." Pp. 5–29 in M. Kanter (ed.), *Mobility & mobile health.* Springfield, IL: Charles C. Thomas.

MURPHY, JANE M. 1964. "Psychotherapeutic aspects of shamanism on St. Lawrence Island, Alaska." Pp. 53–83 in A. Kiev (ed.), *Magic, faith, and healing: Studies in primitive psychiatry today.* New York: Free Press.

——. 1976. "Psychiatric labeling in cross-cultural perspective." *Science* 191:1019–27.

MYERS, J. K. 1964. "Attitudes toward mental illness in a Maryland community." *Public Health Report* 79:769–72.

MYERS, JEROME K., JACOB J. LINDENTHAL, AND MAX P. PEPPER. 1975. "Life events, social integration, and psychiatric symptomatology." *Journal of Health and Social Behavior* 16:421–27.

MYERS, JEROME, AND BERTRAM ROBERTS. 1959. *Family and class dynamics in mental illness.* New York: Wiley.

NARENS, LOUIS. 1973. "Belief systems of the insane." Social Science Working Paper 31, School of Social Science, University of California, Irvine.

NARROW, W. E., D. A. REIGER, D. S. RAE, R. W. MANDERSCHEID, AND B. Z. LOCKE. 1993. "Use of services by persons with mental and addictive disorders: Findings from the National Institute of Mental Health Epidemiologic Catchment Area Program." *Archives of General Psychiatry* 50:95–107.

NATIONAL CENTER FOR HEALTH STATISTICS. 1978. *Office visits to psychiatrists: National ambulatory medical care survey, United States, 1975–76.* Advance Data, No. 38. Washington, DC: Department of Health, Education, and Welfare.

NATIONAL CENTER FOR HEALTH STATISTICS AND CENTERS FOR DISEASE CONTROL. 1992. "Serious mental illness and disability in the adult household population." Advance Data. Washington, DC: U.S. Government Printing Office.

NATIONAL INSTITUTE OF MENTAL HEALTH. 1985. *Mental health, United States, 1985.* Washington, DC: U.S. Government Printing Office.

——. 1986a. "Characteristics of admissions to the inpatient services of state and county mental hospitals, United States, 1980." Mental Health Statistical Note No. 177. Washington, DC: U.S. Department of Health and Human Services.

———. 1986b. "Use of inpatient psychiatric services by children and youth under age 18, United States, 1980." Mental Health Statistical Note No. 175. Washington, DC: U.S. Department of Health and Human Services.

———. 1987. *Mental health, United States, 1987.* Washington, DC: U.S. Government Printing Office.

———. 1990. *Mental health, United States, 1990.* Washington, DC: U.S. Government Printing Office.

NAVARRO, VICENTE. 1986. *Crisis, health, and medicine: A social critique.* New York: Tavistock.

NEFF, JAMES ALAN. 1984. "Race differences and psychological distress: The effects of sex, urbanicity and measurement strategy." *American Journal of Community Psychology* 12:337–51.

NEFF, JAMES ALAN, AND BAOAR A. HUSAINI. 1980. "Race, socioeconomic status, and psychiatric impairment: A research note." *Journal of Community Psychology* 8:16–19.

———. 1987. "Urbanicity, race, and psychological distress." *Journal of Community Psychology* 15:520–36.

NEIGHBORS, HAROLD W., AND CLEOPATRA S. HOWARD. 1987. "Sex differences in professional help-seeking among adult black Americans." *American Journal of Community Psychology* 15:403–16.

NEWMANN, JOY P. 1984. "Sex differences in symptoms of depression: Clinical disorder or normal distress?" *Journal of Health and Social Behavior* 25:136–59.

NORRIS, FRAN H., AND STANLEY A. MURRELL. 1984. "Protective function of resources related to life events, global stress, and depression in older adults." *Journal of Health and Social Behavior* 25:424–37.

NUNNALLY, J. C., JR. 1961. *Popular conceptions of mental health.* New York: Holt, Rinehart & Winston.

O'BRIEN, BERNIE. 1984. *Patterns of European diagnoses and prescriptions.* London: Office of Health Economics.

ÖDEGAARD, O. 1932. *Emigration and insanity: A study of mental disease among the Norwegian born population of Minnesota.* Copenhagen: Levin & Munksgaards.

OLMSTED, DONALD W., AND KATHERINE DURHAM. 1976. "Stability of mental health attitudes: A semantic differential study." *Journal of Health and Social Behavior* 17:35–44.

OLMSTED, DONALD W., AND DOROTHY L. SMITH. 1980. "The socialization of youth into the American mental health belief system." *Journal of Health and Social Behavior* 21:181–94.

O'MALLEY, PATRICK M., JERALD G. BACHMAN, AND LLOYD D. JOHNSTON. 1988. "Period, age, and cohort effects on substance use among young Americans: A decade of change, 1976–86." *American Journal of Public Health* 78:1315–21.

OMARK, RICHARD C. 1979. "The dilemma of membership in Recovery, Inc., a self-help ex-mental patients' organization." *Psychological Reports* 44:1119–25.

———. 1982. "Cycles and balance: Personality change versus organizational maintenance." *Psychiatric Quarterly* 54:109–22.

OXFORD ANALYTICA. 1986. *American perspective.* Boston: Houghton Mifflin.

PADILLA, AMADO M., AND RENE A. RUIZ. 1973. *Latino mental health: A review of the literature.* Rockville, MD: National Institute of Mental Health.

PARRY, GLENYS. 1986. "Paid employment, life events, social support, and mental health in working-class mothers." *Journal of Health and Social Behavior* 27:193–208.

PARSONS, TALCOTT. 1951. *The social system.* New York: Free Press.

PEARLIN, LEONARD I., AND JOYCE S. JOHNSON. 1977. "Marital status, life-strains and depression." *American Sociological Review* 42:704–15.

PEARLIN, LEONARD I., MORTON A. LIEBERMAN, ELIZABETH G. MENAGHAN, AND JOSEPH T. MULLAN. 1981. "The stress process." *Journal of Health and Social Behavior* 22:337–56.

PEARLIN, LEONARD I., AND CARMI SCHOOLER. 1978. "The structure of coping." *Journal of Health and Social Behavior* 19:2–21.

PERRUCCI, ROBERT. 1974. *Circle of madness: On being insane and institutionalized in America.* Englewood Cliffs, NJ: Prentice Hall.

PERRUCCI, ROBERT, AND DENA B. TARG. 1982. "Network structure and reactions to primary deviance of mental patients." *Journal of Health and Social Behavior* 23:2–17.

PHILLIPS, D. L. 1963. "Rejection: A possible consequence of seeking help for mental disorders." *American Sociological Review* 28:963–72.

———. 1964. "Rejection of the mentally ill: The influence of behavior and sex." *American Sociological Review* 29:679–87.

———. 1966. "Public identification and acceptance of the mentally ill." *American Journal of Public Health* 56:755–63.

———. 1967. "Identification of mental illness: Its consequences for rejection." *Community Mental Health* 3:262–66.

PIERCE, ALBERT. 1967. "Economic cycle and the social suicide rate." *American Sociological Review* 32:457–62.

PILGRIM, DAVID, AND ANNE ROGERS. 1993. *A sociology of mental health and illness.* Buckingham, UK: Open University Press.

PORTES, ALEJANDRO, DAVID KYLE, AND WILLIAM W. EATON. 1992. "Mental illness and help-seeking behavior among Mariel Cuban and Haitian refugees in south Florida." *Journal of Health and Social Behavior* 33:283–98.

PRINCE, RAYMOND. 1964. "Indigenous Yoruba psychiatry." Pp. 84–120 in A. Kiev (ed.), *Magic, faith, and healing: Studies in primitive psychiatry today.* New York: Free Press.

QUERY, JOY M. N. 1980. "The factory hospital: A ten year study of chronic patients." *American Journal of Orthopsychiatry* 50:156–59.

RABKIN, JUDITH G. 1974. "Public attitudes toward mental illness: A review of the literature." *Schizophrenia Bulletin* 10:9–33.

RADO, S. 1949. "Pathodynamics and treatment of traumatic war neurosis (tramatophobia)." *Psychosomatic Medicine* 43:363–98.

RAINER, JOHN D. 1985. "Genetics and psychiatry." Pp. 25–42 in H. Kaplan and B. Sadock (eds.), *Comprehensive textbook of psychiatry,* Vol. 2, 4th ed. Baltimore: Williams & Wilkins.

RAMON, SHULAMIT. 1994. "Community mental health services for the continuing-care client." Pp. 173–230 in J. Hollingsworth and E. Hollingsworth (eds.), *Care of the chronically and severely ill: Comparative social policies.* New York: Aldine de Gruyter.

RAPPAPORT, J., AND G. LASSEN. 1965. "Dangerousness-arrest rate comparisons of discharged patients and the general population." *American Journal of Psychiatry* 121:776–83.

———. 1966. "The dangerousness of female patients: A comparison of the arrest rate of discharged psychiatric patients and the general population." *American Journal of Psychiatry* 123:413–19.

RAY, OAKLEY. 1978. *Drugs, society, and human behavior.* 2nd ed. St. Louis: Mosby.

REIGER, D., J. BOYD, J. BURKE, D. RAE, J. MYERS, M. KRAMER, L. ROBBINS, L. GEORGE, M. KARNO, AND B. LOCKE. 1988. "One-month prevalence of mental disorders in the United States." *Archives of General Psychiatry* 45:977–86.

REISS, S. 1972. "A critique of Thomas S. Szasz's Myth of Mental Illness." *American Journal of Psychiatry* 128:71–84.

RIDENOUR, N. 1961. *Mental health in the United States: A fifty-year history.* Cambridge, MA: Harvard University Press.

RIEF, D. 1961. *Freud: The mind of the moralist.* New York: Doubleday.

ROBERTS, ROBERT E. 1980. "The prevalence of psychological distress among Mexican Americans." *Journal of Health and Social Behavior* 21:134–45.

ROBERTS, ROBERT E., AND STEPHEN J. O'KEEFE. 1981. "Sex differences in depression reexamined." *Journal of Health and Social Behavior* 22:394–400.

ROBIN, STANLEY S., AND MORTON O. WAGENFELD. 1977. "The community mental health worker: Organizational and personal sources of role discrepancy." *Journal of Health and Social Behavior* 18:16–27.

ROBITSCHER, JONAS. 1976. "Moving patients out of hospitals—in whose interest?" Pp. 141–75 in P. Ahmed and S. Plog (eds.), *State mental hospitals.* New York: Plenum.

ROGLER, LLOYD H., AND AUGUST B. HOLLINGSHEAD. 1965. *Trapped: Families and schizophrenia.* New York: Wiley.

ROSE, ARNOLD. 1956. "Neuropsychiatric breakdown in the garrison army and in combat." *American Sociological Review* 21:480–88.

ROSEN, G. 1968. *Madness in society.* Chicago: University of Chicago Press.

ROSENBERG, EMILY J., AND BARBARA S. DOHRENWEND. 1975. "Effects of experience and ethnicity on ratings of life events as stressors." *Journal of Health and Social Behavior* 16:127–29.

ROSENBERG, MORRIS. 1984. "A symbolic interactionist view of psychosis." *Journal of Health and Social Behavior* 25:289–302.

ROSENBERG, M., AND R. SIMMONS. 1972. *Black and white self-esteem: The urban school child.* Washington, DC: American Sociological Association.

ROSENFIELD, SARAH. 1980. "Sex differences in depression: Do women always have higher rates?" *Journal of Health and Social Behavior* 21:33–42.

———. 1982. "Sex roles and societal reactions to mental illness: The labeling of 'deviant' deviance." *Journal of Health and Social Behavior* 23:18–24.

———. 1989. "The effects of women's employment: Personal control and sex differences in mental health." *Journal of Health and Social Behavior* 30:77–91.

———. 1992a. "The costs of sharing: Wives' employment and husbands' mental health." *Journal of Health and Social Behavior* 33:213–25.

———. 1992b. "Factors contributing to the subjective quality of life of the chronically mentally ill." *Journal of Health and Social Behavior* 33:299–315.

ROSENHAN, DAVID L. 1973. "On being sane in insane places." *Science* 179:250–58.

ROSS, CATHERINE E., AND JOAN HUBER. 1985. "Hardship and depression." *Journal of Health and Social Behavior* 26:312–27.

ROSS, CATHERINE E., AND JOHN MIROWSKY. 1979. "A comparison of life-event-weighting schemes: Change, undesirability, and effect-proportional indices." *Journal of Health and Social Behavior* 20:166–77.

ROSS, CATHERINE E., JOHN MIROWSKY, AND WILLIAM C. COCKERHAM. 1983. "Social class, Mexican culture, and fatalism: Their effects on psychological distress." *American Journal of Community Psychology* 11:383–99.

ROSS, CATHERINE E., JOHN MIROWSKY, AND JOAN HUBER. 1983. "Dividing work, sharing work, and in-between: Marriage patterns and depression." *American Sociological Review* 48:809–23.

ROSS, CATHERINE E., JOHN MIROWSKY, AND PATRICIA ULBRICH. 1983. "Distress and the traditional female role: A comparison of Mexicans and Anglos." *American Journal of Sociology* 89:670–82.

ROTTER, J. B. 1966. "Generalized expectancies for internal vs. external control of reinforcement." *Psychological Monographs* 80:1–28.

RUBIN, LILLIAN BRESLOW. 1976. *Worlds of pain: Life in the working class family.* New York: Basic Books.

RUCH, LIBBY O. 1977. "Multidimensional analysis of the concept of life change." *Journal of Health and Social Behavior* 18:71–83.

RUSHING, WILLIAM A. 1971. "Individual resources, societal reaction, and hospital commitment." *American Journal of Sociology* 77:511–26.

———. 1978. "Status resources, societal reactions, and type of mental hospital admissions." *American Sociological Review* 43:521–33.

———. 1979a. "The functional importance of sex roles and sex-related behavior in societal reactions to residual deviants." *Journal of Health and Social Behavior* 20:208–17.

———. 1979b. "Marital status and mental disorder." *Social Forces* 58:540–56.

RUSHING, WILLIAM A., AND JACK ESCO. 1977. "Status resources and behavioral deviance as contingencies of societal reaction." *Social Forces* 56:132–47.

RUSHING, WILLIAM A., AND SUZANNE T. ORTEGA. 1979. "Socioeconomic status and mental disorder: New evidence and a sociomedical formulation." *American Journal of Sociology* 84:1175–1200.

ST. JOHN, NANCY. 1975. *School desegregation: Outcomes for children.* New York: Wiley.

SALZINGER, KURT. 1973. *Schizophrenia: Behavioral aspects.* New York: Wiley.

SAMPSON, HAROLD, SHELDON MESSINGER, AND ROBERT TOWNE. 1961. "The mental hospital and marital family ties." *Social Problems* 9:141–55.

SARBIN, T. R., AND J. D. MANCUSO. 1970. "Failure of a moral enterprise: Attitudes of the public towards mental illness." *Journal of Consulting and Clinical Psychology* 2:159–73.

SCHEFF, THOMAS. 1964. "The societal reaction to deviance: Ascriptive elements in the psychiatric screening of mental patients in a midwestern state." *Social Problems* 11:401–13.

———. 1974. "The labelling theory of mental illness." *American Sociological Review* 39:444–52.

———. 1975a. *Labeling madness.* Englewood Cliffs, NJ: Prentice Hall.

———. 1975b. "Reply to Chauncey and Gove." *American Sociological Review* 40:252–57.

———. 1984. *Being mentally ill.* 2nd ed. Chicago: Aldine.

SCHEPANK, HEINZ, HERMANN HILPERT, HERMANN HONMANN, et al. 1984. "Das Mannheimer Kohortenprojekt—Die Prävalenz psychogener Erkrankungen in der Stadt." *Zeitschrift für Psychosomatische Medizin und Psychoanalyse* 30:43–61.

SCHEPER-HUGHES, NANCY. 1979. *Saints, scholars, and schizophrenics: Mental illness in rural Ireland.* Berkeley and Los Angeles: University of California Press.

SCHMIDT, K. E. 1964. "Folk psychiatry in Sarawak: A tentative system of psychiatry of the Iban." Pp. 155–89 in A. Kiev (ed.), *Magic, faith, and healing: Studies in primitive psychiatry today.* New York: Free Press.

SCHUTT, RUSSELL K., TATJANA MESCHEDE, AND JILL RIERDAN. 1994. "Distress, suicidal thoughts, and social support among homeless adults." *Journal of Health and Social Behavior* 35:134–42.

SCHWAB, JOHN J., AND MARY E. SCHWAB. 1978. *Sociocultural roots of mental illness: An epidemiologic survey.* New York: Plenum.

SCHWARTZ, SHARON, BRUCE P. DOHRENWEND, AND ITZHAK LEVAV. 1994. "Nongenetic familial transmission of psychiatric disorders? Evidence from children of Holocaust survivors." *Journal of Health and Social Behavior* 35:385–402.

SECHEHAYE, MARGUERITE. 1964. "Autobiography of a schizophrenic girl." Pp. 164–84 in B. Kaplan (ed.), *The inner world of mental illness*. New York: Harper & Row.

SEGAL, STEVEN P., AND URI AVIRAM. 1978. *The mentally ill in community-based sheltered care*. New York: Wiley-Interscience.

SELIGMAN, M. E. P. 1975. *Helplessness: On depression, development and death*. San Francisco: Freeman.

SELYE, HANS. 1956. *The stress of life*. New York: McGraw-Hill.

SENNETT, RICHARD, AND JONATHAN COBB. 1972. *The hidden injuries of class*. New York: Random House.

SHAH, SALEEM A. 1975. "Dangerousness and civil commitment of the mentally ill: Some public policy considerations." *American Journal of Psychiatry* 132:501–5.

SHARPE, L., B. J. GURLAND, J. L. FLEISS, R. E. KENDELL, J. E. COOPER, AND J. R. M. COPELAND. 1974. "Some comparisons of American, Canadian, and British psychiatrists in their diagnostic concepts." *Canadian Psychiatric Association Journal* 19:235–45.

SHEHAN, CONSTANCE L., MARY ANN BURG, AND CYNTHIA A. REXROAT. 1986. "Depression and the social dimensions of the full-time housewife role." *Sociological Quarterly* 27:403–422.

SHIELDS, J., L. HESTON, AND H. GOTTESMAN. 1975. "Schizophrenia and the schizoid: The problem for genetic analysis." Pp. 167–97 in R. Fieve, D. Rosenthal, and H. Brill (eds.), *Genetic research in psychiatry*. Baltimore: Johns Hopkins University Press.

SHILOH, AILON. 1971. "Sanctuary or prison—responses to life in a mental hospital." Pp. 9–24 in S. Wallace (ed.), *Total institutions*. Chicago: Aldine.

SHNEIDMAN, EDWIN S. 1975. "Suicide." Pp. 1774–85 in A. Freedman, H. Kaplan, and B. Sadock (eds.), *Comprehensive textbook of psychiatry*, Vol. 2, 2nd ed. Baltimore: Williams & Wilkins.

SIDEL, RUTH, AND VICTOR W. SIDEL. 1982. *The health of China*. Boston: Beacon Press.

SIEDOW, HELMUT. 1985. "Zur Lager der Sozial Psychiatrie." *Mensch Medizin Gesellschaft* 10:75–76.

SIMMONS, ROBERTA G. 1978. "Blacks and high self-esteem: A puzzle." *Social Psychology* 41:54–57.

SIMON, RITA J., AND DAVID E. AARONSON. 1988. *The insanity defense*. New York: Praeger.

SIMON, RITA J., AND WILLIAM C. COCKERHAM. 1977. "Civil commitment, burden of proof, and dangerous acts: A comparison of the perspectives of judges and psychiatrists." *Journal of Psychiatry & Law* 5:571–94.

SIMPSON, GEORGE M., AND PHILIP R. A. MAY. 1985. "Schizophrenia: Somatic treatment." Pp. 713–24 in H. Kaplan and B. Sadock (eds.), *Comprehensive textbook of psychiatry*, Vol. 1, 4th ed. Baltimore: Williams & Wilkins.

SKINNER, B. F. 1971. *Beyond freedom and dignity*. New York: Knopf.

SNOW, LOUDELL F. 1978. "Sorcerers, saints, and charlatans: Black folk healers in urban America." *Culture, Medicine, and Psychiatry* 2:69–106.

SNYDER, SOLOMON H. 1977. "Biochemical factors in schizophrenia." *Hospital Practice* 12:133–40.

———. 1980. *Biological aspects of mental disorder*. New York: Oxford University Press.

SPIRO, H. R., I. SIASSI, AND G. CROCETTI. 1973. "Ability of the public to recognize mental illness: An issue of substance and an issue of meaning." *Social Psychiatry* 8:32–36.

SPITZER, ROBERT L., AND PAUL T. WILSON. 1975. "Nosology and the official psychiatric nomenclature." Pp. 826–45 in A. Freedman, H. Kaplan, and B. Sadock (eds.), *Comprehensive textbook of psychiatry*, Vol. 1, 2nd ed. Baltimore: Williams & Wilkins.

SROLE, LEO, T. S. LANGNER, S. T. MICHAEL, P. KIRKPATRICK, M. K. OPLER, AND T. A. C. RENNIE. 1975. *Mental health in the metropolis: The Midtown Manhattan study*. Books 1 and 2. Rev. and enlarged ed. L. Srole and A. Fischer (eds.). New York: Harper & Row.

SROLE, LEO, T. S. LANGNER, S. T. MICHAEL, M. K. OPLER, AND T. A. C. RENNIE. 1962. *Mental health in the metropolis: The Midtown Manhattan study*. Vols. 1 and 2. New York: McGraw-Hill.

STAFFORD-CLARK, DAVID, AND ANDREW C. SMITH. 1978. *Psychiatry for students*. 5th ed. London: Allen & Unwin.

STAR, SHIRLEY. 1952. "What the public thinks about mental illness." Paper presented at the National Association of Mental Health meetings, Chicago, Illinois, November.

———. 1955. "The public's idea about mental illness." Paper presented at the National Association for Mental Health meetings, Chicago, IL, November.

STARR, PAUL. 1994. *The logic of health care reform*. Rev. and enlarged ed. New York: Penguin.

STEADMAN, HENRY J. 1981. "Critically reassessing the accuracy of public perceptions of the dangerousness of the mentally ill." *Journal of Health and Social Behavior* 22:310–16.

STEADMAN, HENRY J., AND JOSEPH J. COCOZZA. 1974. *Careers of the criminally insane*. Lexington, MA: Heath.

STONE, ALAN A. 1975. *Mental health and law: A system in transition.* Washington, DC: National Institute of Mental Health.

STOUFFER, SAMUEL A., EDWARD A. SUCHMAN, LELAND C. DE VINNEY, SHIRLEY A. STAR, AND ROBIN M. WILLIAMS, JR. 1949. *The American soldier.* Vol. 1. Princeton, NJ: Princeton University Press.

STRAUSS, ANSELM. 1969. *Mirrors and masks.* San Francisco: Sociology Press.

STROUP, A., AND R. MANDERSCHEID. 1988. "Male–female admission differentials in state mental hospitals, 1880–1980." *Journal of the Washington Academy of Sciences* 78:259–70.

STURM, LOUELLA. 1973. *The mental hospital nightmare.* New York: Exposition Press.

STYRON, WILLIAM. 1990. *Darkness visible: A memoir of madness.* New York: Random House.

SUTHERLAND, EDWIN H. 1939. *Principles of criminology.* 3rd ed. Philadelphia: Lippincott.

SUTHERLAND, EDWIN H., AND DONALD R. CRESSEY. 1974. *Criminology.* 9th ed. Philadelphia: Lippincott.

SUTHERLAND, N. S. 1977. *Breakdown.* Briarcliff Manor, NY: Stein & Day.

SUTTON, JOHN R. 1991. "The political economy of madness: The expansion of the asylum in progressive America." *American Sociological Review* 56:665–78.

SWANK, R. L. 1949. "Combat exhaustion." *Journal of Nervous and Mental Diseases* 109:475–508.

SWANSON, GUY E. 1972. "Mead and Freud: Their relevance for social psychology." Pp. 23–43 in J. Manis and B. Meltzer (eds.), *Symbolic interaction,* 2nd ed. Boston: Allyn & Bacon.

SWARTZ, MARVIN, BERNARD CARROLL, AND DAN BLAZER. 1989. "In response to 'Psychiatric Diagnosis as Reified Measurement.' " *Journal of Health and Social Behavior* 30:33–34.

SYTOKOWSKI, PAMELA A., WILLIAM B. KANNEL, AND RALPH B. D'AGOSTINO. 1990. "Changes in risk factors and the decline in mortality from cardiovascular disease." *New England Journal of Medicine* 322:1638–41.

SZASZ, THOMAS S. 1968. *Law, liberty, and psychiatry.* New York: Collier.

———. 1970. *The manufacture of madness.* New York: Dell.

———. 1974. *The myth of mental illness.* Rev. ed. New York: Harper & Row.

———. 1987. *Insanity.* New York: Wiley.

TAYLOR, IAN, PAUL WALTON, AND JOCK YOUNG. 1973. *The new criminology: For a social theory of deviance.* London: Routledge & Kegan Paul.

TAYLOR, VERTA, ALEXANDER G. ROSS, AND D. L. QUARANTELLI. 1976. "Delivery of mental health services in disasters: The Xenia tornado and some implications. Monograph 11. Columbus: Disaster Research Center, Ohio State University.

TEPLIN, LINDA A. (ed.). 1984. *Mental health and criminal law.* Beverly Hills, CA: Sage.

TESSLER, RICHARD, AND DAVID MECHANIC. 1978. "Psychological distress and perceived health status." *Journal of Health and Social Behavior* 19:254–62.

THIELEN, HILMAR. 1986. "Ideology and psychotherapy." Pp. 545–70 in D. Light and A. Schuller (eds.), *Political values and health care: The German experience.* Cambridge, MA: MIT Press.

THOITS, PEGGY A. 1982. "Conceptual, methodological, and theoretical problems in studying social support as a buffer against life stress." *Journal of Health and Social Behavior* 23:145–59.

———. 1983. "Multiple identities and psychological well-being: A reformulation and test of the social isolation hypothesis." *American Sociological Review* 48:174–87.

———. 1984. "Explaining distributions of psychological vulnerability: Lack of social support in the face of life stress." *Social Forces* 63:453–81.

———. 1985. "Self-labeling processes in mental illness: The role of emotional deviance." *American Journal of Sociology* 91:221–49.

———. 1986. "Multiple identities: Examining gender and marital status differences in distress." *American Sociological Review* 51:259–72.

———. 1987. "Gender and marital status differences in control and distress: Common stress versus unique stress explanations." *Journal of Health and Social Behavior* 28:7–22.

———. 1994. "Stressors and problem-solving: The individual as psychological activist." *Journal of Health and Social Behavior* 35:143–59.

THOMAS, MELVIN E., AND MICHAEL HUGHES. 1986. "The continuing significance of race: A study of race, class, and quality of life in America, 1972–1985." *American Sociological Review* 51:830–41.

TIERNEY, KATHLEEN J., AND BARBARA BAISDEN. 1979. *Crisis intervention programs for disaster victims: A source book and manual for smaller communities.* Rockville, MD: National Institute of Mental Health.

TITCHENER, JAMES L., AND FREDERIC T. KAPP. 1976. "Family and character change at Buffalo Creek." *American Journal of Psychiatry* 133:295–99.

TORREY, E. FULLER. 1973. *The mind game: Witch doctors and psychiatrists.* New York: Bantam.

TOWNSEND, JOHN MARSHALL. 1975a. "Cultural conceptions and mental illness: A controlled comparison of Germany and America." *Journal of Nervous and Mental Disease* 160:409–21.
———. 1975b. "Cultural conceptions, mental disorders and social roles: A comparison of Germany and America." *American Sociological Review* 40:739–52.
———. 1976. "Self-concept and the institutionalization of mental patients: An overview and critique." *Journal of Health and Social Behavior* 17:263–71.
———. 1978. *Cultural conceptions and mental illness: A comparison of Germany and America.* Chicago: University of Chicago Press.
TRIMBLE, JOSEPH E. 1987. "Self-perception and perceived alienation among American Indians." *Journal of Community Psychology* 15:316–33.
TUDOR, WILLIAM, JEANNETTE TUDOR, AND WALTER R. GOVE. 1977. "The effect of sex role differences on the social control of mental illness." *Journal of Health and Social Behavior* 18:98–112.
———. 1979. "The effect of sex role differences on the societal reaction to mental retardation." *Social Forces* 57:871–86.
TURNBULL, S. R. 1977. *The samurai: A military history.* New York: Macmillan.
TURNER, BRYAN. 1988. *Status.* Milton Keynes, UK: Open University Press.
TURNER, R. JAY. 1981. "Social support as a contingency in psychological well-being." *Journal of Health and Social Behavior* 22:357–67.
TURNER, R. JAY, AND WILLIAM R. AVISON. 1992. "Innovations in the measurement of life stress: Crisis theory and the significance of event resolution." *Journal of Health and Social Behavior* 33:36–50.
TURNER, R. JAY, AND JOHN W. GARTRELL. 1978. "Social factors in psychiatric outcome: Toward the resolution of interpretive controversies." *American Sociological Review* 43:368–82.
TURNER, R. JAY, AND FRANCO MARINO. 1994. "Social support and social structure: A descriptive epidemiology." *Journal of Health and Social Behavior* 35:193–212.
TURNER, R. JAY, AND SAMUEL NOH. 1983. "Class and psychological vulnerability among women: The significance of social support and personal control." *Journal of Health and Social Behavior* 24:2–15.
TWEED, DAN L., AND LINDA K. GEORGE. 1989. "A more balanced perspective on 'Psychiatric Diagnosis as Reified Measurement.' " *Journal of Health and Social Behavior* 30:35–37.
UEHARA, EDWINA S. 1994. "Race, gender, and housing inequality: An exploration of the correlates of low-quality housing among clients diagnosed with severe and persistent mental illness." *Journal of Health and Social Behavior* 35:309–21.
ULBRICH, PATRICIA M., GEORGE J. WARHEIT, AND RICK S. ZIMMERMAN. 1989. "Race, socioeconomic status, and psychological distress: An examination of differential vulnerability." *Journal of Health and Social Behavior* 30:131–46.
UMBERSON, DEBRA, CAMILLE B. WORTMAN, AND RONALD C. KESSLER. 1992. "Widowhood and depression: Explaining long-term gender differences in vulnerability." *Journal of Health and Social Behavior* 33:10–24.
VANFOSSEN, BETH E. 1981. "Sex differences in the mental health effects of spouse support and equity." *Journal of Health and Social Behavior* 22:130–40.
VAUGHN, C. E., AND J. P. LEFF. 1976. "The influence of family and social factors on the course of psychiatric illness: A comparison of schizophrenic and depressed neurotic patients." *British Journal of Psychiatry* 129:125–37.
VEROFF, JOSEPH, RICHARD A. KULKA, AND ELIZABETH DOUVAN. 1981. *Mental health in America.* New York: Basic Books.
VINOKUR, A., AND M. L. SELZER. 1975. "Desirable versus undesirable life events: Their relationship to stress and mental distress." *Journal of Personality and Social Psychology* 32:329–37.
VONNEGUT, MARK. 1975. *The Eden express.* New York: Praeger.
WAGENFELD, MORTON O., AND STANLEY S. ROBIN. 1976. "Boundary busting in the role of the community mental health worker." *Journal of Health and Social Behavior* 17:112–222.
WARHEIT, GEORGE J., CHARLES E. HOLZER III, AND SANDRA A. AVERY. 1975. "Race and mental illness: An epidemiologic update." *Journal of Health and Social Behavior* 16:243–56.
WARHEIT, GEORGE J., CHARLES E. HOLZER III, ROGER A. BELL, AND SANDRA A. AVERY. 1976. "Sex, marital status, and mental health: A reappraisal." *Social Forces* 55:459–70.
WARHEIT, GEORGE J., CHARLES E. HOLZER III, AND JOHN J. SCHWAB. 1973. "An analysis of social class and racial differences in depressive symptomatology: A community study." *Journal of Health and Social Behavior* 14:291–99.

WEBB, STEPHEN D., AND JOHN COLLETTE. 1977. "Rural-urban differences in the use of stress-alleviative drugs." *American Journal of Sociology* 83:700–707.

WEINER, HERBERT. 1985. "Schizophrenia: Etiology." Pp. 650–86 in H. Kaplan and B. Sadock (eds.), *Comprehensive textbook of psychiatry*, Vol. 1, 4th ed. Baltimore: Williams & Wilkins.

WEINER, RICHARD D. 1989. "Electroconvulsive therapies." Pp. 1600–09 in H. Kaplan and B. Sadock (eds.), *Comprehensive textbook of psychiatry*, Vol. 2, 5th ed. Baltimore: Williams & Wilkins.

WEINFELD, MORTON, JOHN J. SIGAL, AND WILLIAM W. EATON. 1981. "Long-term effects of the holocaust on selected social attitudes and behaviors of survivors: A cautionary note." *Social Forces* 60:1–19.

WEINSTEIN, FRED, AND GERALD M. PLATT. 1973. *Psychoanalytic sociology: An essay on the interpretation of historical data and the phenomena of collective behavior.* Baltimore: Johns Hopkins University Press.

WEINSTEIN, RAYMOND M. 1979. "Patient attitudes toward mental hospitalization: A review of quantitative research." *Journal of Health and Social Behavior* 20:237–58.

————. 1981. "Attitudes toward psychiatric treatment among hospitalized patients: A review of quantitative research." *Social Science and Medicine* 151:301–14.

————. 1983. "Labeling theory and the attitudes of mental patients: A review." *Journal of Health and Social Behavior* 24:70–84.

WEISSMAN, MYRNA M. 1979. "Environmental factors in affective disorders." *Hospital Practice* 14:103–9.

WEISSMAN, MYRNA M., AND G. L. KLERMAN. 1977. "Sex differences and the epidemiology of depression." *Archives of General Psychiatry* 34:98–111.

WEISSMAN, MYRNA M., AND E. S. PAYKEL. 1974. *The depressed woman.* Chicago: University of Chicago Press.

WELNER, AMOS, SUE MARTEN, ELIZA WOCHNICK, MARY A. DAVIS, ROBERTA FISHMAN, AND PAULA J. CLAYTON. 1979. "Psychiatric disorders among professional women." *Archives of General Psychiatry* 36:169–73.

WENGER, D. L., AND C. R. FLETCHER. 1969. "The effects of legal counsel on admissions to a state mental hospital: A confrontation of professions." *Journal of Health and Social Behavior* 10:66–72.

WETHINGTON, ELAINE, AND RONALD C. KESSLER. 1986. "Perceived support, received support, and adjustment to stressful life events." *Journal of Health and Social Behavior* 27:78–89.

WEYERER, S., AND H. DILLING. 1984. "Prävalenz und Behandlung psychischer Erkankungen in der Allgemeinbevölkerung." *Der Nervenarzt* 55:30–42.

WHATLEY, CHARLES D. 1959. "Social attitudes toward discharged mental patients." *Social Problems* 6:313–20.

————. 1964. "Employer attitudes, discharged mental patients and job durability." *Mental Hygiene* 48:121–31.

WHEATON, BLAIR. 1978. "The sociogenesis of psychological disorder: Reexamining the causal issues with longitudinal data." *American Sociological Review* 43:383–403.

————. 1980. "The sociogenesis of psychological disorder: An attributional theory." *Journal of Health and Social Behavior* 21:100–24.

————. 1983. "Stress, personal coping resources, and psychiatric symptoms: An investigation of interactive models." *Journal of Health and Social Behavior* 24:208–29.

————. 1985. "Models for the stress-buffering functions of coping resources." *Journal of Health and Social Behavior* 26:352–64.

WHITT, HUGH P., AND RICHARD L. MEILE. 1985. "Alignment, magnification, and snowballing: Processes in the definition of symptoms of mental illness." *Social Forces* 63:682–97.

WIERSMA, D., R. GIEL, A. DE JOND, AND C. SLOOF. 1983. "Social class and schizophrenia in a Dutch cohort." *Psychological Medicine* 13:141–50.

WILDE, WILLIAM A. 1968. "Decision-making in a psychiatric screening agency." *Journal of Health and Social Behavior* 9:215–21.

WILDMAN, RICHARD C., AND DAVID RICHARD JOHNSON. 1977. "Life change and Langner's 22-item mental health index: A study and partial replication." *Journal of Health and Social Behavior* 18:179–88.

WILKINSON, GREGG S. 1973. "Interaction patterns and staff response to psychiatric innovations." *Journal of Health and Social Behavior* 14:323–29.

———. 1975. "Patient-audience social status and the social construction of psychiatric disorders: Toward a differential frame of reference hypothesis." *Journal of Health and Social Behavior* 16:28–38.

WILLIAMS, ANN W., JOHN E. WARE, JR., AND CATHY A. DONALD. 1981. "A model of mental health, life events, and social supports applicable to general populations." *Journal of Health and Social Behavior* 22:324–36.

WILLIAMS, DAVID R., DAVID T. TAKEUCHI, AND RUSSELL K. ADAIR. 1992a. "Marital status and psychiatric disorders among blacks and whites." *Journal of Health and Social Behavior* 33:140–57.

———. 1992b. "Socioeconomic status and psychiatric disorder among blacks and whites." *Social Forces* 71:179–94.

WILSON, O. MEREDITH. 1976. "The normal as a culture-related concept." Pp. 21–35 in J. Masserman (ed.), *Social psychiatry: The range of normal in human behavior*, Vol. 2. New York: Grune & Stratton.

WILSON, WILLIAM JULIUS. 1987. *The truly disadvantaged*. Chicago: University of Chicago Press.

WING, J. K. 1967. "Institutionalism in mental hospitals." Pp. 219–38 in T. Scheff (ed.), *Mental illness and social processes*. New York: Harper & Row.

WONG, NORMAN. 1989. "Theories of personality and psychopathology: Classical psychoanalysis." Pp. 356–98 in H. Kaplan and B. Sadock (eds.), *Comprehensive textbook of psychiatry*, Vol. 1, 5th ed. Baltimore: Williams & Wilkins.

YARROW, M., C. SCHWARTZ, H. MURPHY, AND L. DEASY. 1955. "The psychological meaning of mental illness in the family." *Journal of Social Issues* 11:12–24.

YATES, ALAYNE. 1987. "Current status and future direction of research on the American Indian child." *American Journal of Psychiatry* 144:1135–42.

ZANDER. 1976. "Civil commitment in Wisconsin: The impact of Lessard v. Schmidt." *Wisconsin Law Review* 1976:503–41.

ZITRIN, A., A. S. HARDESTY, E. I. BURDOCK, AND A. K. DROSSMAN. 1976. "Crime and violence among mental patients." *American Journal of Psychiatry* 133:142–49.

Name Index

Subject Index